Dancing Your Way to Fertility: How I Had the Babies of My Dreams and How You Can Too—Plus The Ultimate Fertility Success Program!

Other Books by the Author:

The Turning 40 Portrait
Early Morning Coffee: Laugh Out Loud Stories about My Life as a Mom
Tree House Cupcake Girls
Your Perfect Wedding
Diary in the Bed
Izzy and the Ice Skating Bakery
Stop Bullying Forever
Tonight at the Fire pit
The Amber Series
The Sammy Series
The Hope Chest
Its Not Your Fault Adam
Cat Tales: My Family and The Cats We Have Loved
Ask The Love Lady
Transference
Sarah and The Sunrock
Sunday at Grandma's
Sunday With Uncle Charlie
Tonight at Salisbury Beach

Visit www.paulafuocodavis.com to learn more!

Dancing Your Way to Fertility
Paula Fuoco Davis
PaulaMediaandEntertainment.com, Nashua, NH
ISBN:
Edition Notice
Date of Publication
Number of Printings: First printing
Year of publication: 2016

Copyright 2016 Paula Fuoco Davis. All rights reserved.

No part of this book may be reproduced in any written, electronic, audio recording, or photocopying form without written permission of the publisher or author. The exception would be in the case of brief quotations embodied in critical articles or reviews and pages where permission is specifically granted by the publisher or author.

Although every precaution has been taken to verify the accuracy of the information contained herein this book, the author and publisher assume no responsibility for any errors or omissions. No liability is assumed for damages that may result from the use of information contained within this book and whatever electronic forms of communication or other forms of communication the information in this book may take or be conveyed in.

The information provided within this book, in whatever form it is conveyed, translated or read, is for general informational purposes only. The publisher and author do not in any way guarantee, no representations or warranties, express or implied, the completeness, accuracy, reliability, suitability or availability with respect to the information, products, services, or related graphics contained in this book for any purpose.

Any use of the information in this book is at your own risk.

By reading this book, you agree to comply with the following:

This book's author, publisher, its affiliates or employees are not to be held responsible for any inaccuracies, omissions, editorial errors or any consequences resulting from the information provided.

By continuing to read this book, you indicate acceptance of these terms. Those who do not accept these terms should not read, access, use, interact with, view or listen to this book.

The material within this book is not intended to be a definitive set of instructions. Readers who fail to consult with appropriate health authorities assume the risk of any injuries.

The author and publisher of this book are not responsible for errors or omissions or resulting injury from anything written in this book.

The entire content of this book is not intended as a substitute for a medical diagnosis or treatment by qualified medical professionals. Please consult your physician for personalized medical advice.

Always seek the advice of a qualified healthcare provider with any questions regarding a medical condition, diagnosis, or treatment. Never disregard or delay seeking professional medical advice or treatment because of something you have read or seen in this book.

This book does not promise a cure for infertility, or any guarantee regarding fertility.

The author and publisher shall have no liability or responsibility to any person or entity regarding any loss or damage incurred, or alleged to have incurred, directly or indirectly, due to the material contained in this book. Before taking any supplements, foods, vitamins, herbs or any other food or substance mentioned in this book, consult your health care provider for a thorough evaluation. A qualified physician should make a decision regarding foods, vitamins, herbs and other items that can enter the body based on each person's medical history and current prescriptions.

Note: all who choose to read this book should consult a doctor before taking any of the advice, information, outlined in this book. Before taking any supplements, herbs, vitamins, foods discussed in this book, all readers should consult with a physician about how these may interact with any medications they are currently taking. This book, the author and publisher, in no way promises or guarantees any cure or remedy for infertility or any other reproductive problem or challenge.

The reader should seek advice from a medical professional and a mental health professional before attempting anything in the book.

This book is not intended to be a substitute for the medical advice of a licensed physician. The reader should consult with their doctor in any matters relating to his/her health.

The author and publisher expressly disclaim responsibility for any adverse effect that may result from the use or application of the information contained in this book.

As an express condition to reading this book, and associated products, you must agree to the following terms. If you disagree with any of these terms, please do not read this book. Your use of this book, its website or products means that you are agreeing to be legally bound by these terms.

You agree to hold this book, LLC, its owners, agents, and employees harmless from any and all liability for all claims for damages due to injuries, including attorney fees and costs, incurred by you or caused to third parties by you, arising out of the information discussed in this book.

We make no representation or warranties with respect to the accuracy or completeness of the contents of this book and we specifically disclaim any implied warranties of merchantability.

This book does not contain all information available on this subject. This book has not been created to be specific to any individual's or organizations' situation or needs. This book should not be considered as the ultimate source of subject information. This book contains information that might be dated.

All material in this book is provided as information only and may not be construed as medical advice or instruction. No action or inaction should be taken based solely on the contents of this book. Instead, readers should consult appropriate health professionals on any matter relating to their health and well-being.

Reliance on any information provided by the author and this book is solely at your own risk.

The material in this book is provided for informational purposes only and is not intended as medical advice. The information contained in this book should not be used to diagnose or treat any illness, disorder, disease or health problem. Use of the programs, advice, and information contained in this book is at the sole choice and risk of the reader.

The resources and information made available in this book are provided for informational purposes only, and should not be used to replace the specialized training and professional judgment of a health care or mental health care professional.

The author and publisher cannot be held responsible for the use of the information provided. Please always consult a physician or a trained mental health professional before making any decision regarding treatment of yourself or others.

If you are currently in treatment or in therapy, please consult your therapist, psychiatrist or mental health professional before you use any of the information contained in this book.

If you feel suicidal or depressed, contact a Crisis Hotline or seek help at a hospital, Emergency Room, treatment center, or with a physician, qualified mental health care provider, or through a law enforcement agency or social services.

This book and its contents (including any information available from the book located on websites or excerpted) is for informational and entertainment purposes only and is not intended to replace or substitute for any professional, medical, legal, mental health or any other advice.

In addition, the author and publisher make no representations or warranties and expressly disclaims any and all liability concerning any treatment or action by any person following the information offered or provided within or through this book. If you have specific concerns or find yourself in a situation in which you require professional or medical advice, you should consult with an appropriately trained and qualified specialist.

Please consult your physician, mental health professional or therapist before you utilize the materials that can be purchased from this book.

If you do not agree to be bound by all of these terms, do not read this book.

We make no representation or warranties with respect to the accuracy or completeness of the contents of the book and we specifically disclaim any implied warranties of merchantability for any particular purpose.

All material in this book is provided for your information only and may not be construed as medical advice or instruction. No action or inaction should be taken based on the contents of this information. Instead, readers should consult appropriate health professionals on any matter relating to their health and well-being.

The information in this book does not and is not intended to replace professional medical or nutritional advice.

The information contained in this book should not be considered complete and does not cover all diseases, ailments, physical conditions or their treatment. It should not be used in place of a call or visit to a medical,health or other competent professional, who should be consulted beforeadopting any of the suggestions in this book or drawing inferences from it.

The information about drugs, herbs, vitamins, foods, drinks, and any other food sources contained in this book is general in nature.

They do not cover all possible uses, actions, precautions, side effects, or interactions of the medicines mentioned, nor is the information intended as medical advice for individual problems or for making an evaluation as to the risks and benefits of taking a particular drug, vitamin, herb, supplement, or food.

This book and the operator(s) of this site specifically disclaim all responsibility for any liability, loss or risk, personal or otherwise, which is incurred as a consequence, directly or indirectly, of the use and application of any of the material on this site.

If you do anything recommended in this book without the supervision of a licensed medical doctor, you do so at your own risk because the information, remedies or exercise in this book may not be U.S. Food and Drug Administration (FDA) approved.

The medical information in this book is provided "as is" without any representations or warranties, express or implied.

You must not rely on the information in this book as an alternative to medical advice from your doctor or other professional health care provider.

If you think you may be suffering from any medical condition or before starting any new treatment you should seek immediate medical attention. Proper medical attention should always be sought for specific ailments.

Never disregard professional medical advice, delay in seeking medical treatment or discontinue medical treatment due to information obtained in this book

Any information provided in this book is not intended to diagnose, treat or cure infertility or any other illness, disease or medical condition.

Books may be purchased by contacting the publisher and author at books@paulamediaandentertainment.com.

Books may be purchased in quantity and/or special sales by contacting the publisher, PaulaMediaandEntertainment.com or by email at books@paulamediaandentertainment.com.

Library of Congress Catalog Number:
ISBN:0997145900
   1. Infertility 2. Fertility 3. Health

   First Edition

This book is dedicated to my mother, Sarah Fuoco for being the best mother in the world. You embody what motherhood is in every way. I have always loved and will always love sitting across from you at the kitchen table talking. There is no place I rather be. I loved as a child seeing your white car waiting to pick me up from school, our Monday trips to the mall, visits to Friendlys, and every moment inbetween. You were kind when I didn't deserve it, and more loving and amazing then I could have ever hoped for. I am grateful you are my Mom. How could I not want to be a mother after having a mother like you? You gave me everything and more and I can't thank you enough for being everything to me.

My father, Joseph Fuoco, for taking such good care of me and Mom, and working so hard and responsibly to make life beautiful for us. You were a fun Dad, smart, generous and loving. How can I even begin to thank you for all you have given me? Thank you for paying for all my vitamins as I went through infertility treatments. For this, I could never say thank you enough. You are a beautiful person.

My beautiful children, Amber and Sammy, who God sent as an answer to all my prayers. You were worth every part of this journey, every needle, every minute..all so worth it because having you both has been the most wonderful part of my life. You both fill my days with more joy than you can imagine. Amber, from the day you were born, I saw you as gold from heaven. You are the perfect girl for me. I like and love everything about you. Thank you for all the conversations—you are never boring and I needed that in my life so much. Thank you for loving books and being such a great writer that you constantly surprise me with your ability— and thank you for sitting on my lap for hours as a baby and toddler and letting me read to you. Those moments were pure joy. Sammy, (whose friends also know as Brandon) from the moment you were born, you were glistening with a perfect sweetness. You were the boy I needed in my life always. Thanks for playing baseball with me. You, like your sister, are like gold to me. You are understanding, smart, handsome and fun—who would have ever imagined I would have a son so good at basketball? Amber and Sammy, thank you for everything....all the great car rides to Grandma's where you put up with my changing the radio station every five minutes and everything else. You are both amazing, beautiful, and so smart. I am beyond privileged to be your mother.

Most of all, I dedicate this book to Jehovah God, the one who answers all prayers. Thank you, thank you, thank you Jehovah. Without you, I could not have survived this. Without the privilege of prayer, I would not have been able to walk this road. Without you, all this would have never happened. Thank you for listening, for always being there, and for helping me have the babies of my dreams. I could never thank you enough. There is no God like you, and you deserve every bit of praise and honor always.

My best friend, Leah Page Mortimer, who walked with me and helped me every step of the way. You were there during my darkest times, offering hope, acceptance, love, understanding. Yes, you are a genius! And for all the times you said exactly what I needed to hear, thank you.

My husband, Christopher Davis, for being there and walking this hard road with me. You were brave and kind, a true hero, and without you, I would not have my kids. There is no one else I would have rather walked this road with. You helped me give birth to these beautiful children and I can't thank you enough.

Table of Contents

Introduction:	25
Infertility: A Training Ground for Motherhood	31
Ten Things About Infertility That Nobody Will Tell You—But You Need to Know Right From The Start	33
The Ultimate Fertility Success Program: Getting Your Body Ready	35
12 Cleanses To Help Restore Your Fertility	39
Liver Cleanse	39
Heavy Metal Cleanse	42
Yeast Cleanse	43
Adrenal Cleanse	44
Colon Cleanse	47
Kidney Cleanse	50
Parasite Cleanse	53
Uterine Cleanse	56
Blood Cleanse	59
Lymph System Cleanse	61
Thyroid Cleanse	64
Balancing Your Hormones and Improving the Quality of Your Eggs	69
How to Improve Your Egg Quality	75

Strengthening and Preparing Your Organs for Maximum Fertility	81
Vagina	81
Ovaries	83
Thyroid	83
Spleen and Digestive System	89
Pituitary Gland	89
Hypothalamus and thymus	91
Pineal Gland	91
Pancreas	92
Important Ways to Enhance and Strengthen Your Fertility	94
Vegetable Based Drinks	94
Increase Circulation to Your Reproductive System	96
Restore Good Bacteria In Your Body	97
Exercise Mildly	97
Medications	98
Electromagnetic Energy	98
Sleep	100
Chemicals In The Environment	101
Sunlight	103
Water	104
Deep Breathing	104
Cervical Mucous	104
Conditions That Threaten Your Fertility	105
Iron Deficiency	105
Weight	106
Body Energy Flow	106
Teeth and Gum Infection	107
Spine	107
Acidity	108
Infection	109
Allergies	109
Celiac Disease	109
Body Temperature	110
Alternative Holistic Treatments	110
Acupuncture	110
Bio Cleanse	112

Lymphatic Massage, or Manual Lymphatic Drainage	112
Applied Kinesiology	113
Cranio-sacral therapy	114
Blood Type	114
Homeopathy	114
Ayurvedic Medicine	115
Traditional Chinese Medicine	116
Naturopathic Doctors	116
Tests to Request At the Fertility Clinic	117
Vitamins and Other Supplements To Prepare Your Body For Pregnancy	118
Powerful Foods to Help Heal Your Infertility	122
BONUS: Your Personal Food Journal	145
More Ways to Maximize Your Fertility	146
Getting Your Guy Ready: The Ultimate Male Fertility Preparation Program	150
Tests for Men	151
Cleanses for Men	152
Holistic and Alternative Health Treatments To Consider	153
Vitamins and Supplements	153
More Things Your Guy Can Do To Improve Fertility	156
Fertility-Enhancing Foods For Men	159
Conditions To Have Checked	163
Chapter 3: How to Prepare For the Journey Through Infertility	164
Chapter 4: Emotions That Can Come From Suffering With Infertility	187
Chapter 5: Coping With The Ups and Downs Of Infertility	192

Chapter 6: The People In Your Journey and Some of the Rude Comments
You May Hear Along the Way 222

Chapter 7: A Note About Husbands and How to Not Let Infertility Ruin
Your Marriage 229

Chapter 8: Choosing The Right Doctor 233

Chapter 9: Common Mistakes You Need To Know About 239

Chapter 10: Bye Bye Stress! 241

Chapter 11: Freeing Your Body From the Traumas and Painful ... 256
Life Experiences That Might be Destroying Your Fertility

Chapter 12: Letting Go Of Your Secret Thoughts and Hidden Beliefs
That Might Be Holding You Back From Getting Pregnant 256

Chapter 13: 50 Creative Projects To Help Tap Into Your Creative ... 283
Reproductive Energy

Chapter 14: Making Your Home Into A Fertility Nesting Center ... 294

Chapter 15: Journal Your Way to Pregnancy 306

    Journal Writing Through Your Subconscious 306

    Your Daily Happiness Journal 324

    Life and Birth Affirmation Journal 327

    My Child & I Journal 329

Chapter 16: Keeping Track Of Your Emotions 330

Chapter 17: Visualize Your Way to Your Baby 343

Chapter 18: Fertility Affirmations 355

Chapter 19: Your Personal Fertility Vision Statement 363

Chapter 20: Letters To Yourself 368

Chapter 21: The Emotion of Deserving	391
Chapter 22: Start Living Authentically	395
Chapter 23: Welcoming Your Mother Within	398
Chapter 24: Hitting Bottom	400
Chapter 25: Remember Who You Are	412
Chapter 26: What I Did Right....What I Did Wrong...What You Can Learn From My Stupid Mistakes	436
Chapter 27: Advice and Ideas for Fertility Clinics	482
Part II: Secondary Infertility: My story of secondary infertility	487
Chapter 28: Coping with Shots and Injections	493
Chapter 29: How To Protect A Cherished Pregnancy	494
Chapter 30: How to Maximize Your Chances for Conception Before and After An IVF	577

I suffered and cried, but in the end my dream came true.

I want the same to happen to you.

I tried to put in this book everything I wish someone told me, so my journey would not have been so painful, and maybe I would have been successful a little bit sooner.

I wish you all the success you deserve.

Acknowledgements

Dr. Robert Deutsch for all you did to help me through my journey, and for being in my opinion, one of the greatest chiropractors and doctors in the world. Few understand the human body like you do and with your knowledge and insight, you do medical miracles everyday. It is truly a privilege to be your patient and know you. You are truly the best.

Eileen Beasley for helping me release so much pain and becoming the person I wanted to be. Your kindness and gentleness will never be forgotten.

Dr. Myung Kim, you are probably one of the best acupuncturists in the world and you helped me so much. I thank you a million times over. You are truly a master at what you do.

The reproductive center I went to, including Christine, ultrasound technician, for patiently helping me through many difficult ultrasounds and most of all, for being patient and kind during that first ultrasound where I could have given up. You gave me the time I needed and helped me grow, so that eventually, the ultrasounds were not difficult at all. I will always be grateful for your professionalism and your kindness. Thank you also to Carol for always holding my hand and being such a great support during my IUIs.

Dr. Samuel Pang and Dr. Goldstein, for never calling my eggs bottom of the barrel, for being kind, always trying and helping me. Dr. Goldstein, thank you for giving me a chance when others wanted to give up on me.

Leah Page Mortimer, again, for everything.

Peter Rockett, for the night I called you, worried as usual that I might never get pregnant, and when I asked you if you thought I would get pregnant, you, as you always are, were loving and positive. "Of course you will get pregnant kid," you said without hesitation. You offered words of hope, and dared to be positive, when you could have shot down my dreams. I will always cherish you.

Judy Ahern Salsich, for looking at me one day at work and saying you could picture me having a daughter with cork-screw curls. I needed those words so much that day and you provided them. Working beside you for 11 years was truly a privilege, as is just knowing you. You taught me so much. I will always cherish you and wish I could see you daily. You are one of the best mothers I have ever met, and your wisdom, kindness and intelligence to match is profound.

Chelsea Lowe, for always listening and on a very sad day, telling me to go home and drink some nice warm tea. I still think about and recall your advice almost daily. You are kind and smart, an amazing writer, and a friend I cherish. We still talk about the monkey you sent as a present when Sammy was born, and we will always love Bananas Foster.

Richard and Janice Campioni, my beautiful neighbors, thank you for being part of my pregnancy. I am glad you were next door to me through all of this.

My grandmother, Maria Fuoco, for your good advice and being there the night I announced I was pregnant. I love and miss you always.

My parents, Joseph and Sarah Fuoco, again, for every everything.

To Nature Sunshine and its products and Sarah Montagna who introduced me to them. You were a big help Sarah. Thank you.

Mary, the nurse, at Holy Family Hospital, who knelt beside me and asked if I wanted to pray, as I was preparing for the caesarean.

Rosalyn Minassian, for praying for me while you were in Armenia waiting for your little girl. You gave me much wise advice over the years.

Dr. Michel Lirrette, truly the best OB/GYN in the world. There is no one else I would have wanted as my doctor. You made giving birth a fun and beautiful experience. You are kind and smart and it was a privilege to have you as my doctor. I thank God you were my doctor. Your beautiful personality and skillful knowledge will always be remembered and appreciated.

To Cindy Michaud St. Laurent, and her children, for visiting me the day my daughter was born and being the best friend anyone could wish for. Since ninth grade you've walked beside me and I am eternally grateful for that.

Andy Preston Horton, for everything, including always having the right word at the right time.

For everybody at WGBH Channel 2 I worked with during my battle with infertility, for listening to all my stories and helping me. You were all amazing and I thank you all for being there. Just having all of you to talk to on a regular basis lightened my load.

Paula Fuoco Davis: has been a a writer since she was in fourth grade and her beloved teacher Mrs. Klein knelt down and told her 'you could be a writer' after writing an essay about water. For more than 30 years, she worked as a newspaper reporter and journalist for The Lawrence Eagle-Tribune, The Nashua Telegraph and New Hampshire magazine. She covered education, social issues and features. She founded and is editor of Commitment.com, an online site for women and authored more than 25 books. She is a survivor of infertility and wants others to have every single bit of information she didn't have. She has loved writing this book.

24

Dancing Your Way to Fertility

Dancing Your Way to Fertility

My doctor looked at me point blank and said without a trace of mercy that my eggs were "bottom of the barrel."

Bottom of the barrel... Her words rang in my head like a cruel pronouncement.

I was 37 years old and desperately wanted a second child. My doctor didn't believe I could have one.

I had been through this before. To have my daughter, I endured 10 IUIs, several operations and too many nights of crying to count.

So I left her office: desperate, heartbroken, and wildly, frantically panicked. The words 'your eggs are bottom of the barrel' kept repeating in my head. Despite everything I've gone through, I always had hope. My insides were screaming: 'I can't live with this.' I was so shaken, I could barely drive home. Her words nearly broke my will and spirit to try again.

For some reason, on the way home, I stopped at a natural foods market. Walking around the supermarket, amidst all the healthy foods and supplements, I began to question what the doctor told me. Was the poor quality of my eggs something that could be improved? Was I unhealthy on some undetectable level that was impacting my fertility? I went home and called my ever-wise mother. She gave me great advice: dump that doctor and try again.

I did exactly what Mom said.

I decided I would do everything I could to restore and heal my fertility, and not be hindered by my age, regardless of what the doctor said.

Over time, I learned that there was hope for me and others like me—and just because a doctor says you can never get pregnant does not mean your body, if given the right elements, cannot heal from infertility.

My devastation and despair turned to determination, and everything I learned, I put in this book. As a newspaper reporter for more than 25 years, I utilized my skills as a journalist to get to the root of fertility problems, the physical and the emotional.

I am now also a fertility success certified life coach.

I wrote this book for those of you suffering with infertility, who like me who have been told that your eggs are too old, that your body is too unhealthy, weak, or damaged, that there is little hope.

I wrote this book for all of you who feel that having a child is some type of impossible dream, that you are the victim of some pathologically cruel biological problem.

I wrote it for you brave survivors of infertility who dream of starting a family, but find the road long, cruel, uphill, and not always forgiving of slight mistakes and accumulated years.

Together, we will work to heal everything in your body and mind that could be stopping you from getting pregnant. Consider me your personal fertility success coach.

I will help you identify all the physical and emotional obstacles that might be standing in the way of your having the children you desire. Then-one-by-one, we are going to knock these obstacles out of your body and your life.

I created the Ultimate Fertility Success Program, which I believe is one of the most comprehensive body-mind makeover plans available to fertility patients today.

The Ultimate Fertility Success Program includes 12 cleanses that will detoxify your body and expand your fertility potential. It will also show you how to improve the quality of your eggs—something previously not thought possible—and balance your hormones.

It includes a chapter on strengthening, preparing, and emotionally and spiritually healing every organ in your body that impacts your fertility.

Then we will look at the foods you eat, the lifestyle you live, and vitamins and herbs that will give you a fair and fighting chance to enjoy vibrant fertility. You may be eating, thinking and experiencing life in a way that is depleting your reproductive organs, and you didn't even know it.

The program is designed to change the track you are on so you can become more healthy, vibrant and fertile—as you deserve to be!

For your guy, I've included The Ultimate Male Fertility Preparation Plan, that includes little known information to help your guy enhance his fertility.

We will address all the obvious and not so obvious blocks to your fertility, because some fertility problems are difficult to diagnose and there are not yet diagnostic tools available to detect the slight shifts, blocks, and traumas in the body that can prevent or delay pregnancy.

The traumas and painful emotions we experience can lodge themselves in our cells, interrupting our body's natural healthy energy flow.

This book will help you examine all aspects of your life, from your childhood and family experiences, to your deepest thoughts and beliefs about pregnancy and motherhood, so that you are fully aware of your subconscious feelings and beliefs and every part of you can work together to have the babies of your dreams.

I will share with you the information you need to unblock and destroy the emotional and spiritual traumas, thoughts and fears that could secretly be preventing your body from having a baby.

I've included 50 art, writing, music and dance activities you can do in your home to help you unlock your creative reproductive powers and release negative energy patterns in your body.

Everything in this book can be used in conjunction with an IVF, IUI or other assisted reproductive technologies. We will discuss how to prepare for an IUI and/or IVF, and how to treat yourself the days following these procedures to maximize your chances of getting pregnant.

I have included my own story of battling infertility that I hope you will find useful and inspiring.

As a bonus, I'm including:

• Your Fertility Food Tracker Diary: Its simple, easy to use and will help you track what fertility foods you are giving your body each day.

I've also included several other free journals. These include:

• Journal Writing Through Your Subconscious: to help you discover what your deepest consciousness truly thinks about fertility, motherhood and parenting.

• Your Daily Happiness Journal: to help you gain access to your inner positive-feeling antenna that is ever alert to everything good within you and around you.

• Life Affirmation Journal: designed to help you take note of all the ways birth and life take place in the world around you each day, and how you are intrinsically part of the world's never-ending reproductive cycle.

• My Child & I Journal: where you can share your dreams of a future with your children by your side.

• Emotional Tracking Journal: to help you understand what triggers your positive and negative emotions each day.

This book will also discuss how to:

• Deal with negative comments from friends and relatives, as well as your own internal negativity.

• How to not let infertility ruin your marriage.

• How to choose the right doctor and clinic.

• Ways to reduce stress in your life.

• Writing exercises that will give you a chance to go deep within to unearth and destroy all the self-defeating beliefs and traumas that might be buried deep in your tissues that could be destroying your fertility.

• More than 100 affirmations and visualizations.

• A personal fertility vision statement, that I have written as a certified life coach. It is used to help motivate and get you past the blocks and obstacles to your fertility. You can listen to and read it each day.

- Letters you can send yourself, or just leave around the house, when you need a lift or a reminder of how strong and powerful you really are.

- How to start enjoying a close loving friendship with your body, so your body becomes your best friend and teammate.

- How to turn your home into a fertility nesting center.

- Coping with the unfairness of it all.

- Ways to protect your baby once you are pregnant

And all my mistakes (which were many) you can learn from.

This is, most importantly, a book of hope…and about taking action to have the children you deserve and are worthy of.

That doctor who claimed my eggs were 'bottom of the barrel' was wrong. Less than a year later, I gave birth to my beautiful son.

Someday, I would like to send her a picture of my boy and write in blazing letters across the picture: "Is this what bottom of the barrel looks like?"

Infertility: A Training Ground for Motherhood?

In times past, women have always endured sacrifice and trial as part of motherhood. Now, due to a host of factors such as age, health and environment, women are put through a severe test of their maternal stamina even before they conceive their child.

This road, this test, this initiation, will test all of you--and it will make you one of the strongest, most capable, confident, resourceful, perseverant mothers a child could ever have. Experiencing infertility gives you a lifetime pass to enjoy motherhood in a way few ever get to enjoy it, because with the difficulties of this disease come confidence and appreciation.

This journey will demand all the best parts of you. It will demand you persevere when you want to give up. It will demand patience and persistence when frustration and helpless surrender might feel like a more natural path. It will demand that every survival skill you possess be brought forth and utilized. It will demand sacrifice, self-preservation, and a willpower beyond what you knew you had, but what intrinsically you knew you were capable of.

If you are not fortunate, you may have your heart broken in 1000 pieces.

If you are fortunate, you could still have your heart broken in 1000 places.

When you give birth to your baby none of it will matter. Your heart will heal, the scars will seem insignificant, and all the tears, disappointments and devastations will seem like bunny rabbits and balloons on a summer's day.

No big deal.

If you do not give birth to a baby, but decide to adopt, become a foster parent, a teacher, coach, counselor or play a very active role in the life of a young niece, nephew, neighbor, or cousin, you will be ready and able to mother these children and impact a younger generation in a way more powerful than you ever imagined.

You have probably been through the best training course for motherhood possible: you understand pain, you understand the potential for joy, you are willing to do the work to get the child you want, and you've proven you can take the bad stuff that comes with going after the good stuff. In doing this, you will join a group of super cultivated mothers, women ready to nurture and love the next generation, and have more than proven their worth to do this.

Infertility hurts.

Winning over infertility can be a painful process that demands resolve and sacrifice.

It is an initiation rite, of sorts, an involuntary one, of course. No one should have to go through this to have a baby and no one would voluntarily choose this road. Nonetheless, it is a reality for many of us, and it will prepare you for motherhood in a grand and inspiring way that someday you may even feel thankful to have experienced.

It is a long road and an unfair one, but at the end of the road, you could be holding the baby of your dreams, just as the same as someone who made love one night and woke up pregnant the next morning.

Then nothing at all will matter but your baby.

Ten Things About Infertility That Nobody Will Tell You--But You Need To Know Right From The Start

1. You are going to hear no. Expect to hear it at times, but don't let hearing it keep you down or stop you from going after your dream.

2. You are going to have to put some aspects of your life on hold. It will be worth it, but be prepared to spend your time, energy and money on getting pregnant and putting certain aspects of your life on hold.

3. You are going to hear negative comments, sometimes even from the people you love. Don't pay attention to what they say. This can work out for you, despite what anyone says or thinks about your health or situation.

4. This is a journey you might sometimes take alone. Don't be surprised if sometimes even your husband can't be there for you the way you need him to. If that happens, don't waste your time getting angry--just keep going.

5. The doctor you choose and the reproductive clinic they are associated with matters—choose a good one. You want a doctor who is open to trying new medications and procedures and who answers your questions and listens to what you have to say.

6. You are going to have to eat and take care of your body in a way you never have before. Get ready to make spinach, garlic and pumpkin seeds your new best friends.

7. You are going to have to be strong and stay positive, even when nothing positive is happening. You are going to have to get ready to harness every little bit of inner strength you've ever had.

8. You are also going to fall apart sometimes. Just expect it.

9. It is going to feel rotten to be invited to baby showers, children's parties, and see pregnant women at the supermarket. When that happens, just remember: someday, it could very well be you having that baby shower, hosting the children's parties and being that beautiful pregnant lady at the supermarket. And you never know: that mother with the beautiful baby that made your heart ache? She might have once been a fertility patient too.

10. You are going to have to work hard and be flexible. It is important to understand that a lot of work may be required to beat infertility. Infertility treatments require going to lots of appointments, and doing whatever you can to improve your health. This journey takes effort and push. Accepting the hard work involved will make it easier, and hopefully empower you to do what is available to heal your infertility. While beating infertility can be really hard work, the reward it well worth any effort you have to make.

Chapter 1: The Ultimate Fertility Success Program: Getting Your Body Ready

Are you ready to be pregnant? Have you been told that you cannot get pregnant for unexplainable reasons? Have you been trying for a baby for a long time and you are weary, tired and very, very sad?

Infertility is one of the most difficult journeys a woman can take.

But, starting today, know this: Infertility is not a final statement on your ability to have the family you dream of—infertility is a medical condition that, with the right treatments, is often temporary and can be cured.

So starting today, see your infertility as a temporary condition that is a signal that your body is off-track and needs something to heal it.

Infertility clinics often give patents a diagnosis of "unexplained infertility", but infertility is never a result of unexplainable, mysterious problems. Infertility is always a result of specific problems or deficits in the body—problems that are sometimes hard to detect in the way that Western medicine diagnoses ailments.

When your body does not conceive easily and naturally, there is disease, dysfunction and malfunction occurring on some level, even if it is a level so very subtle that it cannot be detected on standardized tests.

Some of the fertility problems your body may be experiencing may be hard to find because there are not machines or diagnostic tools yet available to detect slight shifts, blocks, traumas in the body that can prevent or delay pregnancy.

So just because a doctor says you can never get pregnant does not mean your body, if helped, cannot heal from infertility—but here's the catch—you have to do the right things to get back your infertility.

By turning your body from acidic to alkaline, from a diseased toxic state to one that is cleansed, from a body full of inflammation to one that is healthy.

Sometimes, our body can get onto a disease track, and it then must be pushed and healed back over to a track of health.

In this chapter, we'll discuss a comprehensive body makeover program that will change the track you are on and help you become more healthy, vibrant and fertile—as you deserve to be!

You can go to an infertility clinic and take advantage of all the latest and best treatments and medications available, which I recommend, and at the same time embark on a course of holistic, alternative healing to maximize your chances of getting pregnant and having the babies you dream of.

The first step to overcoming infertility is to change the track your body is on from:

• A state of disease and dysfunction to one of health

• An acidic state to an alkaline state

• A state of clogged toxins in the body, to one of a cleansed body
with all your organs cleansed and able to function at their highest level possible.

What can set the body down a wrong course? Unhealthy foods, low-quality drinking water, chemicals or toxins in our environment and in products we use, stress, traumas and painful life experiences that tire and weaken our organs.

Sometimes we live, eat, think and experience life in a way that can deplete our reproductive organs in ways that we are completely unaware of.

Picture yourself driving down the highway in the wrong lane. Imagine switching to another lane in order to get to your desired destination.

That is your goal right now--to get your body off the wrong road of toxic build-up to a cleansed road, from a road of tired organs to cleaned out revived organs.

Your job is to change the state of your body, by digging deep to uncover the root causes of your infertility.

Here are 10 things you can do immediately to get your body back on a healthy ready-to-conceive track:

1. Buy a juicer or a fruit/vegetable drink mixer. Learn as much as you can about making healthy vegetable and fruit drinks. Make this a daily part of your routine, whether it is simply juicing a bag of spinach or making a spinach/blueberry/flaxseed drink.

2. Find a reputable, licensed acupuncturist in your area and start going once, twice or even three times a week.

3. Visit a local health or nature food store and purchase a liver cleanse. You may want to do this more than once. This is to be done before you are in the midst of an IUI or IVF cycle.

4. Visit a supermarket and stock up on garlic, spinach, pumpkin seeds, sunflower seeds, kale, yams, and pineapple.

5. Schedule 20 minutes in your day to sit outside in the sunshine. Pick a place that feels comfortable—even if it is just putting a chair out in your front yard, a driveway or at a local park.

6. Find an excellent, highly reputable chiropractor in your area who is somewhat familiar with issues of infertility who can adjust your spine.

7. Start eating as much spinach and garlic as you can.

8. Get more sleep. Make sure your room is completely dark and get to bed earlier.

9. Stop drinking coffee and eating sugar.

10. Stop all trans fats that are in your diet. Cut down on white flour products too.

As always check with a physician before pursuing any course of treatment.

To begin:

- **Start by having a complete physical:** Go to your primary care physician and request a complete work-up.

You need to find out if you have:

- Gallstones

- Blood problems or disorders, such as anemia

- Ask for a complete work-up of your thyroid, liver and kidneys. This includes a thyroid stimulating hormone test and a comprehensive metabolic panel.

- Get tested for allergies, as you could be eating a food that weakens your body, such as gluten.

- Have your white blood cell count checked. This might help in determining if there is an undetected infection in your body.

The aim of the physical is to find out if there is an area in your body that has been overlooked, because one weak area can throw off the rest of the body.

- **Visit Your Dentist:** Get a complete dental check-up to be sure there are no lingering or untreated infections in your mouth.

Cleansing and Detoxifying Your Body

12 Cleanses To Help Restore Your Fertility

The next step in changing the state, or condition, of your body is cleansing and detoxifying. The importance of detoxifying your body should never be underestimated. In this chapter, we'll look at 12 cleanses that can help restore and maximize your fertility potential.

Please note: cleanses should be done before you start infertility medications or treatments, because you do not want them to interfere with medications or a pregnancy, if there is even a slight chance you could be pregnant. Cleansing can be compared to overturning and fertilizing the soil before planting the seed.

If you are just starting infertility treatments, you may want to choose just one or two cleanses, so as not to delay treatment.

If you've been trying to get pregnant for a long time with no success, you might want to consider doing various cleanses to strengthen your body.

Here are some cleanses to consider:

• A Liver Cleanse

Never never NEVER underestimate the importance of having your liver cleaned and detoxified. The liver is a highly influential organ that plays a key role in fertility and is one of the most important organs in your body. The liver governs approximately 500 metabolic processes and many studies have shown that the oestrogen receptors in the liver are critical for maintaining fertility.

I cannot say enough about the importance of having a clean, de-toxified liver in the quest to get pregnant.

An ineffective liver allows toxins to seep into the ovaries and endocrine system.

If your liver is congested, it cannot adequately remove toxins and fats from the body.

Instead, they will continue to recirculate through your system—causing hormonal disturbances and imbalances. It also means your ovaries will be flooded with toxic substances that your liver was suppose to clean—and your ovaries are the source of your eggs. These impurities will result in poor egg quality—all because your liver was too congested to do its job. So if you want to improve the quality of your eggs, make sure your liver is as clean and detoxified as possible.

Once the liver is cleansed, the entire endocrine and reproductive system becomes free of toxins and impurities, so they can begin functioning at a higher capacity.

What causes a sluggish, tired liver? Stress, poor diet, medication, toxins in the environment, low-quality food, coffee, sugar, white flour products and low quality drinking water, are among a few of the culprits. The older we get, the more our liver needs to be cleaned out because of the junk that we have taken into our body over the years.

A liver cleanse will help kick your body into high gear, increasing energy and vitality to all your organs.

Liver cleanses can be found online and at most health and natural food stores. You may want to do a 30-day cleanse more than once. Please note: A liver cleanse should never be done while you are taking infertility medications, as it could interfere with the effectiveness of the medication. It is something to do BEFORE you begin any infertility treatments or medication, and is never to be done if you could be pregnant.

In addition to a liver cleanse, here are some other ways to detoxify, cleanse and strengthen your liver:

• Milk thistle is a wonderful herb for cleansing the liver. Read the directions on the bottle carefully as to amounts taken.

• Lemon is a great liver cleanser. About 20 minutes before breakfast in the morning, squeeze the juice from one or two fresh lemons into some warm water and drink.

• Beets are excellent liver cleansers. You can eat them cooked or juice them. To juice beets, peel and cut into small wedges that can easily fit in your juicer. Juice the beets with some apple, spinach or kale.

• Chlorophyll is a highly esteemed liver cleanser.

• Artichokes are powerful liver protectors because they contain a flavonoid called silymarin, which is an antioxidant that protects the liver from toxicity.

• Foods that are good for your liver include: spirulina, garlic, carrots, romaine lettuce, apples, grapefruit, chicory, mustard greens, dandelion greens, avocados, walnuts, turmeric and parsley.

• Cabbage can also be juiced and is effective in cleaning the liver.

• Amino acids, derived from healthy sources of protein, are key to the liver working at maximum capacity. Foods that contain these amino acids include: nuts, such as pumpkin seeds, squash seeds and almonds; lean meats, eggs, and beans, such as lentils and garbanzo.

• In Chinese medicine, infertility is often linked to Liver chi stagnation, a result of stress, overwork, and the effects of coffee and alcohol. Irritability, headaches and frustration are just some of the physical and emotional symptoms of liver chi stagnation. Acupuncturists and herbalists can work on unblocking energy stagnation in the liver.

- According to Chinese medicine, emotional and lifestyle cures for liver stagnation include being assertive, making clear decisions and enjoying lots of fun, laughter and relaxation. Holding on to anger, feeling stuck and depression impair the liver by stagnating the energy. Letting go, moving on, and exercising control over one's life, can help in healing the liver.

• Heavy Metal Cleanse

Every day, we come into contact with heavy metals that can disrupt our fertility. As much as possible, you'll want to start paying attention to the metals you may be unintentionally bringing into your body through the products you use and your lifestyles choices. Cosmetics, drinking soda straight from a can, deodorants that contain aluminum, solvents in dry cleaning, exposure to radiation, all contain metals that can find their way into our body, causing metabolic disruptions in organs, such as our heart, brain, kidneys and liver.

Because heavy metals are so common in our world, most of us have them in our systems.

There are a variety of heavy metal cleanses available online and in health food stores. You may want to do this cleanse more than once. This is, however, a cleanse to be done before you start infertility treatments and medications.

Along with a heavy metal cleanse, here are some additional ways to cleanse your body of heavy metals:

- Garlic is known to help reduce metal levels in the body. It contains the antioxidant allicin. You can eat garlic raw, include it in your cooking or juice it. To juice, simply peel the garlic, juice, and drink combined with lemon juice and water. Have a big glass of water nearby to help reduce stomach discomfort.

- Milk thistle is an herb that can also help remove heavy metals from the liver.

- Cilantro is a powerful herb that is known for binding heavy metals and whisking them out of the body.

- Alpha Lipoic Acid and Gluthatione are powerful supplements for helping cells remove heavy metals from the body.

- Chlorella is a fresh water algae loaded with chlorophyll. Buy it in powder form and mix with water for fast absorption. It can also be taken in capsule or tablet form.

- A steam bath can help remove metals.

- Burdock is a potent blood purifier and can remove heavy metals from the body. It also helps purify the liver.

- Onions contain the antioxidant quercetin, which helps remove heavy metals from the body. Add to your salads daily or juice them.

• A Yeast Cleanse

Yeast, also known as candida, can impact your fertility by causing your internal vagina's flora to become unbalanced, making it difficult for sperm to reach the uterus.

Candida is a common yeast that lives in our gut, and an overgrowth of it can lead to leaky gut syndrome, which wreaks havoc with many of the body's systems, including the endocrine system, that plays a huge role in reproduction and fertility

Yeast can also impact estrogen levels in the body, causing thyroid problems and hormonal imbalances. Yeast problems can come from frequent or long-term use of antibiotics, birth control pills, or eating foods with a lot of sugar. Getting rid of yeast is an important step in rebalancing your body so it can heal itself.

Some ways to rid your body of yeast:

- Do a yeast or candida cleanse, that can be bought online, at health food store or nature food store.

- Acidophillus can help control candida.

- Flaxseed is known to help control yeast.

- Garlic is an enemy of yeast. Take garlic capsules, juice garlic and eat lots of raw garlic.

- Avoid sugar and white flour foods. These can include sugary juices, desserts, breads, crackers, pre-packaged meals, soda. Be alert to foods with hidden sugar, such as salad dressings or ketchup. Avoid alcohol, chocolate, cakes and carbonated beverages.

- Eat plain yogurt.

- Consider taking probiotics in a supplement form.

- Enzyme supplements are available that are made specifically to fight yeast.

- Replace your regular salt with Celtic salt or kosher salt.

• Adrenal Cleanse

Adrenal fatigue, also known as adrenal burn-out, impacts many women suffering with infertility. If you are having trouble getting pregnant, this could be one of the not-so-obvious and sometimes difficult to diagnose reasons behind your infertility.

The adrenals are a very important to your fertility because they are part of the endocrine system, which is responsible for producing and balancing more than 50 hormones in your body. When the adrenals are weak or not working at full capacity, the body's entire endocrine system and hormones can become imbalanced.

Adrenal burn-out occurs when the adrenals are stressed and pushed to the point where they begin producing excessive amounts of cortisol and adrenaline, which results in progesterone in the body producing too many stress hormones.

The adrenals become too sluggish, and then the other endocrine glands are not signaled to release their hormones, which results in the entire communication system in the endocrine glands breaking down.

Emotional trauma, living in a constant state of fight or flight, chemical toxins, lack of sleep, anxiety, stress, depression, poor diet, infections, and some prescription drugs, can all cause adrenal burn-out.

If the adrenals are exhausted, you may not produce enough progesterone, which is the pro-gestational hormone needed to get pregnant and carry a pregnancy to term.

Here are some ways to help strengthen your adrenals:

• Take a Vitamin C supplement. The adrenal gland uses vitamin C at a higher rate than other cells in the body.

• Don't let your blood sugar levels get too low. Eat regular meals and never skip breakfast. Keep your blood sugar levels normal by eating healthy foods throughout the day.

• Stop drinking coffee or drink no more than one cup of coffee a day. Caffeine depletes the body of B vitamins, which the adrenals need. Stop trying to energize and push your body by drinking another cup of coffee. Instead, eat fruits and vegetables that will provide your body with healthy forms of energy.

• Drink lots of high-quality water.

• Consider taking a Vitamin B complex, Vitamin E and an adrenal gland supplement.

• A high-quality liquid trace mineral supplement can help support the adrenal glands. Note: Although you may want to drastically reduce your intake of this supplement once you are pregnant, or consult with a doctor on the levels of minerals that are safe and healthy to take during pregnancy.

- Make lifestyle changes that reduce stress in your life. Do you need to change jobs? Relocate? Take a hard and honest look at the way you live your daily life. Start including more activities in your life that eliminate stress and reduce a fight-or-flight way of living. These include: deep breathing, massage, daily walks by a lake, ocean or in a beautiful park.

Consider more time for prayer, journal writing, and positive visualization.

- Foods that help adrenals include spinach, garlic, onions, green leafy vegetables and brown rice.

- Almonds and cashews, which are high in magnesium, are very healthy for the adrenal system.

- Eat more seeds, such as sunflower and pumpkin seeds.

- Avoid white flour products, soda, sugary fruit juices or anything that makes blood sugar levels rise rapidly.

- Alternative health therapies, such as applied kinesiology, myofascial release, and craniosacral therapy can restore a weakened adrenal system.

- Getting more sleep and better sleep can help restore the adrenal glands. So, go to bed earlier, preferably aim for a 9 to 10 o'clock bedtime, and try to stop all technology and electronic stimulation about an hour before bed for a better quality sleep.

- Sea salt, celtic salt or regular salt in moderate amounts can help the adrenal system provided that you don't suffer from high-blood pressure.

- Healthy fats like olive oil, coconut oil, ground flax seed or flax seed oil are excellent for burnt-out and exhausted adrenals.

- Adrenal exhaustion can sometimes be caused by hidden food allergies. Find out if you are allergic to wheat, corn or dairy products.

• A Colon Cleanse

Cleansing your colon can significantly improve your overall health and fertility. A colon that is diseased, inflamed or full of yeast, mold, fungus or parasites can cause a general malaise in the body and lower the body's pH balance, making it more acidic – and acid creates a hostile environment for reproductive health.

A colon that is weighed down by years of buildup can also press on the uterus and surrounding reproductive organs.

Those who have undergone colon cleanses will attest to the dramatic improvements in how they feel afterwards. By ridding your body of decaying matter, you could very well be turning back the hands of time. Colon cleansing, sometimes called colon hydrotherapy, can rid the body of chemicals and toxins that affect the egg and sperm.

Colonic irrigation and herbal cleansings help remove toxins, parasites and mucus that have built up in the colon. By flushing out impacted waste, passing stool is easier and transit times are improved. Removing impurities goes a long way in helping the body absorb nutrients, and enhancing energy levels.

Some doctors believe that poor bowel management is at the root of many health problems, and many diseases are a result of toxins built-up in the intestinal tract that are not eliminated. A digestive tract that has a build-up of unhealthy, slow moving foods that stick to the intestinal walls result in an overburdened colon full of decaying fecal matter and foods are acid-forming.

Yeasts, molds, fungus, bacteria, parasites and fecal materal can then enter the blood stream, causing what is known as leaky bowel syndrome. This results in a reduction of nutrients the body is able to absorb, and in turn impacts fertility.

Have your colon cleansed, at a licensed, reputable establishment with a long-time track record.

This can be an uncomfortable process, but in cleaning out your colon, you will be bringing new youth to your body.

You can also clean your colon with colon cleansing products available online, or at a natural foods store or supermarket.

Note: once there is even a chance that you are pregnant, stop all colon cleanses. This is something to be done only BEFORE there is any chance you are pregnant. If there is any possibility that you are pregnant, do not continue with any type of colon cleanse.

Here are some other ways to cleanse and detoxify your colon:

• Foods that help keep the colon clean include apples, blackberries, blueberries, raspberries, figs, dates, avocados, spinach, Swiss chard, oatmeal, flax, and chickpeas.

• Foods to avoid include sugar, white flour, and hormone/antibiotic-filled meats that assault the body.

• Fennel and garlic are known to kill bacteria and parasites in the colon, thus improving colon function.

• Cayenne pepper and garlic are also known colon cleansers.

• Flaxseeds and psyllium husk seeds help clean the colon.

• Herbs like Slippery Elm and Cascara Sagrada also are used in many colon detoxification cleanses.

• Eat large amounts of fiber.

• Ginger and garlic can help with healthy bowel movements, along with some olive oil in the morning. Leafy greens and healthy fibers can also aid in elimination.

• Apples and carrots, which contain a large amount of water, go far in cleansing the colon.

• Consider juicing apples, carrots, spinach, and other green vegetables as a way to help cleanse the colon.

• Be aware of your bowel movements. Make sure you are having at least one healthy bowel movement a day. Don't hold in a bowel movement if you feel it coming.

• Drink lemon, honey or maple syrup and cayenne pepper several times a day. Drink with or without food for several days as a way to cleanse the colon.

• Reduce the amount of processed foods, fast foods, pizza and foods with additives that you eat.

• While detoxifying your colon, start taking probiotics as a way to replenish your intestinal flora.

• Eat a diet with a lot of high fiber vegetables, such as dark leafy greens,

• Drink a lot of high-quality water each day. Inadequate hydration can lead to a build-up of toxins in the colon.

• Juice or make a drink with vegetables daily.

• Include essential fatty acids in your diet, such as ground flax seed, evening primrose oil, cod liver oil and coconut oil.

• Eat foods rich in healthy fats, such as avocados, olive oil and nuts.

• Include more olive oil in your diet, because it reduces bile acid and increase enzymes that regulate cell turn over in the lining of the intestines.

- In Chinese medicine, the colon is one of the two organs in the metal element, and has the function of eliminating what is unnecessary or toxic in our bodies. On the emotional level, the colon enables us to let go of the garbage directed at our bodies and spirit. To heal the colon, it is important to 'let go' of negative experiences that may have tainted our self-worth.

For issues that are unresolved, write them on paper and burn them, thus releasing their content. Breath slowly and deeply each day. As you breath, feel the negativity, impurity and pain leave your body, and breath in energized, purified air. If you are chronically constipated, it may be that you are having a hard time letting go of something in your life, such as a past hurt, rejection or trauma. Allow yourself to accept and be open to new experiences in your life. As much as you can, make room for new, transforming experiences in your life.

• Kidney Cleanse

According to Chinese herbal medicine, one of the most common causes of infertility is a problem with or a deficiency in the kidney. In fact, in Chinese medicine, a kidney deficiency is the most common diagnosis in infertility.

In Chinese medicine, the kidney is considered the main root of our Qi (chi) which regulates reproduction and is considered the seat of procreation, the vitality center of the body. A weak Qi, or kidney function, affects the quality and development of eggs, and impacts the ovaries and uterus.

A kidney deficiency is often a result of poor diet and stress.

Here are various ways to cleanse and strengthen the kidney:

- Make sure you are working on cleansing and detoxifying the liver, because a healthy, clean liver results in a healthy, strong kidney.

- Find an acupuncturist who is experienced in working with kidney deficiency and its impact on fertility.

- Stop all coffee or limit coffee intake to no more than a cup a day.

- Avoid carbonated beverages, artificial sweeteners and excessive amounts of dairy products.

- Limit red meat.

- Reduce sugar and sodium in your diet. Stop potato chips, crackers, cheese spreads, deli meats and instant potato mixes.

- Kidney problems are often the result of stress, chronic anger and shame, so it is important to release and free yourself from these feelings. Journal writing, prayer, forgiveness of yourself and others, are all steps that can begin the healing process.

- Dandelion tea is known to help flush toxins from the kidney.

- Cod liver oil contains high levels of Vitamin D that strengthen the kidneys.

- Foods that regenerate the kidney include chestnuts, strawberries, walnuts, raspberries; black, kidney and mung beans, fennel, onions, beetroot, garlic, ginger, cloves, red bell peppers, cabbage, cauliflower, dandelion, blueberries, red grapes, and wild salmon.

- Add lots of flaxseed, pumpkin, and sunflower seeds to your diet.

- Walnuts and chestnuts enhance the kidney's function.

- Spirulina, kelp, chlorella, and wheatgrass are good for the kidney.

- Eat lots of asparagus and other deep green leafy vegetables.

- The herb Nettle is known to strengthen the kidney.

- Drink lots of water.

- Limit alcohol intake. Do not overtax your kidney with too much alcohol.

- Juice cabbage, parsley, cucumbers and ginger.

- Eat more apples, cranberries, olive oil, and onions.

- Stay away from high-sodium foods.

- Milk thistle is a great nutrient for the kidney.

- Staying hydrated is very important to flushing out toxins in the kidney.

- Eat large amounts of watermelon for a few days.

- A Chinese herbalist can provide herbal formulas to clean the kidney.

- Burdock tea helps removes waste from the kidneys.

- Dandelion tea is known to help cleanse the kidneys.

- Ginger root and turmeric tea is good for the kidneys and can be made by boiling some turmeric powder with peeled ginger root.

- Grapes and cranberries. Grapes help flush uric acid and other waste products from the kidney. Cranberries contain quinine, which the liver converts to hippuric acid, which in turns helps remove urea and uric acid from the kidneys.

- Apples are often used as a home remedy for kidney stones.

- Garlic is a natural diuretic that helps flush out kidneys.

- Cucumbers are a natural diuretic that can dissolve kidney and bladder stones.

- Onions can help pass kidney stones.

- Kidney beans and peas contain arginine, an amino acid that helps cleanse the kidney of ammonia.

- Make sure you are getting enough Vitamin C, Vitamin E, calcium and B-6.

- Keep your blood pressure, blood glucose level, and cholesterol levels in healthy ranges, so your kidneys are not overtaxed.

- According to natural healers, the emotion that seems to impact the kidney the most is fear. Some believe that chronic fear and anxiety in childhood impacts the health of the kidneys later in life. To release fear, begin to embrace your life with courage. Welcome life! Do not push it away or hid from it.

In Chinese medicine, the ability to use our will power to express our unique creativity is also dependent on good kidney energy. With a strong kidney qi, we will have the resolve to overcome fear and pursue goals. A weak kidney results in a shaky sense of purpose and one who is easily distracted. Feeling stuck and not letting go is also sometimes the emotional root of kidney disease. The kidneys can store deep sadness, which can in turn result in illness. It is important to work on letting go of anger, fear, and traumatic, painful memories. Bring balance into your life in whenever way you can. Enjoy natural beauty and lots of rest. Spend more time enjoying natural bodies of water, such as lakes, oceans, and rivers. Keep a bowl of water with flowers nearby.

- Get a foot massage. Ask the massage therapist to stimulate and massage the kidney point on the foot that will revitalize the kidney qi.

• Parasite Cleanse

Another facet of cleansing is eliminating parasites in your body. Parasites can impact hormone levels and some nutritionists feel that parasites can also weaken a man's sperm quality.

Symptoms of parasites include brain fog or mental fuzziness, toe fungus or athletes foot, constant illness, rectal itching, especially at night, endometriosis, anxiety and depression.

Sleep problems, immune disorders, teeth grinding, eczema, hives, and chronic fatigue can also be the result of parasites.

Common tests that can discover whether or not you have parasites include a comprehensive digestive stool analysis, candida testing and a gastric acid self-test.
Doctors can also test for parasites through x-rays.

To avoid getting parasites, do not eat raw fish or sushi and be sure to cook all fish very well. Avoid undercooked meat. Wash all fruits and vegetables thoroughly. Be very careful when eating at salad bars. Do not let animals lick you in the face or mouth. Be aware of foods you eat when you visit other countries.

Health food stores and various health-related web sites have various parasite cleanses to choose from, and this is often a first and best step to rid the body of parasites. Make sure to drink lots of water while cleansing.

Along with doing a parasite cleanse, here are some tips on ridding your body of parasites:

• Pineapple is an effective agent in ridding the body of parasites. Pineapple contains the digestive enzyme bromelain that can help clear tapeworms.

• The probiotics in yogurt are also known to kill parasites.

• Avoid sugar. Parasites are known to feed off sugar—so the less that is in your system, the less they are able to flourish within your body.

• Avoid or reduce white flour products.

• Apple cider vinegar, which is high in B-vitamins, can help neutralize the body's pH balance and improve digestion.

• Probiotics can help restore gut bacteria wiped out by parasites. Do not take a probiotic, however, within an hour of taking apple cider vinegar.

• Cinnamon is a natural remedy for parasites.

• Include more garlic in your diet. Juice it, eat it, include it in your meals, whenever you can.

• Olive oil can help remove parasite waste.

• Trichomoniasis is a vaginal infection that is seen to play a role in infertility. Ask to be tested for this.

• Chlorphyl can help eliminate parasites.

• Papaya seeds are a natural method for removing parasites. Blend them with honey or coconut oil for seven days in a row, as a parasite cleanse. Make sure to drink lots of water while cleansing.

• Pumpkin seeds are effective in killing roundworms or tapeworms. Oven roast lightly. They are more effective if eaten on an empty stomach.

• Eat pomegranates alone as they are known for destroying worms in the intestinal tract.

• Cloves and turmeric can help fight parasites.

• Sweet potatoes and squash can increase resistance to parasites because of their high Vitamin A content.

• Raw onions and garlic provide sulfur containing amino acids that are anti-parasitic.

• Thyme and thyme tea can help clear the body of parasites.

- Cayenne pepper helps repel parasites.

- A colonic irrigation, also known as a colon cleaning, can also help kill parasites.

• Uterine Cleanse

You want to do everything possible to create the best and healthiest environment for your growing baby, and that means doing what is needed to create a healthy uterine lining for implantation of your embryos.

Conditions like hormonal imbalance, low circulation, or an unhealthy diet can impact the uterus. Other factors that impact the condition of the uterus include: stagnation of blood flow to the uterus, uterine fibroids, scar tissue from a cesarean, abdominal surgery, a D&C after a miscarriage, endometriosis, or a pelvic inflammatory disease caused by a sexually transmitted disease.

Here are some ways to cleanse and strengthen your uterus:

- Goldenseal root cleanses the uterus.

- Dong Quai, an herb, increases blood flow to the uterus and builds the uterine lining. It also tones and strengthens the uterus by regulating hormonal balance, improving uterine tone and is a blood tonic that helps circulation. It also relieves congestion and pain in the reproductive system.

- Damiana, an herb, encourages circulation and blood supply to the uterus.

- Red Raspberry Leaf or Red Raspberry Root has long been used as a uterine tonic to regulate and tone uterine muscles. It can be taken as a supplement or a tea.

- Eat or juice dandelion leaves, spinach, beets, garlic and lemon.

- Nettle Leaves is a uterine cleanser.

- L-Arginine promotes synthesis of nitric oxide, which increases blood flow to the uterus and ovaries.

- Eating foods rich in zinc can help strengthen the uterus. These include pumpkin seeds, sesame seeds and spinach.

- Some health practitioners recommend propping one's legs up against a wall 15 minutes a day to encourage increased blood flow to the uterus.

- Avoid soy and peas.

- Acupuncture can help bring more blood to your uterus. Let your acupuncturist know you are working on fertility and would like to improve your circulation to your uterus.

- Eat blood nourishing foods, such as spinach and dates.

- Pomegranates and pomegranate juice can help build uterine lining.

- Chinese medicine adheres to the belief that it is important to keep the uterus and belly warm while trying to get pregnant. They suggest not drinking or eating anything too cold, wearing socks and keeping one's feet warm at night. Do not go barefoot or wear flip-flops.
However, this does not mean overheating your body with a water bottle or doing anything that could overheat a growing fetus.

- Write a letter to your womb. Let whatever wants to be said come up and be said. Express whatever you are feeling, whether it is anger, fear or lack of self-love. Do not repress any of your feelings. Allow yourself the freedom to speak your truth, whatever it is.

- Practice deep breathing into your uterus and repeat the affirmation: I receive, I receive, I receive. I receive my baby, I receive my baby, I receive my baby.

- Your uterus deserves acknowledgement, respect and unconditional love. It needs to be told it is strong enough, good enough and worthy enough to receive a baby.

- A Native American fertility tradition is to wear a long skirt with no underwear, and sit on the ground to release whatever wounds are within you into the earth. As you do this, imagine your womb is a beautiful flowering place full of energy and light. Let the earth's energy flow up to your uterus, so it can draw from the healing energy of the earth.

- Pineapple contains a proteolytic enzyme called bromelain which reduces inflammation and breaks up proteins that prevent embryo implantation. Eating pineapple core a few days before and after an IVF cycle can help implantation. But stop eating pineapple immediately after any IVF or IUI or if you think if there is any chance you might be pregnant. While pineapple helps implantation, it is definitely not recommended for pregnancy.

- Eat lots of blueberries. Research shows they contain anthocyanins that help maintain the lining of the uterus.

- Brazil nuts contain selenium, that can thicken the uterine lining and help with implantation.

- Foods with omega-3 fatty acids can improve blood flow to the uterus, such as salmon, flaxseed oil, pumpkin seeds, walnuts, and olive oil.

- See a massage therapist who is familiar with massage to help increase circulation to the uterus and unblock the reproductive system. Look for a massage therapist experienced in deep tissue massage or massage that is used to clear blocked energy in the organs.

Acupressure, myofacial release and reflexology can also offer massage that brings blood and oxygen to the reproductive organs.

- Ask your uterus these questions: have you ever felt judged? Blamed? Abused? What do you need to heal? What can I do to help you feel loved and nurtured? Write the answers that come up from within you.

- Visualize your uterus as a cozy, warm, loving and safe place for your baby. Repeat, write and sing these affirmations:
-my uterus is healthy and just right for my baby
-my uterus welcomes my baby
-my uterus is a safe and welcoming place for my baby
-my uterus is a healing, balanced, and loving home for my baby
-I love you uterus. Thank you for taking good care of my baby.
-Uterus, you are enough. You are enough to hold my baby.
-Dear uterus, I honor and respect you.

- Supplements recommended to help implantation include zinc, Vitamin C, selenium and iron.

- Important To Note: herbs used to strengthen and cleanse your uterus must be stopped once there is any chance you are pregnant or while taking infertility medications.

• Blood Cleanse

You want to cleanse your blood of toxins and chemicals as much as possible, because chemicals and toxins in your bloodstream can impact the health of your eggs and various organs that impact fertility.

Here are some ways to cleanse and detoxify your blood:

- Chlorophyll is known to cleanse the blood of impurities.

- Juice or eat cilantro, parsley and beets. Beet juice is a strong blood purifier.

- Drink lemon and water

- Burdock Root is revered by natural practitioners as one of the most effective blood cleansers and purifiers. It strengthens the liver and increases urination to help the kidneys remove toxins from the blood.

- Yellow Dock Root enriches and purifies the blood

- Dandelion promotes bile production that breaks down fats in the body, and destroys harmful microbes found in digested food that can enter the bloodstream.

- Goji berries are a powerful antioxidant that alkalize the blood.

- Consider digestive enzymes between meals or before bed

- Red clover is a blood purifier.

- Apple cider vinegar helps cleanse the blood.

- Echinacea is known for enhancing the immune system and cleaning the blood of pathogens.

- Drink lots of pure water

- Garlic is a strong blood purifier. Juice it, eat it, crush cloves of garlic in water and drink it, or chew on raw garlic each day.

- Turmeric purifies the blood

- Teas made from Oregon Grape Root and Sarsaparilla Root rid the blood of waste products.

- Broccoli, cabbage, cauliflower and watercress are all blood purifiers. Some recommend juicing cauliflower as a great way to clean your blood.

- Parsley is a natural blood cleanser.

- Cayenne pepper improves the circulatory system by cleaning out the channels that the blood flows through.

• A Lymph System Cleanse

The lymph is a very important, but often overlooked, system in the body that impacts fertility. It is so important that some health practitioners believe that a clogged, sluggish, toxic lymph system accounts for many illnesses in the body.

The lymph system is a complex system of vessels and ducts that move fluid and toxins out of the body. A sluggish lymph system means the body is not disposing of waste properly. This affects fertility because the lymphatic system plays a key role in the circulation of hormones, and a stagnant lymphatic system can impact the feedback system of these hormones.

A cleansed lymph system can help revive sluggish, congested ovaries and reduce acid levels in the vagina.

Lack of exercise, a sedentary lifestyle, stress, chronic digestive imbalances, and a high-sodium diet, can make the lymphatic system sluggish and ineffective.

Symptoms of a sluggish lymph system include feeling tired and fatigued, getting sick a lot, being overweight, having fatty deposits of cellulite, acne, rashes, as well as having lots of food sensitivities and allergies.

Some believe that fibromyalgia and chronic fatigue syndrome are a result of a clogged lymph system.

Here are some ways to cleanse the lymph system:

• To help the flow of your lymph system, drink plenty of high-quality water each day. Staying well hydrated is key to a healthy lymph system.

• Eliminate, as much as you can, sugar, soda and fruit juices from your diet.

- Always remember that the lymph system has no pump, so it is up to you to help keep your lymph flowing by drinking lots of water and moving your body. Exercises such as jumping on a mini-trampoline, dancing, walking or swimming are helpful. Jumping helps the lymphatic circulation by stimulating the millions of one-way valves in the system. If you are laid up due to a surgery or illness, it is important to find ways to move the lymph system, such as a lymph massage of a self-massage.

- Do deep breathing exercises.

- Eat lots of green vegetables to purify the blood and lymph.

- Essential fatty acids are important to the lymph. Walnuts and flaxseeds give the lymph system the fatty acids it needs. Almonds, sunflower seeds, pumpkin seeds, Brazil nuts, coconut oil and flaxseed oil also provide essential fatty acid.

- Use a natural bristle brush to brush your skin in circular motions, upward from the feet to the torso, before showering.

- Avoid processed foods that have artificial preservatives, flavors, colors, stabilizers, which includes many packaged and fast foods. These can also include hot dogs, canned foods, cereals, packaged dinners and luncheon meats.

- Avoid fatty foods and white breads.

- Raw fruit is a powerful lymph cleanser.

- Cranberries and cranberry juice can also help emulsify fat in the lymph system.

- Foods that help the lymph system include beets, onions, garlic, avocados, seaweed, kelp, kombu, kale, radish and mustard greens.

- Juice one green drink a day.

- Eat lots of citrus fruits, like lemons and limes.

- Take chlorophyll to help purify your lymph system.

- Consider an apple cider vinegar cleanse that combines honey, garlic and apple cider in a blender.

- Herbs such as Echinacea, Goldenseal and Astragalus can lessen congestion and swelling in the lymphatic system.

- One of the ways to cleanse your lymph system is a lymphatic massage, sometimes called manual lymphatic drainage.

Lymph massage is a very gentle form of deep tissue massage that moves the lymph under your skin, freeing trapped toxins and improves lymph flow in the body. It combines a gentle pressure with soft pumping movements in the direction of the lymph nodes in the body. You can find this type of practitioner by searching 'lymphatic drainage massage with your city/town/' or by searching holistic practitioners in your area, who might be able to direct you to someone who does this type of massage.

- Massaging under your arms can be helpful in relieving congestion. Place your fingertips under your armpit. Then gently push inward, towards the center of your body. Repeat this circular motion.

- Acupuncture is very helpful to the lymph system.

- Drink a cup of red clover tea each day.

- Laugh from your belly, which helps pump your lymphatic system.

- Avoid white flour products, white rice, bread and pasta, as much as possible.

- Eating foods high in potassium can improve your lymph system. These include bananas, raisins, dates, spinach and orange juice.

- Sip hot water throughout the day.

- Beets are healthy for the lymph system.

- Cayenne pepper can boost a sluggish lymph system and reduce mucous congestion.

- Stop using underarm deodorants that contain aluminium and clog the natural excretion of toxins from the lymph system.

- Stop wearing tight bras.

- Letting yourself feel your congested emotions encourages natural detoxification of the lymph system. Allow yourself to feel. Let yourself express your grief through crying, moving anger out of your body, talking, writing or whatever way your body chooses. Honor and express your emotions.

• Thyroid Cleanse

Your thyroid is a key organ that impacts your fertility.

To keep your thyroid healthy:

- As much as possible, eliminate gluten from your diet.

- Alkalize your body as much as possible, through green vegetables, green drinks and green smoothies.

- Drink warm lemon water throughout the day to loosen toxins in the digestive system.

- Foods that can help the thyroid include: Spirulina, Brazil nuts, sunflower seeds, black walnuts.

- Iodized table salt

- Chlorophyl and coconut oil are known to strengthen the thyroid.

- Avoid all soy products

- Herbs to consider include Irish moss and Kelp.

My Diary: Throughout this book, I will share my experience of infertility. This was the first essay I wrote at the start of my journey.

Today is my first day of writing a journal on my road to victory over infertility. I am writing this book for women like me who have been told that their eggs are too old, that our bodies are too old, weak, or damaged, that there is little hope. I am writing this book for women who feel that having a child is some type of impossible dream, that they are the victim of some pathologically cruel biological problem.

I am writing this book for women who, like me, dream of starting a family, but find the road long, cruel, uphill, and not always forgiving of slight mistakes and accumulated years.

I am 36 years old. Last week, a doctor that seemed very kind when I first met her told me that my eggs were the 'bottom of the barrel.' I have been seething with pain and engulfed in sadness ever since.

'Bottom of the barrel' the very image leaves me feeling hopeless. I cannot yell at her. I cannot criticize her. For if I do, the clinic may label me 'psychologically unfit' to undergo further infertility treatments. So I stay quiet. I watch my words. I must adhere to and accept as normal their warped and perverse idea that pulling hope away is truly in the best interest of the patient, when with all my heart I know that it is only hope and faith that will ultimately give me the baby I so desperately want. What kind of monsters are they? I so want to walk into that clinic, tell that monster doctor disguised as a kind, caring medical professional off, and never step foot in there again. But then what? I have no choice but to bite my tongue, and wait until it is my turn to walk in there with a beautiful baby and say, "hello, do you want to see what bottom of the barrel looks like?' That is when my victory will be complete.

For now, I wait and suffer and try to erase their hopeless images from my head.

In this book, I will recount my experience with infertility.

I will tell you now that this book will end with my successfully creating the family I dream of. I say this with confidence, for I believe God created us with a body that can heal and thrive and grow past illness, and that doctors do not understand the miracle of faith and the miracle of hope.

And for that doctor who tried to destroy my hope, I dedicate this book to you and anyone else who believes in stomping on a women's hope.

I don't always believe in being realistic—in putting my faith in only what I can see. Sometimes holding on to a dream takes being strong enough to push aside the skeptics, the cynics, the naysayers and delving into the world of hope--a world that takes a lot of strength to hold on to when everything around you is crumbling.

I begin this day by swimming. I am trying to get as healthy as possible. In the world of infertility, at 36, I am labeled old, but I don't feel old. Well, yes, maybe I do feel old. Withered inside at times. I just went through a harrowing IVF that ended with my becoming pregnant, only to lose the baby within two weeks of conception.

Cruel. That is how I feel right now about the past two weeks: cruel. They dubbed this pregnancy a chemical pregnancy, relegating it to something that almost didn't happen, didn't really happen, never existed. Thus was taken my right to feel sad or mourn, as it wasn't a pregnancy and it wasn't a miscarriage, but it was in a way, or is it? Nothing...dismiss it...mourning stamped invalid.

Most of all, I dedicate this book to God, who is the
strength of my life. Without the privilege of prayer, I could not endure the hell of infertility. When the load was too heavy, it was only through prayer to God that I kept one foot in front of the other and kept trying.

So together, I begin this journey with you, a fellow infertility victim and survivor. I pray that we all see victory, in whatever form we wish it to come. For those of you wanting a child, I pray for your victory.

For those of you who have come to the point that adoption is a joyful option, I pray for you. I pray that we all can have the families we want and deserve, for family is a blessing and a gift, and all women deserve to receive this treasure of security, companionship, love and purpose.

Balancing Your Hormones and Improving the Quality of Your Eggs

• Balancing Your Hormones

If our hormones are not balanced, our fertility is compromised on every level. Our hormones, produced by our glands and tissues, are chemical communicators that deliver messages to our body. These messages are then released into our blood, where they travel to other tissues and send signals initiating various activities within our body and brain.

Hormones affect how we think and feel.

Our hormones are impacted by stress, fluid changes in the body, vitamin and mineral levels, infections, exposure to environmental toxins and body fat. Blood sugar imbalances, a toxic liver, folic acid deficiency, inflammation in the ovaries, breast and joints, and unhealthy gut flora can all be a result of unbalanced hormones.

Other symptoms of a hormonal imbalance can include insomnia, headaches, migraines, anxiety, foggy thinking, hot flashes, mood swings, thinning hair, bloating, rapid heartbeat, and allergies. Our hormones are impacted by stress, fluid changes in the body, vitamin and mineral levels, infection and exposure to environmental toxins and body fat.

It is important to support and strengthen the entire endocrine system. Hormones are coordinated by this system, which includes the hypothalamus, pituitary gland, adrenal gland, thyroid, parathyroid, pancreas, pineal gland, thymus and ovaries. The foods you eat, the stress levels you experience, the chemicals in your environment, all impact the endocrine system, and in turn, your hormones.

Progesterone is a key hormone in fertility and you want to do whatever you can to make sure you have adequate progesterone levels in your body. Progesterone plays an important role in conception and maintaining a healthy pregnancy. It works to balance the effects of estrogen.

It helps maintain the lining of the uterus, which makes it possible for a fertilized egg to attach and survive.

It also makes cervical mucous accessible to the sperm, preventing immune rejection of the developing baby and normalizes blood clotting. Progesterone is produced by the corpus luteum in the ovaries and by the adrenal glands.

One of the main causes of a progesterone defiency is too much estrogen in the body. Estrogen dominance is extremely dangerous to one's fertility. It can result from eating a lot of commercially raised meat and dairy products that contain large amounts of estrogen. Chemicals called xenoestrogens are often in these food sources and they mimic the hormone estrogen and disrupt the delicate balance between estrogen and progesterone. Other excess hormones and hormone-like substances found in our environment, food and water also impact progesterone levels in the body. Pollution, stress, processed foods, soy products, and endometriosis, can cause an overload of estrogen. Allergies like asthma, hives, dry eyes, weight gain, irregular periods, and foggy thinking are symptoms of estrogen dominance.

A low thyroid, recurrent early miscarriages, sleep disturbances, and heart palpitations, can sometimes be symptoms of progesterone deficiency.

Other hormones important to fertility include estradiol, or estrogen, that are produced by the follicles and corpus luteum, also known as the remnant egg sac in the ovaries. The luteinizing hormone, known as the LH surge, produced in the anterior pituitary gland, triggers ovulation and the development of the corpus luteum. It works in conjunction with the follicle stimulating hormone (FSH) that is also released and synthesized by the anterior pituitary gland. The FSH hormone regulates the reproductive process and signals the follicles in the ovary to begin maturing in preparation for ovulation.

Tests that can track your hormone levels include progesterone, estradiol, FSH, LH, prolactin, testosterone, sex hormone binding globulin, glucose tolerance test, thyroid panel and a blood lipid panel.

Here are some ways to balance and maintain healthy fertility hormone levels in your body:

• Reduce your exposure to xenohormones, which can be found in car exhaust, plastics, solvents, adhesives, pesticides, and emulsifiers found in soap and cosmetics and PCD's from industrial waste.

• Consider the herb Chaste Tree Berry, also known as Vitex Extract, that can balance hormones and strengthen the pituitary and ovary glands. This herb can correct hormonal communication in the body and hormonal problems at their source.

• Progesterone shots. You may want to talk to your doctor about progesterone shots if you had recurrent miscarriages or just want help maintaining your pregnancy. This is something to consider requesting if your doctor has not initiated it and if you exhibit the symptoms of a progesterone deficiency.

• Natural progesterone cream. Check with your doctor and discuss the amount to use.

• Vitamin B6 is known to help maintain optimal levels of progesterone and is key in progesterone production. Vitamin B also helps the liver break down estrogen. Food sources of Vitamin B6 can be found in walnuts, lean red meat, poultry, bananas, spinach, and potatoes.

• Turmeric, thyme and oregano are all considered helpful in raising progesterone levels.

• Vitamin C is known to considerably increase progesterone production.

• Zinc is key for producing adequate levels of progesterone in the body. That is because Zinc is a mineral that prompts the pituitary gland to release follicle stimulating hormones, which in turn promote ovulation and stimulate the ovaries to produce estrogen and progesterone. Along with a zinc supplement, natural sources of zinc include lean red meats, wheat germ, chickpeas, pumpkin and squash seeds, watermelon and dark chocolate.

- Practice stress-reduction techniques, as stress can considerably reduce progesterone levels in the body.

- Do you have low cholesterol? This can mean you are not making enough pregnenolone, which is used to make progesterone.

- Are your adrenals healthy? They house DHEA that is essential to the production of progesterone. One way to improve your adrenal health is to improve your natural circadian rhythm and get more sleep.

- Maintain a healthy digestive tract. If you have a damaged digestive tract, you won't have the raw materials within your body to absorb the nutrients in your food that helps the body produce hormones.

- You may want to consider testing for parasites, candida, or pathogens which can impact your hormonal balance.

- Maca, a root vegetable in the radish family, can balance hormones and nourish and balance the endocrine system. It protects the body from stress damage. Maca is a nutritionally dense super food that contains high amounts of minerals, vitamins, enzymes and all of the essential amino acids. Maca also stimulates and nourishes the hypothalamus and pituitary glands, which are the "master glands" of the body. It is available in powder form or capsules,

- Coconut oil stimulates the thyroid and provides omega-3's that help balance hormones. Other healthy fats essential to hormone health include flax oil, evening primrose oil and olive oil.

- Magnesium is known to break down excessive estrogens in the system and assist in balancing hormones. Kelp and cashews are rich in magnesium. Other sources of magnesium include black beans, spinach, okra, watermelon seeds, sunflower, pumpkin seeds and squash seeds.

- Garlic is an important nutrient for the endocrine system.

- Ginkgo and ginseng help regulate hormones

- Consider supplements such as Vitamin C and Vitamin B.

• Getting more sleep helps balance hormones.

• Flaxseed contains lignans and fiber, which help remove excess estrogen from the body.

• Hormone imbalances can be a result of obesity. Fat cells can create hormonal imbalances. If you think you are overweight, consider trying to lose some of the weight to help your hormonal system.

• Red Clover, an herb, protects the body from xenohormones.

• Black Cohosh, an herb, is well-known for its effect on hormone functioning.

• Do a liver cleanse. The liver plays a key role in to hormonal balance. Milk thistle, dandelion leaf and burdock root are all potent liver cleansers.

• Royal jelly is rich in amino acids and contains acetylcholine, which is needed to transmit nerve messages from cell to cell.

• Ashwagandha root supports endocrine system function and helps to regulate hormones.

• Be aware of chemicals in your diet, water, and environment that can throw your hormones out of balance.

• Drink only filtered water. Avoid water with fluoride. Fluoride is known to weaken the thyroid, one of the key organs responsible for your hormones.

• Be aware of products that may contain aluminium, including deodorants, anti-perspirants, and cosmetics.

• Be careful of meats coated with nitrate salts.

• Do not eat foods from plastic containers. Whenever possible, use glass and stainless steel.

- Avoid vegetable oil, canola oil, soybean oil, margarine, shortening and other chemically altered fats.

- Drink whole milk, not skim milk

- Licorice is a hormone balancer.

- Natural sources of iodine can help regulate hormones. These include kelp, cranberries and strawberries.

- Improve indoor air-quality with plants.

- Limit caffeine.

- Other supplements to consider for hormonal balance include calcium, Vitamin E and grapeseed extract.

- Address your hormonal imbalance on the emotional level. Are you feeling trapped? Unloved? Stuck? Angry? Are you living in a way that is true to who you are? Let your body tell you why your hormones are imbalanced.

- Foods To Help Balance Hormones

- Pumpkin seeds and Brazil nuts.

- Avocados and acai

- Spinach, kale, parsley, broccoli, asparagus and other leafy greens.

- Sweet peppers.

- Pears and peaches are known to help regulate hormones. They are used often in traditional Chinese medicine.

- Shiitake and reishi mushrooms, chia seeds, seaweed and spirulina.

- Avocados block estrogen absorption and promote progesterone production.

How to Improve Your Egg Quality

Good news—you can improve the health and quality of your eggs.

In the past, we were told we were all born with a certain number of egg cells that run out as we age. We were led to believe that egg cells were the only cells in the body that did not regenerate, but instead were a finite number. We are finding out THIS IS JUST NOT TRUE. Recent research has shown that women can produce new eggs throughout their reproductive years.

You may have been told that your eggs are not healthy or that your eggs are too old.

Here's the great news: there is much you can do to enhance the health of your eggs.

It was commonly believed that the only factor that determined egg health and quality was age. Several new studies have shown that stress, hormones and environmental toxins all impact our egg health.

Your egg's health is a key cornerstone of a healthy fertility, because the health of your eggs can affect whether or not fertilization, implantation and ultimately a healthy pregnancy and birth will occur.

Here are some things you can do to improve your egg health:

• Coenzyme Q10: Coenzyme Q10 is an excellent way to improve the quality and energy within your eggs. In several studies, the supplement Coenzyme Q10 has been shown to improve egg quality. It boosts energy production in the oocytes, which are cells in the ovary. Providing additional energy in the form of Coenzyme Q10 is needed when there is decreased energy production in the ovaries due to aging. It is also a source of fuel for the mitochondria, which produces energy within the cells and with age, can begin to weaken. Along with taking a Coenzyme Q10 supplement, natural sources of CoQ10 include almonds, spinach, sardines, broccoli, strawberries, and walnuts.

- Green Tea: Green Tea contains hypoxanthine which provides follicular fluid that helps eggs mature, along with polyphenols that are powerful antioxidants that prevent chromosomal abnormalities, and repair oxidative damage within the body. However, green tea can reduce the body's absorption of folic acid, so you may want to increase your dosage of folic acid at the same time.

- Start eating foods high in antioxidants that will protect your eggs from free radical damage. Free radicals can damage both the egg cell health and the cell's DNA. Foods high in antioxidants that can combat free radicals include blueberries, cranberries, garlic, Granny apples, artichokes, spinach, kale, broccoli, plums, walnuts, and oregano.

- Include Maca in your diet, which is a root-like cruciferous vegetable and the only plant known in the world that can grow and thrive at a high altitude in harsh weather. Maca contains 31 different minerals and 60 different phytonutrients. It nourishes the endocrine system, aids the pituitary, adrenal and thyroid glands, and helps balance hormones and increases energy and stamina in the body.

Maca controls estrogen levels in the body, which is very important because if estrogen levels are too high or low, it can prevent a woman from becoming pregnant or carrying full term. Excess estrogen levels can also cause progesterone levels to become low. Make sure that when you purchase Maca, it contains the root, not just leaves and stem. Once, you are pregnant, you need to stop Maca immediately—it is to be taken only to prepare your body to become pregnant.

- L-Arginine is an amino acid that has been shown to increase ovarian response, endometrial receptivity and pregnancy rates.

- Royal Jelly

- Omega-E fatty acid

- New research has shown that melatonin can improve egg quality. Consider taking a melatonin supplement, because new research has shown that the hormone melatonin may help improve egg quality.

- Vitamin B

- DHEA

- Spirulina

- Red raspberry leaf

- Flaxseed

- Coconut oil

- Olive oil

- Grapeseed extract

- Pomegranate

- Kelp

- Bee pollen

- Improve the blood flow and oxygenation to your ovaries. Oxygen rich blood flow to the ovaries is essential for good egg health.
A lack of good blood flow can be due to lack of exercise, dehydration and thick blood. To increase blood flow to the ovaries, drink at least 8 glasses of pure, high-quality water each day. Make sure the water is NOT bottled in plastic. Do light exercise, such as walking. Massage your uterus and ovaries. You might want to look for a massage therapist experienced in abdomen massage

- Hormonal balance is key to proper egg health and cleansing your system of excess hormones can help. You can do this by doing a liver cleanse, especially if you suffer from an overabundance of estrogen.

- Work on improving your uterine health. Some herbs that can help include Burdock Root, Milk Thistle Seed, Dandelion Root, Yellow Dock Root, Licorice Root and Goldenseal Root to cleanse the uterus.

- If your FSH levels are high, consider Vitex, a shrub native to Greece and Italy whose berries have been used in herbal medicine for centuries. Vitex has an amazing ability to balance fertility hormones and is considered one of the most useful herbs in fertility. It helps support and regulate the pituitary gland, inhibits follicle-stimulating hormones, lengthens the luteal phase, and increases progesterone levels.

- Reduce stress as much as you can in your life.

- In Chinese medicine, ovarian health is linked to kidney health. Do a kidney cleanse and eat foods that support and strengthen your kidney.

- Start acupuncture treatments once, twice or three times a week.

- Be aware of the two most common allergens that can impact your body, gluten and dairy.

- Avoid environmental contaminants.

- Avoid dietary fats.

- Be aware of insulin levels and eat in a way that reduces blood sugar level spikes.

- Avoid white flour products

- Repeat affirmations like "my eggs are healthy and can create a beautiful baby."

• Foods and Substances To Avoid

To maximize your egg health, you want to reduce your exposure to xenohormones, which are substances not found in nature that have hormonal effects on the body. These toxic substances can be absorbed through the skin and build up in the body over time. Sources of xenohormones include solvents and adhesives, including paint, varnish, nail polish and in dry cleaning, car exhaust, all plastics, meat from non-organic livestock, pesticides, herbicides and fungicides, emulsifiers in soap and cosmetics, bug sprays, lawn sprays, and pesticides.

Avoid cosmetics and soaps made with petrochemical emulsifiers.

Do not use mineral oil on your body. Do not microwave your food in plastic. Stop wearing polyester clothing.

• Do not use air fresheners, fabric softeners, spermicide, feminine care products.

• Avoid cigarettes, coffee, alcohol, sugar, non-organic meats and dairy products

• Avoid soda

• Avoid diet foods, processed foods, trans fats and GMO foods.

• Do not eat corn

• Very little to no gluten if possible

• No soy

• Avoid all monounsaturated fats

- **Foods To Enhance Your Egg Health and Quality**

- Broccoli, berries, dark leafy vegetables, salmon, pumpkin seeds

- Sesame seeds

- Turmeric

- Dark green leafy vegetables, such as kale, spinach or chard

- Start making your own super fertility smoothie, with ingredients like spinach, strawberries, spirulina, Maca Root, bee pollen, royal jelly, and flax seed.

Strengthening and Preparing Your Organs

As you prepare to be pregnant, it is important to strengthen the various organs in your body.

• Your Vagina

You want to make your vagina a welcoming environment. A healthy vagina produces healthy cervical mucus, a key to conception. Healthy bacteria in one's vagina can enhance fertility, while an acidic or unhealthy vagina can be a barrier to fertility. Medications, illness, excessive douching, severe emotional stress, or clothing that holds in body heat and moisture, can upset the balance of a healthy vagina. You want to help make your vagina a welcoming environment.

Here are some ways to promote a healthy vagina:

• Wear cotton underwear for good air flow. This prevents the development of damp conditions that promote yeast and unhealthy bacteria. Avoid underwear made from synthetic fabrics, silk, lace and other materials that don't breath freely.

• Do not use douches or feminine sprays that can wash out healthy bacteria that helps the vagina stay clean and infection-free. Avoid scented creams, scented pads, scented tampons and wipes.

• Go to a doctor to see if you have bacterial vaginosis, which is an overgrowth of bacteria inside your vagina and should be treated.

• Check to see if you have any vaginal abnormalities that can impact fertility, such as fusion of the labia or an imperforate hymen.

• It is important not to ignore yeast infections and vaginal infections, such as vulvovaginitis.

• Sexually transmitted diseases, such as Chlamydia and gonorrohea, need to be treated.

- When you wash your vagina, use hot water rather than strong soaps. If you choose to use soap, make sure you thoroughly rinse your vaginal area with warm water so no trace of soap is left behind. Using harsh soaps can lead to infection, and irritation.

- Eat garlic. It has properties that kill yeast.

- Do not use lubricants of any kind.

- Aim to make your vagina less acidic and more sperm friendly. Ideally, your pH range should be at 6.5 to 7.5. If your body is acidic, your cervical mucus will also be acidic, thus creating a hostile environment for sperm.

- Avoid vegetable oil.

- Avoid saliva.

- Avoid glycerin.

- Minimize your intake of sugar, alcohol and white flour products.

- The gut flora, or bacteria in your gut, colonize your vagina. Eat sufficient probiotics or yogurt with bifidus and acidophilus cultures. Yogurt has lactobacillus acidophilus, or "good bacteria." Avoid sugary yogurt.

- L-Arginine increase production of mucus during ovulation.

- Calcium helps the pH balance of the cervical mucus be less acidic and more sperm friendly.

- Grapeseed extract protects the sperm and helpsthe cervical mucus sperm be more sperm-friendly.

- Vitamin C increases the amount of water in your cervical mucus, thus helping produce more cervical mucus.

- Avoid foods that make your blood acidic, such as processed foods, red meat and hydrogenated oils.

- Evening Primrose Oil helps increase cervical mucus production.

- Red clover and Siberian ginseng also help support vaginal health.

• Ovaries

The ovaries rely on fat for fertility and hormonal balance. Vitamins A and E found in foods such as olive oil and avocados support reproductive health. The antioxidants found in fruits and vegetables, especially those with a deep orange color, are known to strengthen the ovaries. These include sweet potatoes, cantaloupe, oranges, orange bell peppers. Vitamin B6 is also important to ovarian health. If you are deficient in B6, your body may produce more estrogen than you need, which disrupts the menstrual cycle and can prevent your ovaries from releasing eggs on a consistent basis. Foods rich in Vitamin B6 include avocado, spinach, broccoli, beans and potatoes.

• Thyroid

Undiagnosed thyroid problems can sometimes be at the root cause of infertility or recurrent miscarriages. To start, visit your primary care doctor and have your thyroid tested to find out the amount of the thyroid hormone your thyroid is secreting. Request a thyroid stimulating hormone test (TSH) with the full panel of thyroid levels, including thyroid antibodies and thyroxine. Ask for the numerical result for the TSH level. Some doctors believe that if a woman has a TSH level higher than 2.0, it may indicate that she will have problems getting pregnant.

Hypothyroidism, or an underactive thyroid, and hyperthyroidism, known as over-active thyroid, are sometimes pinpointed as the cause of infertility.

Both hypothyroidism and hyperthyroidism can cause imbalances which impact your ovaries. The ovaries are very sensitive to changes in thyroid levels and even seemingly small declines in thyroid levels can adversely impact ovarian function. Some symptoms of a thyroid dysfunction include cold hands and feet, weight gain and depression.

If you have an underactive thyroid, it means your thyroid gland doesn't produce enough of certain hormones. Low levels of thyroid hormones can interfere with the release of eggs from your ovaries.

That's because the hypothalamus and pituitary glands can sometimes sense an underactive thyroid gland and try to kick things back to normal by increasing the levels of hormones in the body.
 Low levels of the thyroid hormone can interfere with ovulation, which impairs fertility.

Along with being treated by a doctor who specializes in thyroid problems, here are some other things you can do to help your thyroid condition:

• Eat foods high in vitamin A, such as yellow vegetables and dark green vegetables.

• Foods that contain iodine nurture the thyroid, such as kelp and seaweed. Seaweed can be added to soups, salads or just eaten plain. Other foods rich in iodine include: asparagus, bananas, carrots, garlic, onions, spinach, and tomatoes.

• Coconut oil is known to be excellent for boosting thyroid function.

• Foods rich in zinc nourish the thyroid, such as oatmeal, chicken and spinach.

• Raisins are rich in copper, which help the body produce thyroid hormones.

• Soy should not be eaten at this time, because soy can interfere with thyroid hormones.

• The amino acid Tyrosine, found in beef and chicken, help support the thyroid.

• Beet tops, leafy greens, and parsley are helpful in supporting thyroid function.

• Dark green leafy vegetables that are rich in minerals also boost the thyroid.

• Foods to avoid include cauliflower, brussel sprouts, canola oil, soy, peanuts, cabbage and kale, which have goitrogens that are high in sulfur have been known to impede thyroid gland function. A note of caution here, however, those with an overactive thyroid may find these foods helpful. It is recommended you meet with a physician or nutritionist to discuss which foods are best for you, depending on your thyroid condition.

• Avoid coffee, caffeine products and excessive amounts of alcohol.

• Keep your blood sugar levels steady, as fluctuating blood sugar levels can negatively impact the thyroid.

• Avoid artificial sweeteners, such as aspartame.

• Include a good quality sea salt or Celtic salt in your diet, instead of white table salt.

• For an underactive thyroid, consider foods like sea kelp, chicken, dates, molasses, and parsley.

• Reduce your intake of sugar as much as you can.

• Alternative therapies that can help the thyroid include acupuncture and lymph drainage massage, in which the thyroid and lymphatic system are massaged so as to loosen any blocks.

• Avoid drinking out of plastic and soda cans. Instead, drink only out of glass, stainless steel or BPA free plastic bottles.

• Include lots of natural fats in your diet, such as olive oil, flaxseed and avocados.

Vitamin and mineral supplements considered helpful to thyroid function include:

- B-complex

- Vitamin C

- Omega 3s that are found in fish, flaxseed and walnuts, which are the building blocks for the hormones that control immune function and cell growth.

- A multi-mineral formula in liquid form, since minerals are key to glandular health.

- Calcium/magnesium are also known to help the metabolic process.

- High-quality natural thyroid supplements. Note: you may want to seek the advice of a well-trained nutritionist on what type of supplements are appropriate for those who are trying to get pregnant, and what dosage is appropriate once you are pregnant or on infertility medications.

- You might want to consider a glutathione supplement and include in your diet foods that contain glutathione, such as asparagus, broccoli, peaches, spinach, garlic and grapefruit.

- Pay attention to your food allergies and sensitivies.

- Reduce gluten in your diet or if you can, go entirely gluten free.

- Take a probiotic, because for the thyroid to be healthy and function well, it needs and depends on having a sufficient supply of healthy gut bacteria.

- Pay attention to adrenal burn-out or fatigue, because there is a strong connection between the thyroid and adrenal glands. Think of the thyroid and adrenals as Frick and Frack—if you have a problem with hypothyroidism, you are probably suffering with some level of adrenal fatigue or burn-out too.

- Include seaweed in your diet.

- Avoid excessive forms of radiation if you can.

- Do a heavy metal cleanse. Heavy metal exposure is sometimes linked to thyroid problems. In addition to a heavy metal cleanse, begin eating or juicing garlic and cilantro, and include such as taking Milk Thistle, turmeric and chlorella in your diet.

- Eat more foods that contain selenium, such as salmon, sunflower seeds, onions and brazil nuts.

- Stress and emotional traumas, such as a job loss or marital problems, can weaken thyroid function. Explore creative ways to reduce stress, such as joining a chorus, taking gentle walks in a beautiful area, or take a painting or drawing class. Deep breath.

- The thyroid gland is located in the throat, the center of our communication with the world. Holistic practitioners often view low thyroid function as a result of a blocked throat chakra, a result of feeling like you can't speak your truth. It is important to learn new and creative ways of finding and using your voice, such as singing, writing and creating art. Stop 'swallowing' your feelings. Speak your truth instead. Create an expression center in your home, where you feel safe to freely say what you want to say and let your deepest feelings be known.

- Avoid drinking tap water.

- Do not use non-stick cookware.

- Stop using perfume for now, especially in the neck area.

- Eat foods that contain tyrosine, an amino acid the body needs to manufacture thyroid hormones, such as avocados, almonds, bananas, pumpkin seeds and lentils.

- Include more sea vegetables in your diet, such as kelp and kelp granules that can be sprinkled over your salads.

- Stay outside in the sunshine at least 20 minutes a day.

- Evening primrose oil is rich in amino acids which nourish the thyroid gland.

- Consider taking the herbs Nettle and Bladder Wrack.

- Discontinue using deodorants and body lotions that contain parabens, chlorates and pesticides.

• Your Spleen and Digestive System

The spleen is an important organ involved in the hormonal cycle and is responsible for certain types of progesterone production. It also governs many of the energetic processes in the body. Balancing your digestive system and spleen can help you achieve the right balance of floras in your system to increase your fertility.

The spleen also impacts the thyroid hormone and progesterone production. Some link menstrual difficulties to a spleen imbalance.

Some ways to strengthen and balance your spleen and digestive system include:

- In Chinese medicine, the emotion associated with the Spleen is worry. It is important for spleen health to learn to say no without reason or excuse and make a concerted effort to take care of yourself each day.

- Consider digestive enzymes, with hydrochloric acid, available at health food stores.

- Consider probiotics to increase 'good gut bacteria.'

- Avoid sodas and drink lots of water instead. Lack of water is sometimes the cause of poor digestion.

- Chew your food slowly

- Include ground flaxseed in your diet.

- Increase fiber in your diet, with foods like apples, figs, prunes and dates.

- Acupuncture has been reported to encourage healthy digestion.

- Avoid sugar, white flour products, raw cold foods, soy and dairy products.

- Try to walk each day. Exercise helps move the spleen energy.

- Eliminate possible food allergens in your diet.

- Boost friendly bacteria in your body.

- Massage your stomach to help reduce stress and aid digestion.

• Pituitary Gland

The pituitary gland is sometimes called the master gland of the body, because all the other endocrine glands depend on its secretion for stimulation. It is a tiny gland located at the base of the brain and is sometimes referred to as the thermostat of the body because it controls the other hormone secreting glands. High protein foods help the pituitary gland release its hormones, because the building blocks of proteins are amino acids.

Emotionally, problems with the pituitary gland can come from not respecting your inner wisdom and/or pretending to be someone your not.

Supplements that can help the pituitary gland include:

- Bee pollen
- Spirulina
- Magnesium
- Potassium
- Dandelion
- Omega-3 oil
- Chia seeds

Other ways to help the pituitary gland include:

- Manganese is important to a healthy pituitary gland. Foods that contain manganese include citrus fruits, greens and egg yokes.

- Walk at least 20 minutes a day in sunlight. This will encourage the pituitary gland to produce helpful levels of ovary-stimulating hormones. You also might want to consider a Vitamin D supplement.

- L-Arginine is an amino acid that promotes the section of HGH.

- Fenugreek stimulates the release of HGH while giving your energy levels a kick.

- Get more sleep

- In traditional Chinese medicine, the emotional aspect of pituitary gland health involves bonding with others, sharing words and ideals. Think about and journal about this aspect of your life. Do you feel you are adequately and healthily bonding with others? Are there people in your life where you can take down your 'walls' and share your words and ideals?

- Include meat and protein in your diet.

• Hypothalamus and thymus

The hypothalamus regulates the pituitary gland and secretes hormones that control the thyroid, adrenals, ovaries and testes.

Here are some ways to support your hypothalamus:

- A handful of sunflower seeds each day can boost the hypothalamus. Sunflower seeds contain B1 or thiamine, which is crucial for hypothalamus health.

- Eat foods rich in Vitamin C, including red bell peppers, oranges, lemons.

- Seaweed

- Pumpkin seeds

• Pineal Gland

The pineal gland controls the circadian rhythms in the body, as well as melatonin and pinoline production.

The pineal gland manufactures melatonin, a hormone that plays a key role in fertility, because it controls the timing and release of many key reproductive hormones. In Chinese medicine melatonin is linked to healthy liver energy, considered very important to reproductive health. Having adequate amounts of melatonin in your body has been shown to improve pregnancy rates. Because we live in a light-saturated culture due to TVs, cell phones, computer screens and street lights, we are often robbed of the melatonin we need for a restful night's sleep. Sleep disturbances are a recipe for hormonal imbalance.

Here are some ways to strengthen the pineal gland:

• Fluoride is the number one enemy of a healthy pineal gland. The mineral boron, found in beets and dried plums, can help remove fluoride from the human body.

• Coffee, alcohol and tobacco weaken the pineal gland.

• Apple cider vinegar strengthens the pineal gland.

• Oregano and garlic are considered helpful to pineal gland health.

• Consider a Melatonin supplement.

• Sunlight acts as a food for the pineal gland

• Chlorophyll-rich superfoods, like spirulina and chlorella, detoxify the pineal gland

• Add natural food sources of iodine to your diet, such as seaweed

• Foods that strengthen the pineal gland include watermelon, coconut oil, spinach, asparagus and broccoli.

• Pancreas

Keeping your pancreas healthy and your blood sugar levels stable will help stabilize your hormones when you are trying to get pregnant. When blood sugar levels are high, we suffer spikes that weaken our adrenal glands. Sugar frazzles the hormones and leaves our endocrine system exhausted. When our sugar levels drop, our adrenals release both cortisol and adrenaline in an attempt to restore our sugar levels back to an even kneel, leading to hormonal imbalance.

The reason these sugar spikes impact our fertility is that progesterone, which is the main hormone required for ovulation, and cortisol compete for the same receptor binding sites in the body. Cortisol, however, will always win this showdown. When these hormones battle, it disrupts the entire endocrine system, which in turn, disrupts all the sex hormones, including oestrogen, progesterone, and the androgen DHEA.

To keep your hormones in tip-top shape, reduce your sugar intake.

Here are some ways to keep your pancreas healthy and your blood sugar levels stable:

• Eat foods that nourish your pancreas, such as blueberries, sunflower seeds, almonds, cherries, broccoli, garlic, red grapes, spinach, sweet potatoes. Prepare these foods ahead of time and carry them with you so you can have them available wherever you go.

• Eat something healthy every three hours.

• Eat lots of spinach, which is high in magnesium and is known to help prevent type 2 diabetes.

• Avocados are also high in magnesium.

• Walnuts, which are high in monounsaturated fat, help stabilize blood sugar levels.

• Get at least eight hours of sleep.

• Almonds can lessen the subsequent rise in blood sugar.

• Avoid soda and artificial sweeteners.

Important Ways To Enhance and Strengthen Your Fertility

• Start Making Vegetable Based Drinks Daily

If you want to cleanse and strengthen your body, by all means go out and buy a juicer or some type of bullet and start making vegetable based drinks on a daily basis. Do it today! Now! As soon as possible! This can change your body in a very big way. Making vegetable drinks is a wonderful and effective way to cleanse, alkalize and strengthen the body—three things you need to do to maximize your chances of getting pregnant.

When you make vegetable drinks, you are putting live food into your body. Many of the nutrients in foods are destroyed by cooking, so when you juice or blend vegetables, you are consuming these nutrients in an undisturbed form. It is one of the easiest, fastest ways to assimilate more nutrients into the body. Fresh, whole foods build healthy cells.

One of the health benefits of vegetable drinks is that it allows cellular cleansing on a deep level. When you are trying to fix an imbalance in the body, large amounts of fruits and vegetables can significantly help the body heal.

Making vegetable drinks helps your body become more alkaline, instead of acidic, which is a great booster in promoting fertility. Juicing will also give your body enhanced vitality.

Have I said enough about the power of daily vegetable drinks? Make yourself a healthy vegetable drink each day and you will feel and see almost immediately what a great healer and fertility enhancer it is.

To start, buy a juicer or bullet that is easy to handle, easy to clean and that you don't find intimidating.

There are lots of good ones on the market.

A side note here: making vegetable drinks does not have to be overly time-consuming and complicated. If some of the recipes call for too many ingredients and overwhelm you, make vegetable drinks with one or two ingredients. Spinach and blueberries, spinach, flaxseed and blueberries, kale and strawberries, are just a few.

For me, a bag of spinach and some blueberries juiced each morning, or some garlic and lemon is often enough to put my body on the right track. Parsley, beets, kale can also be juiced alone. If you find eating fruit easy, I would stick to juicing vegetables that you might not normally consume as often. Many people like a spinach/apple combination that is also easy, quick and very effective.

Some juicing suggestions include:

• Garlic. I know, I know, it sounds horrible, but it really isn't. Peel a few cloves of garlic and juice. Then combine the garlic juice with the juice of one or two squeezed lemons. Then pour in lots of water. I usually drink mine slowly. I have a jug of water ready, because if you start to feel sick from the garlic, slugging down lots of water helps ease the nausea. Garlic does great and wondrous things for the body—so start drinking. I promise—it is not as bad as it sounds!)

Some nutritionists have suggested that garlic can also help prevent miscarriages and enhance both male and female fertility.

• Juice spinach for heightened doses of folic acid. Spinach is one of the vegetables I would recommend juicing almost daily. There are so many health benefits to spinach. Some people like to juice spinach with apples, or with other greens. Find the combination you like.

• Along with spinach, beets, asparagus, garlic and kale are considered among the best vegetables for treating infertility. Pineapple, strawberries and oranges are considered among the best fruits for enhanced fertility. Create vegetable/fruit drinks with these combinations.

- Juice kale, chicory, romaine lettuce, parsley.

- Some vegetables to avoid include celery. It is recommended not to juice celery while pregnant or trying to get pregnant.

- Carrots and beets is a mixture that is very healthy for the liver. Carrots provide huge amounts of Vitamin A to the body in a natural form, which is important because Vitamin A deficiency can prevent eggs from properly maturing.

- Other juice combinations can include:
-beet/carrot/radish/
-spinach/apple
-carrot/apple,parsley
-kale/spinach/apple
-ginger/apple
-apple/pear.
-Pineapple/strawberry/spinach
-Cucumber/spinach/celery/apple
-Kale/spinach/apple/carrot
-Apple/carrot/pineapple/celery/lemon
-Parsley/kale
-Kale/spinach/cabbage/mint
-Kale, pineapple and ginger detox.
-Pineapple, lemon and pomegranate
-Fennel, garlic and cabbage

- Other fruits and vegetables that can be juiced and are known to help fertility include red peppers, dark green leaf lettuce, onions, cabbage, broccoli and dark leafy greens.

- You can also add chia seeds, maca, flaxseeds, spirulina, cayenne pepper, and turmeric to your drinks.

• Increase Circulation to Your Reproductive System

Begin to do self-massage. Since many of us hold stress in our stomach, massaging your stomach can help reduce stress and help your digestion.

Do not do massage if there is a possibility you could be pregnant.
If you are not pregnant, massage your liver, kidney, and ovaries.
Put your legs up against a wall to increase blood circulation to the pelvis and ovaries. You can also increase circulation to your reproductive system by brushing your skin to remove toxins. Or take a very hot shower for five minutes, and then follow with cold water for 30 seconds. Green grapes can also improve circulation. Stretch often. Drinking lemon, cayenne pepper and apple cider vinegar can also increase circulation.

• Restore Good Bacteria In Your Body

One way to become more fertile is to restore good bacteria in your body.

Eating yogurt that has little to no sugar, and contains live active cultures is one way to do this. Avoid or reduce your intake of sugar and caffeine. Olive oil and avocados are known to help restore good bacteria in the body.

Foods high in good bacteria include apples, beets and sour cream.

Eat a diet low in white flour or gluten products.

Start taking a high-quality probiotic supplement.

• Exercise Mildly

When you exercise, do it moderately and mildly, not too strenuous or obsessively. Intense exercise can negatively impact infertility and make you a higher risk for miscarriage. Light exercise is the goal. Nothing too strenuous or intense at this time. Avoid over-exercise.

Some doctors of Chinese medicine believe that activities like mountain biking, aerobics, jogging and weight-lifting are 'yang' activities that force the body to expend too much energy, and steal much-needed power from the reproductive organs.

Light exercises, such as gentle swimming and walking, on the other hand, are considered ideal because they do not take energy away from the body's reproductive organs.

• Stop Unnecessary Medications

At this time, you might want to consider stopping any unnecessary medications that might be clogging up your system and making your liver sluggish. Be very careful, however, because you may be on medications for your mental and/or physical health that are absolutely necessary to your well-being. Do not go off any medicine without first thoroughly investigating the consequences with your physician.

But if you are on a medicine that you no longer need or can comfortably, safely and healthily live without temporarily, removing this medicine from your system might improve the state of your liver and other organs.

This is not a decision to be taken frivolously or lightly in any way, and should only be done with your doctor's consent and full understanding of any ramifications that going off your medicine might involve. If you are on medication for mental health, it is important to continue taking them.

You may also want to avoid or reduce over-the-counter medications at this time, such as ibuprofen.

• Be Aware of Electromagnetic Energy

There is research that suggests that electromagnetic fields can reduce fertility. Don't get panicked about this, but just be aware of how much electromagnetic energy you come in contact with daily.

Here are some steps you can take to reduce your exposure to electromagnetic energy:

- Take all electrical devices out of your bedroom, or at least unplug them before you go to sleep at night.

Remove or unplug radios, TVs, stereos, alarm clocks and computers in your bedroom.

- If you can, reduce your time in front of a computer. Surf the Internet only when you need to. Unplug your computer when not in use.

- Keep your microwave unplugged and stand faraway from it while using it.

- Reduce the time spent on your cell phone. Use your cell phone only for emergencies, and do not keep it in your pocket.

- If you are using a cordless phone, change back to a standard fixed line when you are at home if you can.

- For now, put away electric blankets.

- Keep laptops off your body.

- Unplug electrical appliances while not in use.

- Use manual toothbrushes, not electric.

As much as possible, do things manually—also known as the old-fashioned way—at least for now. Whenever you can, reduce your time on devices that are wireless.

While we need these modern conveniences, reduce your time near them as much as possible. Instead, surround your body with as much natural forms of energy as possible, such sunlight.

• Get More Sleep

Many studies are now suggesting that not getting enough sleep can impact a woman's fertility because sleep has a powerful influence on the body's hormonal system. Those who don't get enough sleep have higher levels of the stress hormone cortisol and adrenocorticotropic, which can suppress a healthy fertility cycle.

Try to get on a regular sleep schedule. No more staying up until 11:30 watching TV or surfing the Internet. If possible, try for a 8, 9 or 10 o'clock bedtime, which gives your body plenty of pre-midnight sleep time.

Some believe that one hour of sleep before midnight is worth two hours after, meaning that the body benefits from pre-midnight sleep enormously Think of our ancestors, who went to bed soon after the sun set. Their body clocks aligned with the natural world, allowing them maximum rest and rejuvenation.

The body reportedly needs seven to nine hours of sleep a night. Chart your sleep schedule to see if you are within this range.

The goal should be getting to bed earlier to ensure more pre-midnight sleep time, and a regular sleep schedule that eliminates any chance that your body might be suffering from sleep deprivation.

Exercising lightly and getting enough sunlight is reported to help encourage healthy sleep patterns. Do not drink anything caffeinated in the afternoon. Stay on a relatively predictable bedtime schedule. Avoid watching TV late at night, or checking e-mail, which can be overstimulating. Some studies have shown that those who consume electronic media just before bedtime experience lower-quality sleep.

To experience higher quality and deeper sleep, consider relaxing activities before bed such as reading, taking a bath, knitting, listening to soothing music, doing a jigsaw puzzle, or drawing or sketching in bed. For me, prayer is my most relaxing bedtime routine.

Keep your bedroom as dark as possible.

A better night's sleep is achieved in total darkness. Block your windows or get room darkening shades. Light at night can impact your pineal gland. Remove or unplug anything in your room that emits light, such as night lights, clock radios or computers. Do not keep chargers in your bedroom.

• Be Aware Of The Chemicals In Your Environment

We all know that toxins and chemicals in our environment are not good for us, and while it is useless to obsess about this or try to control every element of this, there are some things that you can do to reduce the amount of chemical toxins that enter your system while you are trying to conceive.

A note of caution here: don't get too paranoid. Despite the pollution in our environment, millions of babies are born every day in all parts of the
world, smog filled or not. The human body is strong and can handle a lot—worrying about what is out of your control won't do you any good right now.

Your body can handle more than you probably can imagine, and you are not a victim of even the most polluted environment. But when it is in your realm of control, do what you can do to keep your body chemical-free. Think about what you touch and take into your body that is within your realm of control.

Here are some ways to reduce the toxins that enter your system:

• Try not to purchase soaps and cleaning products with the chemical triclocarban, or TCC in it.

• Try to avoid using deodorant when you can, and if you feel it necessary, stick to a natural, aluminium-free deodorant.

• Use regular soap, not anti-bacterial.

• Buy natural cleaning products and laundry detergent.

- Just for now, stop dyeing your hair or using nail polish.

- Avoid products with perfluorooctanoate (PFOA) and perfluorooctane sulfonate (PFOS) that are used to manufacture Teflon non-stick coatings and is in some personal care products. Products known to contain these chemicals include carpet and fabric protectors, microwave popcorn bags and stain-proof clothing.

- Avoid Bisphenol or (BPA) when possible. It is used in plastic water bottles, plastic microwavable plates and utensils, tooth sealants, and soda cans.

- Phthalate is a compound used in perfumes, cosmetics and hairsprays. For now, stop using these products.

- Buy bottled water or put a filter on your tap water at home. You may even want to consider a filter for the water you shower and cook with.

- Avoid painting or being around paint while pregnant.

- Avoid lawn, plant, gardening or insect pesticides.

- Be aware of dry cleaning chemicals and do not have clothes dry-cleaned at this time.

- Be weary of super strength cleaners. When possible, use homemade or natural cleaners. If you do use strong cleaners, wear gloves whenever possible to avoid the chemical seeping into your skin.

- Avoid carpet cleaners and air fresheners if you can.

- Avoid smelling fumes from household cleaners.

- Beware of plastics. Don't microwave and eat from anything plastic while trying to conceive. If you purchase water in plastic jugs, try whenever possible to transfer the water to a glass jug. Plastics can seep into your system and impact your immune system. Do not purchase foods that have to be microwaved in plastic.

- Buy an air purifier for your home.

- Stop using cleaning products with ingredients you cannot identify. Buy only natural cleaning products, with ingredients you can pronounce and understand.

- Just for now, stop using all chemical products on your hair and nails.

- To remove environmental toxins from your body, consider one or more of the following: a liver cleanse, colon cleanse, kidney cleanse, heavy metal cleanse, parasite and/or yeast.

- Find a professional in your area that offers a bio cleanse ionic foot bath, which is an effective way to remove toxins from the body. Some companies sell foot pads that can be used to detox and remove toxins.

- Put more household plants in your house to help filter toxins from the air, or consider a HEPA filter for your home.

- Stay aware of chemicals that you ingest, smell, or put on your skin and can enter your body.

• Get More Sunlight

Both you and your husband/male partner should spend 15 to 30 minutes each day outside in sunlight, as some studies have shown that lack of sunlight can cause a deficiency in Vitamin D, which impacts infertility.

Take walks, or just put some chairs outside and sit for 20 minutes. Many studies have revealed that lack of sunlight can cause male infertility. Exposure to sunlight also stimulates the pineal gland, which increases serotonin, a chemical that produces good feelings in the brain.

• Drink Lots of Good-Quality Water

When trying to conceive, drink lots of high-quality, filtered water. Some recommend 8-10 glasses of water a day or more. Water is critical because 75 percent of our body is made up of water. A water deficiency can impact the liver and kidney.

• Deep Breath

Deep breathing helps your body release toxins, reduce anxiety levels, reduce inflammation, improve digestion and help you feel more relaxed. At least once or twice a day, spend some time consciously deep breathing. Breath through your nose down into your belly, and then exhale through your mouth.

Deep breathing also helps release endorphins and bring fresh oxygen to your cells. Schedule a specific time for deep breathing. You want to get into the habit of doing some deep breathing at the same time everyday, so it becomes part of your routine.

• Enhance Your Cervical Mucous

 Low cervical mucous can result from not enough water intake each day, poor circulation to the reproductive organs, hormonal imbalance and low progesterone levels.

Conditions That Might Be Threatening Your Fertility

Some of these conditions could be among the causes of your infertility.

• Do You Have An Iron Deficiency?

Some studies have found a link between low iron intake and infertility. Low iron, or anemia, can increase the body's risk for being unable to produce healthy eggs. This is because a lack of iron can cause anovulation, or lack of ovulation and in turn, poor egg health. Being low in iron can cause eggs stored in the ovaries to be weak and unviable.

A lack of iron in the body also results in an insufficient number of red blood cells, which are responsible for delivering oxygen to the ovaries and uterus. Ask your physician for a test to see if you are anemic or low in iron. You may want to consider taking a high-quality iron supplement, either in capsule or liquid form, or a multivitamin that has iron in it. Some studies have shown that it is best to take a vegetable based iron, rather than animal based.

• Eat more foods high in iron. These include spinach, beets, molasses, pumpkin seeds, asparagus.

Other iron rich foods include:

• Kale, broccoli, lean red meat, asparagus, parsley, kidney beans, lentils, apricots, and chicken.

• When you get pregnant, make sure your iron levels are sufficient throughout your pregnancy.

• Select an iron supplement that includes nutrients that help iron absorption, which are B12 (folic acid) and Vitamin C.

• Consider Your Weight

Being overweight can cause your body to produce excess insulin, which stimulates the ovaries to produce testosterone male-like hormones. Being overweight can also cause hormonal irregularities and increase one's risk of miscarriage. So if you are overweight, do what you can do lose weight.

When I was trying to get pregnant for a second time, I was told that if I lost weight, my chances for conception would improve significantly. So I went to Friendly's, enjoyed a big five-scoop sundae with lots of hot fudge, and then I joined Weight Watchers. Over the course of seven months, I lost almost 50 pounds. I do believe this helped in my ultimately getting pregnant.

My diet consisted of a lean turkey meat sandwich with healthy bread and mustard, instead of mayonnaise. I also ate a lot of bowls of romaine lettuce and parsley as snacks at work. I was sometimes called a 'rabbit' by my co-workers, and my nightly treat was sugar free, fat free pudding, although I stopped eating this the closer I got to the IVF procedure. I also ate a lot of Weight Watcher's garden vegetable soup.

Cut down on white flour products, sugary juices, sodas and sugar. Write down everything you eat each day. Prepare snacks of cut and washed fruits and vegetables ahead of time each night, so you don't slip during the day. Find a support group or therapist to help if you relied on food to cope with emotional needs, such as loneliness or frustration. Do one thing each day to lose weight.

• Is Your Body's Energy Off Track?

Keeping the energy flow in your body on track is important to good health. In Chinese medicine, infertility is seen as an imbalance of the body's energy levels and that to heal one's infertility it is important to find the imbalances in the body, and then balance the body's organs, hormones, and energy systems.

Restoring balance and getting the body back on track can be done through improved diet, cleansing and detoxifying, releasing stress, and getting consistent acupuncture treatments, along with other holistic methods.

• Do You Have A Tooth or Gum Infection?

Go to your dentist for a thorough cleaning and check-up. A problem with your teeth can weaken the whole body. Do you have any infected teeth? Do you have any cavities that need to be filled? Excessive plaque that needs to be cleaned? Do you need a root canal or a crown? Is there a hidden infection in your teeth that needs to be addressed? It is important that you make sure all infections in your teeth are cleared up and when you begin infertility treatments.

• Is Your Back or Spine Out of Alignment?

Do not underestimate the role your spine plays in your body's mechanics. There are studies that have shown a link between spinal adjustments and increased fertility, because the nerves to the reproductive system run through the spine. When the back is misaligned, the nerves can misfire and cause a hormone imbalance. Getting your spine and body in alignment can help all your organs function at a higher level and increase your energy flow.

Consider finding an experienced chiropractor and getting an adjustment. A chiropractor can identify spinal distortions, also called subluxations, that once corrected can improve infertility. If your spine is properly aligned, your nervous system will have a better chance of working at maximum capacity. Think of what happens when your car is properly aligned--your wheels last longer and other parts of your car work better because they are not having to compensate for an unaligned car. The body works in much the same way.

If your spine is out of alignment, your legs or hips can also be off and weaken the energy and flow in your lower body.

Infections can live in your spine, and if your spine has an infection, it can impact the way your organs communicate with one another.

• Is Your Body Too Acidic?

When you are trying to get pregnant, one of your goals should be to make the environment within your body as alkaline as possible.

Imagine preparing soil for planting—the healthier the soil is, the better chance the seed will have to survive.

More than ever before, your body needs to be alkaline, not acidic. Poor eating habits, lack of exercise, and toxic elements in the environment, can cause your body to become acidic.

Eating lots of acidic foods result in cervical mucus that is an acidic, which is a hostile environment for sperm. Sperm needs an alkaline environment to survive.

You can test the alkaline/acid in your body with pH strips.

To alkalize your body, start your day by drinking a large glass of water with a freshly squeezed lemon.

Foods that alkalize the body include watermelon, apple cider vinegar, artichokes, asparagus, unsalted almonds, coconut oil, lettuce, broccoli, spinach and olive oil.

Chew your food thoroughly.

Foods that help promote an alkaline environment in the body include parsley, garlic, barley grass, green beans, lima beans, zucchini, lemon, beets, asparagus, cabbage, kale, onions, spirulina, flax seeds, sea vegetables, dandelion root, green tea, pumpkin seeds, brussel sprouts. spinach, broccoli, and green leafy vegetables. Figs, apples, grapes, bananas, watermelon, wheatgrass and barley grass are alkaline producing foods.

Meat, bread, carbonated drinks, coffee, sugar, fast foods, sodas, muffins, waffles, pancakes, bacon, sausage often promote high levels of yeast and fungi in the body, leading to higher acid levels.

Allergies, arthritis, acne, heart attacks, and weight problems are often linked to an improper pH balance, or acid, in the body.

If your body is alkalized, you are creating an internal environment conducive to pregnancy.

• Is There Infection In Your Body?

Investigate whether you have any infections in your body. You could have an infection or virus that is weakening you. If so, you may want to consider an antibiotic to get rid of any infections. Juicing and eating lots of garlic can also help fight infections.

• Do You Have Unknown Allergies?

Are you allergic to corn, wheat or dairy products? Food allergies can sometimes be at the root of infertility problems. Schedule an appointment with an allergist to find out if you have any unknown allergies.

Ask yourself: are there certain foods that make me feel tired, weak, achy, and mildly ill after I eat them? Even if you are not diagnosed as allergic to these foods, stay away from foods that leave you feeling weaker than you felt before you ate them.

• Do You Have Celiac Disease?

Researchers are finding that women who are allergic to gluten have higher rates of infertility. Even if you are not diagnosed with celiac disease, reducing the gluten you consume can help make your body stronger and more ready to conceive.

• Is Your Body Cold?

In Chinese medicine, it is believed that the body must be warmed to get pregnant. Avoid iced drinks and very cold foods. Chilled foods cause the body temperature to drop and slows down blood circulation. Do not go barefoot on cold floors. If it is winter and you live in a cold climate, consider wearing warm socks to bed.

Holistic and Alternative Health Treatments To Consider

• Acupuncture

Without a doubt, acupuncture has been shown to help heal infertility and is one of the best and most effective ways to strengthen your reproductive system.

Begin acupuncture treatments as soon as possible. Now! Today! Immediately! Acupuncture is a wonderful and life changing way to get to the root of some of your fertility problems. Numerous studies have shown that acupuncture dramatically helps infertile couples get pregnant and increases the success rate of IVF and other assisted reproductive technologies.

Acupuncture improves ovarian function, hormonal balance, and helps regulate the chemical pathways in the ovaries, pituitary gland and hypothalamus.

Some studies have shown that acupuncture increases your egg health, and keep eggs healthier than they would normally be without treatment.

Acupuncture also increases blood flow to the ovaries and the uterus, which is very important, because enhanced blood flow can help thicken the lining of the uterus.

Acupuncture also helps correct problems in the endocrine system, which includes the thyroid and hypothalamus, key organs in fertility. Acupuncture can strengthen the liver and kidneys, and help activate the brain to release hormones that stimulate the ovaries, adrenal glands and other organs involved in reproduction.

Acupuncture can moves the body over from a track of disease and dysfunction to a track of health. It enhances your energy, removes energy blocks in the body, and shifts energy back on to proper pathways. If there is a blockage in your energy pathway, acupuncture can clear the blockages and allow energy to flow smoothly. By rerouting blocked energy, acupuncture restores the proper balance of yin and yang in the body.

Begin the process of acupuncture and commit to it. To see the benefits of acupuncture takes time and patience. Don't expect to go just once or twice and suddenly have your energy in perfect tune. It takes consistency, but if you stay on track with your weekly treatments, you will eventually see great results.

Try to find someone who has some experience treating infertility patients, but if you can't, that is fine too. If possible, try to go at least twice a week. If you can afford it, go three or four times or as many times as you can.

If money is an issue, you may want to talk with your acupuncturist about getting treatments at a reduced rate. They may be open to giving you a discount if you commit to a certain number of appointments each month, or if you offer to pay up front for five to ten or more appointments at once. Some acupuncturists may discount the treatments for bulk payments. Or some might give you a discount if they know your situation and know you are going to be a long-term customer. In some areas, there are also community acupuncture clinics, also known as group acupuncture, that offer a sliding scale for treatments and are significantly less expensive than one-on-one appointments.

The more acupuncture appointments you can do, the better. Once, during the week I had an IUI scheduled, I went three times to help me conceive, which I ended up doing successfully.

Up until the actual time that you do an IUI or IVF, you can continue acupuncture. There is some disagreement as to whether or not acupuncture should be done once you are pregnant. That is a personal opinion and should be researched and discussed with your acupuncturist. I reserved this wonderful treatment for pre-pregnancy preparation only. If you have an upcoming IVF or IUI, do acupuncture a few times before the procedure.

Bottom line is: you will dramatically increase your chances of if you do acupuncture on a weekly, or preferably, twice weekly basis, for a period of several months.

• Bio Cleanse

An ionic food bath, also known as a bio cleanse ionic detox foot bath, pulls toxins out of the body through the feet. Positive and negative ions are emitted by the ionic foot bath machine, and helps the body rebalance and eliminate toxins in the kidneys, bowel, liver and skin.

A holistic practitioner in your area may have this machine that can remove yeast, parasites, and heavy metals from your liver, kidneys and muscles.

This should only be done as a preparation for infertility treatments, and not once you have started infertility medication or treatments, such as an IUI or IVF. Do not do this if there is any chance you are pregnant. Nor is it safe for anyone with an organ transplant, pacemaker or epilepsy.

• Lymphatic Massage or Manual Lymphatic Drainage

This is a gentle massage that encourages the natural drainage of the lymph from the tissues in the body.

This type of massage is very helpful to your lymph system and is an excellent way to detoxify before an IVF or other types of fertility treatments. Stimulating the lymphatic system helps to drain swollen tissues, enhances the body's immune system, and helps the body's natural waste removal system.

• Applied Kinesiology

Applied kinesiology can provide you with some incredible emotional healing from trauma or sadness trapped in your body.

Our emotions have a physical component and can be energetically trapped in our body, impacting not only our emotional self, but our physical self too.

Sometimes, an event or experience can be so painful, that the emotional trauma of it physically lodges itself permanently in the body. This explains why some memories, betrayals, and traumas can feel so recent decades after they occurred, even when we try to let go and forget them.

In applied kinesiology, a chiropractor or holistic practitioner will use what is referred to a "the gun" or activator to release trauma and emotional pain in your body.

One way to help release trapped traumas in your body is to write a list of all the people, experiences, and events in your life that have hurt you. Give the kinesiologist this list, and ask them to muscle test and locate where these memories have physicall lodged themselves in your body. Once found, the kinesiologist can activate the "gun" to release or free these emotional energy blocks in your body. Once these traumas leave your body, you'll find yourself feeling better, both emotionally and physically. Your body will no longer be weighed down by intensely negative emotions that do impact your organs and entire body system.

• Craniosacral therapy

CranioSacral Therapy is a gentle, hands-on form of body work that releases tension in the layer of tissue called the fascia which surrounds the organs and nervous system. Craniosacral practitioners use light pressure on the skull and lower back to release restrictions on the body's craniosacral system. It is sometimes also done by massage therapists, naturopaths, chiropractors and others who work with the spine, skull and fascia to treat the body's central nervous system. Cranio-sacral can be a powerful tool in releasing past emotional and physical traumas. It can also improve hormone balance and blood flow, and help balance the spinal fluid and nervous system.

• Blood Type Diet

The body has a chemical reaction to the foods you eat, and some holistic practitioners feel there is some benefit to eating in a way that is compatible with your blood type.

If you cannot follow this diet completely, it may help to just be aware of your blood type and take note if you feel more or less energized when you eat foods according to blood type.

There are many books available on eating for your blood type.

• Homeopathy

Homeopathy is a great way to release and unblock emotional traumas or negative patterns that may be affecting your fertility. Homeopathy works on the principle of 'like cures like' and brings the body into balance. Homeopathy uses substances found in nature to give the body the push it needs to begin healing itself.

Homeopathy can be used to treat recurrent miscarriage, irregular ovulation, weakened immune system, and other causes of infertility.

Homeopathy is tailored specifically to each individual's needs according to their symptoms, lifestyle, mental and physical health. Questions like sleep habits, personality, and history will be asked. Treatments are comprised of small doses of what are known as homeopathic remedies.

I did homeopathy when trying to get pregnant for a second time, and within weeks, I could feel some painful emotions leave my body permanently. If trying homeopathy, be sure to select a practitioner experienced in working with infertility.

Common cures include Agnus Castus, also known as Vitex, Sepia 6c for irregular or absent ovulation, Sabin 6c for women who suffer from miscarriages, Phosphorus for treating stress related to infertility and Lycopodium for women who suffer from a dry vagina. The remedies come in tablets, liquid or pellets and are placed under the tongue so they dissolve and are easily absorbed into the system.

• Ayurvedic Medicine

Ayurvedic medicine is a very ancient holistic healing system developed thousands of years ago in India. In Ayurvedic medicine, it is believed that the root causes of infertility include nervous system imbalances, physical and mental stress, disruption of natural biological rhythms, accumulated toxins in the body, poor nutrition, sluggish digestion and a weakened immune system.

In Ayurvedic medicine, it is believed that a person's physical, spiritual and emotional well-being are all interconnected. Foods considered healing to infertility include grapes, pomegranate, seaweed, almonds, walnuts, mangoes, peaches, plums and pears. Spices recommended are cumin, which purifies the uterus in women and the genitourinary tract in men, turmeric, which improves the interaction between hormones and black cumin. Herbs used to help infertility include raspberry leaves, nettle leaves and flaxseed oil.

Herbs used in Ayurvedic medicine to treat infertility include Ashoka, Shatavari, and Kumari.

A fertility-strengthening treatment of a gentle daily warm oil massage of the abdomen in a clockwise motion to support the reproductive organs, followed by a warm bath or shower, is sometimes recommended.

• Traditional Chinese Medicine

When practitioners of Chinese medicine treat infertility, they work to balance the 'foundation' of the body and the qi, or life energy, that flows through the body, through herbal medicine, acupuncture, massage, dietary therapy and exercise. Emotions, sleeping and eating habits, are all looked at in determining the root cause of infertility. They may treat infertility by suggesting increasing blood flow to the reproductive organs, through acupuncture, massage or exercise. Sometimes they treat infertility by recommending patients avoiding dampness and damp foods such as cheese, butter, alcohol, humid environments and moist basements.

In Chinese medicine, healing one's emotions is key to healing infertility. Two of the most common organs related to fertility are the liver and the lungs. The lungs are related to sadness, grief and holding on, while the liver is connected to frustration, stress, desire and anger. Calming the mind through acupuncture and saying positive affirmations can help. Being receptive to conception is also important. To do this, think: warm, enveloping, holding, supportive thoughts.

• Naturopathic Doctors

There are primary care physicians who have also attended naturopathic medical school. They emphasize prevention and self-healing, while focused on identifying the underlying causes of disease. Some of the modalities used in naturopathic medicine to treat infertility include nutrition, homeopathy, hydrotherapy, along with conventional medicine.

Tests You Can Request At the Fertility Clinic

Don't expect or just wait for your doctor to recommend a test or advanced treatment. Request it! If they won't do it, go somewhere else and find a doctor and/or clinic that will accommodate your requests.

Some tests you may want to request include:

- Fibroids or fibroid tumors
- Cysts
- Endometriosis
- Polycystic ovarian syndrome
- Hormone imbalance
- Ovulation problems
- Luteinizing hormone (LH) testing
- Progesterone testing
- Estradiol Level testing
- Hysterosalpingogram
- Laparoscopy to investigate possible scarring, cysts, fibroid tumors or other abnormalities
- Post coital testing
- A thyroid test
- FSH Level
- Fallopian Tube testing, that can include sonohysterogram, hysterosalpingogram, and lapascropy to check if your fallopian tubes are blocked.
- Endometrial biopsy
- Transvaginal ultrasound
- Hysteroscopy: to look for growth or defects in the uterus that cannot be seen with other tests.
- Screen for sexually transmitted diseases

Vitamins and Other Supplements that Can Help Prepare Your Body for Pregnancy

Start with a high-quality prenatal vitamin and a high-quality mineral supplement. If possible, see a reputable nutritionist or holistic health practitioner to start a balanced vitamin and herb regime.

Remember: some vitamins, herbs and supplements need to be stopped the moment you could be pregnant—some are for pre-pregnancy preparation only, and not safe once you have conceived. Other vitamins and herbs should not be taken at the same time you are taking infertility medications.

• A High-Quality Pre-Natal Vitamin

It is most important to start taking a pre-natal vitamin before you are pregnant to give your body the nutrients it needs.

• Omega-3

Some people consider Omega-3 a key part of a fertility health regimen. Omega-3 fats help fertility by regulating hormones, increasing cervical mucus, promoting ovulation and improving the overall quality of the uterus by increasing blood flow to the reproductive organs.

Omega-3 supplements also boost the immune system and reduce natural killer cells that can prevent the embryo's implantation in the uterus.

• Coenzyme 10

This is a supplement both you and your husband should consider taking—and be a supplement that you might consider your new best fertility friend! Recent studies have shown that Co-enzyme Q10 can actually help improve egg quality in older women and improve fertilization rates because it corrects the energy which impacts the division of chromosomes during fertilization.

It can improve the quantity and quality of your eggs, which is key to beating infertility. It is a major cellular antioxidant and can be considered giving your body a high grade fuel to up your cellular energy production process and protect your body from DNA damage. Ubiquinol, the active form of Coenzyme Q10, has demonstrated the ability to improve mitochondrial energy production in aged eggs.

Other studies have shown that it also helps improve sperm density and motility in men. This supplement has been shown to improve the rates of conception and live birth in women who are taking it.

• Folic Acid

You should begin taking folic acid long before you are pregnant in order to build it up in your system. The recommended dosages before pregnancy range from 400 mcg to 600 mcg. When I was trying to conceive, I opted for a higher dose of folic acid.

• Evening Primrose Oil

This oil is known to help produce fertile quality cervical fluid. This should only be taken BEFORE you are pregnant. STOP taking once if there is even a slight chance you could be pregnant. It aids in conception, but is not be taken at all during pregnancy.

• Vitamin C

Known as a great friend to fertility, Vitamin C helps improve hormone levels

• B complex

B6 balances hormone levels and improves low progesterone levels of women affected by luteal phase defect. B12 enhances ovulation and improves the inner lining of the uterus.

- **Vitamin E**

Vitamin E an increase cervical mucus in women, prevent egg defects and increase overall egg health. Some studies suggest it can also lengthen the luteal phase of a cycle.

- **Zinc**

Helps produce mature eggs ripe for fertilization, maintain proper follicular fluid levels, and regulate hormone levels of estrogen, progesterone and testosterone.

- **Bee Pollen**

Stimulates ovarian function, nourishes the ovaries, aids in the production of healthy eggs and normalizes menstrual cycle.

- **Royal Jelly**

High in amino acids, proteins and other vitamins. It balances hormones and supports the production of healthy eggs.

- **Calcium**

A vital ingredient in triggering growth in embryos. The minerals in calcium help create an alkaline environment in the reproductive tract. It also contains the nutrient that the sperm soaks up and gives help in thrusting towards the egg.

- **Iron**

A blood-building nutrient that helps ovulation. Iron deficiency can cause the eggs stored in the ovaries to weaken over time and become unviable. Anemia also makes it impossible for the growing fetus' cells to divide and grow properly.

- **L-Arginine**

Known to enhance ovarian response, endometrial receptivity and pregnancy rates. It also increases cervical mucus.

Powerful Foods To Help Cure Your Infertility

When working towards healing from infertility, never for one moment underestimate the power of the foods you eat.

Right now, this moment, you need to begin seeing everything you eat and drink as either a potential healer of your infertility or a potential destroyer of your fertility.

The foods you eat right now could mean the difference between getting pregnant and not getting pregnant. This is how important the food component of your fertility journey is.

Do not be fooled into thinking that you can drink lots of coffee, eat white flour products, sugar, and processed, fast-foods and it won't impact your body's ability to conceive.

Yes, there are some women who can live off fast food and still get pregnant whenever they choose—but there are also millions of women whose fertility is being stolen by the foods they eat.

To prepare for pregnancy, it is key that you plan, choose and decide to eat as healthy as possible to maximize your body's ability to have a baby.

Don't be trapped into thinking that you can eat the way you've always eaten and still heal your body.

If getting pregnant is not coming easily to you, you need to change your eating habits and let go of archaic ideas about food that could be holding your body back.

Every time you are tempted by that chocolate bar in the vending machine at work, or a cup of coffee, or a cracker with lots of hydrogenated oil, remind yourself that chocolate bar, or that cup of coffee, or that cracker, could be what ultimately prevents you from having a baby.

If you think a bagel, cream cheese and coffee is a healthy way to start to the day, think again.

It is simple: what you eat can make you weak or make you strong. The right foods can heal your infertility and the wrong ones can rob you of your right to be a mother.

Here are some tips that will help you use food as a way to heal your infertility and prepare your body for pregnancy:

To start:

• Stop Or Reduce Your Coffee Consumption

Do you drink coffee? You need to consider stopping. As much as you can, preferably stop all coffee. If you can't stop, drink no more than a half a cup to a cup a day. That's it. Ideally, do everything you can to say goodbye to coffee for now. Coffee is an enemy of your fertility. Every time you are tempted to drink coffee, remind yourself that this cup of coffee could rob you of the ability to give birth to children. Get rid of all caffeine products in your life. Extreme, maybe, but coffee can weaken key organs, such as the liver, and right now, you need to stack the odds in your favor.

Some studies have shown that women who drink high amounts of coffee take up to three times longer to conceive, and even small amounts of coffee can hamper fertility.

To cope with the lack of coffee in your life, you may need to go to bed earlier and eat healthier to compensate for the energy the coffee gave you to get through the day. Coffee cannot be your fuel or main source of energy anymore. Your energy has to come from healthy foods, vitamins, juices, exercise and other genuinely healthy energy-producing sources.

As you detoxify and strengthen your body, your energy will increase and come from your inner core of health—not coffee, an imposter who pretends to hand you energy, but ultimately steals it. Say goodbye to coffee and hello to food sources that genuinely fuel you.

• Eliminate Most Sugars

Do you eat lots of sweets? Realize that donuts, candy, cake, and other foods with sugar weaken your body and can prevent you from becoming pregnant.

Sugar puts your body in a diseased, acidic state. Sugar can cause hormone imbalances, vitamin deficiencies, high insulin levels, and a compromised immune system. While an occasional sweet is okay, overall you'll want to drastically reduce the sugar in your life.
It can be hard to quit eating all sweets entirely. Many of us have sugar cravings, but overall you want to drastically reduce the amount of sugar you consume.

You'll also need to be be aware and carefully examine the foods you eat that may have hidden sugars in them. Read labels carefully as sugar content varies by brand. Always remember: if its packaged, there is a chance it might have sugar in it.

Foods you need to be aware of for potential sugar content include:

- Yogurt
- Cereals
- Canned vegetables
- Canned soups
- Breakfast bars
- Salad dressing
- Condiments
- White flour products.
- Breads and rolls
- Juices
- Fast foods
- Barbecue sauce
- Soda
- Spaghetti sauce
- Energy drinks
- Dried fruit
- Crackers

- Products that list ingredients such as, dextrose, fructose, corn syrup, high-fructose corn syrup, fruit juice concentrate, lactose, sorbitol, xylitol, maltodetrin and turbinado sugar, polydextrose, mannitol, and turbinado sugar. Ingredients ending in 'ose' is often a likely form of sugar.
- Oatmeal
- Protein bars
- Ice tea
- Ketchup
- Frozen meal entrees, even diet ones
- Syrups
- Jelly and jams
- Fruit juice concentrate
- Bouillon cubes
- Bacon
- Luncheon meats

• Consider Reducing Hydrogenated Oils, Also Known As Trans Fats

Another category of food you need to consider cutting from your diet entirely are foods made with hydrogenated oils, also known as trans fats. Several studies have shown that women with fertility problems eat more trans fats or hydrogenated oils than fertile women. Hydrogenated oil is a man-made food substance used widely throughout the food industry because it lengthens the shelf life of many foods and is cost effective.

Trans fats interfere with the metabolic processes in the body, because they take the place of essential fatty acids that perform critical functions. Trans fats clog up the space that natural fats should occupy, making it difficult for essential nutrients to pass in and out of the cells. Bodily functions are altered by these artificial molecules that enter the system.
Various studies have shown that women who eat a diet high in hydrogenated oils are at increased risk for developing endometriosis.

The World Health Organization has tried to outlaw trans fats for decades.

Some say trans fats work against the body, because they cause a cell-by-cell failure that destroys the flexibility of healthy cell membranes—basically tearing the body down from the inside out.

Trans fats increase bad cholesterol, block production of chemicals that combat inflammation and benefit the body's hormonal and nervous systems. Trans fats are also linked to heart disease, stroke and diabetes.

They interfere with the absorption of essential fatty acids and DHA, and weaken cell walls and compromise cellular structure.

That means, if you are trying to get pregnant, you need to dramatically reduce eating foods made with hydrogenated oils, corn oil, vegetable oil, transfats and corn syrup.

Be sure to read food labels carefully so you are aware of what products contain hydrogenated oils.

Fast food restaurants often serve a lot of foods loaded with hydrogenated oils. Cake, pancake, biscuit, and cookie mixes are usually made with hydrogenated oils.

Diet foods that promise 'no fat' often have hydrogenated oils.

Labels that say partially hydrogenated, or hydrogenated, contain trans fats. Even foods that promise to be trans fat free may contain up to 0.5 grams of partially hydrogenated oil, a source of trans fats.

Remember that if you see the word 'hydrogenated' or partially hydrogenated, it means it contains a trans fat. Hydrogenated oils are also trans fats, and that includes hydrogenated coconut or soybean oil.

Read labels carefully because hydrogenated oil content can vary by brand.

Begin to replace hydrogenated oils with healthy oils your body needs, such as olive oil, coconut oil and flax seed oil.

It is best to avoid as many pre-packaged foods that you can at this time. Foods to be aware of can include:

- Commercially baked cakes, cookies, muffins, pies, donuts
- Crackers
- Peanut butter
- Frozen meals
- Frozen bakery items
- French fries
- Whipped toppings
- Margarines
- Shortening
- Cake frosting
- Taco shells
- Microwave popcorn
- Breakfast cereals
- Corn chips and potato chips
- Frozen pizzas and frozen burritos
- Low-fat ice creams
- Pre-made noodle soups and soup mixes
- Bread
- Pasta mixes
- Sauce mixes
- Deep fried foods
- Frozen breakfast foods
- Packaged snacks
- Many different types of candies
- Some salted peanuts
- White bread
- Non-dairy creamers
- Tortillas
- Donuts
- Peanut butter
- Ice cream and low fat ice cream
- Hamburger and hot dog buns
- Movie popcorn
- Frozen pizza
- Refrigerated dough products

- Most fried foods—ask what type of oil the product is fried in
- Piecrust
- Cake mixes
- Pancakes and pancake mixes
- Waffles
- Frozen burgers
- Beef hot dogs
- Refrigerated cookie dough
- Biscuits and sweet rolls
- Refrigerated dough
- Breakfast sandwiches
- Meat sticks
- Crunchy noodles
- Canned chili
- Packaged pudding
- Fish sticks
- Low-fat ice cream
- Frozen burritos
- Noodle soup cups
- Cocoa or hot chocolate mix
- Instant mashed potatoes
- Gravy mixes
- Dips
- Potato chips
- Frozen pot pies
- Sandwiches grilled at a restaurant
- Reduced fat and fat free noodles
- Spreads

• Consider Eliminating Alcohol

At this time, it is best to stop all alcohol. A glass of wine occasionally when trying to get pregnant might not hurt, but nothing more and no hard liquors. Many studies suggest that the higher your alcohol consumption, the less chance you have of conceiving. Alcohol can impair the detoxifying process that occurs within the liver, and if the liver is working hard to metabolize alcohol, it can become run down and sick. Too much alcohol can also contribute to hormonal imbalances.

Alcohol can adversely affect ovulation and affect the body's ability to produce the amino acids necessary for cell development.

• Cut Down On White Flour Products

How many white flour products do you eat each day? Do you start your day with a bagel, donut or white bread toast? If so, get rid of white flour in your life as much as possible. An occasional bowl of spaghetti may be okay, but in general, you want to reduce the white flour products in your life as much as you can. White flour products, including pasta, bagels and bread, are not health builders and will not advance your goal of becoming pregnant. If you feel extremely weak and lethargic after eating white flour products, you may have celiac disease or a wheat intolerance. Symptoms include stomachaches, fatigue, bloating and flatulence. Check labels and brands. Some sources of white flour can include:

- Alcohol
- Crackers
- Cereals
- Corn flour
- Cake and cookie mixes
- Pancake mixes
- Muffin mixes
- Puddings
- Pretzels
- Donuts
- Foods with artificial colorings and preservatives
- Sweet and sour glazes
- Sweet sauces
- Soy sauce
- Ice cream cones
- Foods containing malt
- Powdered or canned soups
- Fast foods
- Gravies

Instead, choose wheat-free products made from rice, oat, rye, and puffed rice cereals.

• Reduce Your Intake Of Diet Foods or Foods with Sugar Substitutes

You may want to consider reducing your intake of diet foods, diet drinks or foods with sugar substitutes or artificial sweeteners. Some experts on fertility recommend avoiding sweeteners listed on labels as aspartame, sucralose, acesulfame potassium, also listed as acesulfame k and ACE, neotame, and saccharin.

Consider cutting back or eliminating diet drinks and powdered drinks that contain any of these sweeteners. These sweeteners may also be in some chewing gums and ice creams.

Some doctors have concluded that these artificial sweeteners interfere with fetal development, and act as 'instant birth control.' Aspartame is considered a endocrine disrupting chemical, by some medical providers.

Artificial sweeteners and sugar substitutes negatively impact the hormones in the pituitary glands, thyroid and ovaries.

Hidden sources of these artificial sweeteners can include:

- Breads
- Jello
- Gelatins
- Toothpaste
- Breath mints
- Drink mixes
- Syrups
- Jellies
- Cereals
- Sugar-free candies

• Reduce or Eliminate Soy

Some studies suggest that high levels of soy act as endocrine disrupters and decrease fertility. The phytoestrogens found in soy interfere with endocrine function and can mimic the female hormone oestrogen, which disrupts the normal production of sex hormones. Soy can decrease the follicle-stimulating hormone (FSH), as well as the leutinizing hormone.

Many soy products are genetically engineered and can reduce the body's ability to absorb minerals. Some soy isoflavones mimic estrogen—which means the body thinks it has estrogen it doesn't have, thus causing hormone imbalances. Some studies have also shown that soy can lead to thyroid problems, such as hypothyroidism.

Soy derivatives are often labeled under different names, including mono-diglyceride, soya, soja, yuba, TSF or textured soy flour, TSP textured soy protein, TVP textured vegetable protein, lecithin, and MSG, yeast extract, soy protein.

Hidden sources of soy include:

- Protein bars
- Meal replacement shakes
- Bottled fruit drinks
- Soups
- Sauces
- Baked goods
- Breakfast cereals
- Chewing gum
- Chocolate
- Bread
- Microwave meals
- Frozen pizzas
- Processed meat
- Soy milk
- Soy beans
- Corn chips
- Canned tuna

• Avoid Fish Known To Potentially Have High Mercury Levels

Due to high mercury levels, some types of fish are best avoided or eaten rarely when trying to get pregnant. These include swordfish, shark, grouper, marlin, orange roughy, tilefish, mackerel, tuna, bluefish, lobster, halibut, croaker and bass saltwater.

The fish with the reported lowest amounts of mercury include calamari, crab, pollock, scallops, salmon, shrimp, clams, and others, but these also need to be eaten in moderation.

• No MSG

Avoid foods that could have monosodium glutamate, also known as MSG. Foods that might contain MSG include potato chips, Chinese food, meat seasonings and packaged soups. MSG can appear on labels as autolyzed yeast, maltodextrin, hydrolyzed pea protein.

• Other Foods To Avoid

- Avoid raw or undercooked meats.
- Avoid raw or undercooked eggs.
- Stay Away From Fast Food
- Avoid Deli Meats

Fertility-Strengthening Foods

• Eat More Vegetables

Here's a simple fact that will increase your fertility: the more vegetables you eat, the more fertile you will be.

Repeat: More vegetables you eat, the healthier and more fertile you will be. Implant that thought in your brain, please, please, please.

Your diet should include a lot of vegetables every single day.

Note the word: a lot.

In fact, most of the foods you eat, starting with breakfast, should be vegetables.

Starting now, the way you eat should revolve around vegetables.

Vegetables should no longer be just a small side dish you include with dinner—they should be the main course, present at almost every meal and every snack you eat. They are the key to healing your body. You need to start looking at vegetables in a way that is not traditional in our culture—as your main source of food.

Vegetables should become part of your breakfast, your snacks, lunch and dinner. You want to find as many ways as you can to dramatically increase the vegetables you eat daily.

For lunch, eat a big bowl of romaine lettuce. Munch on parsley for a snack. Roast some asparagus and olive oil to eat before bed. Bake some sweet potatoes and olive oil for snack. Include spinach in your salads or sandwiches.

Slice up some peppers, carrots, red and green peppers, tomatoes, and seaweeds and place in bags so you have easy-to-eat snacks ready throughout the day.

Don't allow a busy schedule to force you to have to run to the nearest fast food drive-through because you are starving and need to just fill your stomach. At night before bed, prepare a salad of chicory and romaine lettuce. Or just wash some kale or spinach, put in a bag, and have it on your way home from work.

Nibble on broccoli before bed. Include a salad with every meal. Put vegetables on your pizza, in your tomato sauces, soups and stews.

Instead of a sandwich of deli meat, how about a sandwich of tomato and basil, broccoli and cheese, or spinach and tomato?

Eat vegetables the way you would eat fruit—a whole cucumber, a whole tomato, a whole carrot.

Select one or two days a week and eat only vegetables the entire day. Start your day with a green veggie drink or smoothie, add some flaxseed, coconut oil, maca, honey and spirulina.

Make a vegetable breakfast wrap, top an multi-grain English muffin with onions, peppers, and tomatoes. Create dips with vegetables—and then dip your vegetables! Add vegetables to spreads like hummus or mashed avocados. Make vegetable submarine sandwiches, with healthy bread and lots of olive oil.

Juicing or smoothies are a great way to include more vegetables in your diet. Drink a glass of spinach juice each day. Juice parsley, kale, beets, and garlic once or twice a day.

Start including garlic in many of your recipes as you can. Chew on garlic, juice garlic and make garlic part of your daily eating routine.

Remember: from now on, vegetables should make up more than 60 to 70 percent of the foods you eat each day.

Some super fertility vegetables include:

• Spinach is high in iron and folic acid, two important nutrients for reproductive health. Women with low iron intakes are at greater risk for ovulatory fertility.

To enhance absorption of iron from spinach, combine it with a food that contains vitamin C, such as broccoli, strawberries, green peppers or oranges.

• Alfalfa provides the body with a rich source of essential minerals important for reproductive health.

• Broccoli and cabbage contain a phytonutrient that helps with estrogen metabolism.

• Yams and sweet potatoes contain a compound called diosgenins which impacts hormonal patterns and increases ovulation. Yams have massive amounts of vitamin A that improve cervical fluid and follicle development. They are also loaded with beta carotene that helps regulate the menstrual cycle. It also has high amounts of Vitamin B which helps regulate hormones. They also help stabilize blood sugar—and the more stable your sugar levels, the better your ovulation will be.

• Asparagus is also a high fertility food.

• Wheat Grass is one of the best sources of living chlorophyll. It helps balance the PH levels in the body and is high in magnesium, which helps restore sex hormones.

• Spirulina is a great source of the essential acid GLA.

• Chlorella: a green algae that helps the body cleanse and detoxify.

Here is a checklist to help you keep track of the vegetables you eat each day:

Vegetables to eat every day include:

--Spinach
--Yams and Sweet Potatoes
--Peppers
--Broccoli
--Arugula
--Asparagus
--Romaine
--Seaweed
--Garlic
--Cabbage
--Dandelion greens
--Romaine Lettuce
--Red Peppers
--Dark green lettuce
--Kale
--Asparagus
--Beets
--Seaweeds
--Brussel sprouts

• Eat More Fruits

Along with eating as many vegetables as possible, start including more fruits in your diet.

Fruits are packed with antioxidants, which protect the body from cell aging and damage—including cells in the reproductive system, like your eggs.

Start eating one or two bowls of blueberries for breakfast. Blueberries have phytonutrients that have hormone balancing properties that impact ovulation.

Many holistic practitioners recommend eating avocados to boost fertility, because they are a great source of Vitamin E, a huge fertility booster. Avocados help regulate both ovulation and production of cervical mucus. They are rich in folic acid and vitamin B6, which helps prevent luteal phase defect.

Bananas are full of potassium, Vitamin C and fiber, and bromelain which increases sex hormone production.

Slice up some papaya as your bedtime snack, have two or three bowls of strawberries, blackberries, raspberries and blueberries for breakfast, bring apples to work.

Eat fresh pineapple daily, including the pineapple core. Pineapple contains bromelain that aids in implantation. Pineapple is also one the best natural sources of manganese, an important mineral that triggers production of various reproductive hormones. Low levels of this mineral have been reported to be associated with difficulty conceiving. Note: if you are already taking aspirin, be aware that pineapple might thin your blood.

Pomegranates are considered a fertility super food.

Eat lots of fruits that contain Vitamin C, such as oranges, kiwi, blueberries and strawberries, a nutrient key to fertile health.

Fruits to include in your daily diet:

-Plums
-Blueberries
-Strawberries
-Bananas
-Grapes
-Cantaloupe
-Oranges
-Apples
-Mangoes
-Bananas
-Blueberries
-Lemons
-Pomegranate
-Figs
-Apricots
-Prunes
-Peaches
-Blackberries

• Eat More Beans

Beans are an essential food for developing good follicle quality. Black beans are considered by some to be a reproductive tonic. Lentils are also a healthy source of iron that support ovulation and aid fertility. Aduki beans are considered to support the Kidney Qi, which is essential for reproductive function.

• Eat More Nuts

Start including lots of nuts in your diet, such as walnuts, almonds, and brazil nuts. Nuts have high amounts of Omega 3 and Omega 6, which have been known to improve sperm quality and egg quality.

Nuts can enhance pancreas function, thus helping to regulate insulin and blood sugar levels in the body. Almonds contain L-arginine and zinc which are important nutrients to the reproductive system. Walnuts are high in protein and folic acid and are an excellent source of omega-3 fatty acids. Almonds contain high levels of zinc and L-arginine, which are important nutrients to the reproductive system.

• Eat More Seeds

Seeds contain a lot of omega 3s which are key to fertility. Pumpkin seeds which contain zinc, an important nutrient in egg production. Sunflower seeds and sesame seeds provide healthy fats. Black sesame seeds can help enhance liver function and sesame seeds are rich in minerals.

• Healthy Oils

Because fat intake is so vital to fertility, include olive oil, coconut oil and flaxseed oil in your diet. Healthy fats, as opposed to trans fats, can make the body more fertile, reduce inflammation in the body and increase insulin sensitivity.

Olive oil, like avocados, has monounsaturated fat, which helps assist in reproduction. Some people have taken a mixture of olive oil, honey and mustard seed to enhance their fertility.

Flax seed oil helps the hormones hit the receptor cells in a precise way so they can work at their maximum capacity. This helps the membranes in the receptor cells be more flexible, run more smoothly and makes it easier for hormones to bind with. It also encourages healing in the uterus, and is rich in omega fatty acids.

Coconut oil helps maintain hormonal balance for reproduction and helps thyroid function and ovulation cycles.

- **Honey**

Bee pollen stimulates ovarian function. It is also rich in minerals such as copper, potassium, and zinc and also has 20 of the 22 known amino acids. Bee pollen contains natural hormonal substances that stimulate and nourish the reproductive system, stimulate ovarian function and increase the health and biological value of the egg.

- **Wild Salmon**

According to Chinese medicine, salmon is good for nourishing the yin and blood, helping to generate healthy follicles and ample amounts of cervical fluid.

- **Lean Cuts of Meat**

When possible, choose lean cuts of meat. An overload of heavy red meat can work against your fertility.

- **Drink Lots of Good Quality Water**

Drinking a lot of the right water can do so much to enhance your fertility. Water increases cervical fluid which is key in conception. Water can help sperm stay alive for days. Water also facilitates the transport of hormones and plumps up follicles.

The key is that along with drinking a lot of water, you need to drink high-quality water. Do you drink tap water? What is the quality of the water in your community? For now, start buying purified water and use it for all your drinking and cooking needs. Put a filter on your tap water. As much as you can, stop drinking water out of plastic bottles that can contain the chemical bisphenol A, also known as BPA. Keep your water stored in glass containers, rather than plastic.

• Start Your Day Drinking Lemon in Warm Water

Lemon enhances your immunity and increases liver and digestive health.

• Brown Rice

Replace white rice with brown rice for enhanced nutrition. Brown rice is a slow carbohydrate, which means a gradual rise in blood sugar after being eaten.

• Green Tea

For better quality eggs and more viable embryos, consider drinking two or more cups of green tea a day. Green tea contains polyphenols and hypoxanthine, which increase the percentage of viable embryos. Hypoxanthine enhances the follicular fluid that helps eggs mature and be ready for fertilization.

Green tea also contains polyhenols that act as an antioxidant and gets rid of unwanted toxins in the body. Green tea can help repair oxidative damage that occurs in the body due to stress, aging and the environment. Drink in moderation, as it can decrease the body's absorption of iron and decrease the effects of folic acid, so you might want to make sure you taking adequate amounts of iron and folic acid at the same time.

You should reduce the amount of green tea you drink once you are pregnant or if there is even a slight chance you are pregnant. The polyphenols in green tea that help prevent chromosomal abnormalities in your eggs can cause an embryo to miscarry or fail to implant.

• Pomegranates and Natural Pomegranate Juice

Pomegranates help boost fertility by increasing blood flow to the uterus and thickening the uterine lining. They also help balance the hormones estrogen and progesterone.

The antioxidants in pomegranates help prevent DNA damage to eggs and contain folic acid, essential during the early stages of a pregnancy.

• Pineapple Core

Cut the core into round sections and eat after embryo transfers to help implantation. The bromelain found in the core reduces inflammation and improves uterine lining.

• Brewer's Yeast

Brewer's yeast is a great source of B complex, and is rich in minerals like zinc, iron and chromium.

Your Personal Fertility Food Diary

It is important that every day, you keep track of what you eat. How healthy you become is closely related to the foods you take into your body.

There is a direct correlation between your level of fertility, vitality and energy and the foods and liquids you consume.

Ask yourself:

What foods make me feel stronger, brighten my mood, and give me energy?

What foods give me a second wind?

What foods leave me feeling exhausted?

What foods make me tired and cranky?

What live foods do I eat daily?

Breakfast: Say goodbye to cereal and milk, a bagel and coffee, pancakes and maple syrup. Say hello to oatmeal, blueberries and spinach.

Starting your diet with a few teaspoons of cooked spinach, maybe with a pinch or two of romano grated cheese.

Other great breakfast choices: lots of walnuts, avocados and blueberries, a big bowl or romaine lettuce doused with olive oil. A big glass of juiced spinach and kale. A smoothie with spinach, maca, flax seed, blueberries and honey. Or a bowl of walnuts and brazil nuts.

You have to replace all the ideas you've had about traditional breakfast foods, and replace them with foods that are alive, not laden down with corn syrup, sugar and white flour. The standard breakfast foods most of us eat can wreak havoc with our fertility. The goal each morning should be to eat nuts, beans, vegetables. No more lattes, coffees, or anything else caffeinated, white-floured or sugared to kick-start your day.

Lunch: Say goodbye to fast food lunches, deli meat, or lots of poor quality red meat.

Say hello to salads with things like walnuts and chick peas in them. Say goodbye to caffeine and soda to get through the day. No more chips with that tuna fish sandwich. A healthy lunch could include a salad with some chicken in it, homemade vegetable soup, with an apple, a grilled cheese with whole grain bread. A healthy lunch could also include a pumpkin-sunflower seed combination, or slices of pineapple drizzled with honey. A pita pocket filled with parsley, basil and kale, drizzled with olive oil and flaxseed oil.

Snacks: Snacks should include lots of healthy fruits, seeds, nuts, and vegetables. Candy bars, diet drinks or desserts, sugary desserts, chips, all should be eliminated.

Dinner: No white flour, trans fats, fast food, foods that contain msg or trans fats. Think lean proteins, healthy fish, lots of greens, salad, vegetables, nuts, and olive oil.

Your Personal Fertility Food Diary

Green Foods Eaten Today:

Fruits Eaten Today:

Vegetables Eaten Today:

Nuts Eaten Today:

Seeds Eaten Today:

Healthy Oils Eaten Today:

Vegetable and/or Fruit Drinks Made Today:

More Ways To Maximize Your Fertility and Improve Your Chances of Conceiving

• Try Robitussin: Some women swear by Robitussin (guaifenesin) cough syrup because it is believed to help thin cervical fluid.

• Baby Aspirin: Ask your doctor if baby aspirin might be something you should consider. Some research has shown that low doses of aspirin can help increase blood flow to the uterine lining and can enhance ovarian response. Some studies have also shown it reduces the risk of miscarriage.

• You may have heard that when you are trying to get pregnant, intercourse should only take place every few days to help build sperm levels. This is actually untrue. The more you do it, the better – so when you are ovulating, enjoy every moment you have together!

• Do not use any lubricants or oils when trying to get pregnant.

• Find intimate positions that allow for deep penetration.

• After intercourse, remain in bed for 30 minutes.

• Do not urinate 30 minutes after intercourse.

• Go to acupuncture once or twice a few days before an IUI or IVF to balance and strengthen your body.

• If you are already seeing a myofascial release specialist or a kinesiologist, get a treatment a few days before your IUI or IVF to help prepare your body to receive.

• Set aside time and finds places to relax, preferably outside in nature, before and after your IUI or IVF. Can you spend a few days at a local beach or lake right after an IVF? Spending time in sunlight also helps.

• Eat extra healthy foods the week of the IUI and IVF, and, of course, afterwards.

- After an IUI, ask if you can remain on the table for 25 to 40 minutes. Put your legs up against the wall to help the sperm travel to your eggs. Or don't ask permission if you think the answer is going to be no—and just take a really, really long time dressing. They can't force you out.

- Some studies suggest that touching, caressing and other forms of physical stimulation can increase hormones, thus improving chances for conception. Before an IUI or IVF, make out with your husband, touch each another, and get yourself a little bit 'in the mood.'

- Do not urinate 30 minutes after an IUI or IVF.

Diary Excerpt: Adjusting To A New Way of Life

In many ways, starting infertility treatments is like starting a new life—one I wasn't exactly ready for. I tip toed into this process, rather than diving headfirst into it. When I first began, I didn't think a lot about what was happening—all I knew is I wanted a baby and I felt safe that I was in the hands of a reputable fertility clinic. I didn't analyze much or have a well thought-out strategy.

I suppose, looking back, my tip toe approach worked for me, but it was not one I had the luxury of staying with for very long.

I was not prepared for how demanding treatments can be...blood tests at 6 a.m., ultrasounds, more blood tests, shots every night. I was often late for my appointments. I had a hard time juggling my work schedule and the demands of the clinic. I had not yet altered my life enough to include fertility. It felt like an interruption I wasn't yet ready to surrender to.

I felt like the clinic was constantly calling me wanting something...another blood test, one more ultra-sound—didn't they realize that if went to the 6:30 a.m. ultrasound, I would be exhausted by the time I got out of work at 9 o'clock?

Surrender...that is the word that describes the process in many ways. Battling infertility takes battling, but it also takes surrender. For someone like me, I had to progress to the point where the requirements of the clinic had to take priority over my own exhaustion, work schedule, social life, or personal desires.

At a certain point, the only personal desire I had to pay attention to was my desire for a baby.

For the first six months, I was consistently late for most of my appointments. I sometimes didn't show up due to my work schedule or car problems. I did this so many times, I finally got called on the carpet by Dr. P.

"Are you ready for this?" he asked. He told me that if I continued to miss appointments or show up late, the clinic could not continue treating me.

Talk about a wake-up call.

Suddenly, I realized that I had to take this whole process very seriously and live up to whatever it was the clinic asked of me, even when it was hard. I could blow my opportunity to have what I most wanted due to my own irresponsible behavior.

I explained to Dr. P some of the problems caused by my work schedule, and a few car problems that caused me to miss appointments.

He understood, but made it clear that this type of behavior couldn't continue and was not acceptable.

If I wanted their help, I had to be responsible. If I wanted these treatments to work, I had to commit to doing whatever they asked. Whenever they wanted me there, I had to be there.

Looking back, I consider this the first step in my training for motherhood: being responsible isn't an option.

I walked out of that appointment somber and scared.

I wanted a baby, and I would have to put aside whatever was preventing me from getting to my appointments on time.

This was one of the many turning points in my treatment.

Dr. P was forcing me to make a choice: continue life as you know it, without 6 a.m. blood tests, or go through this painful, inconvenient, life-interrupting process in order to get what you want most.

I left knowing I had to change, and this was one of the many times my infertility treatments would push me in ways that I needed to be pushed in order to become the mother I wanted to be.

Chapter 2

Getting Your Guy Ready: The Ultimate Male Fertility Preparation Program

Along with getting yourself prepared for pregnancy, it is important to help your husband and/or partner become as fertile as possible. Don't panic if your guy was diagnosed with a low sperm count. Just as there are many things a woman can do to maximize her fertility, there are also many things a man can do to improve the quality, quantity, and speed of his sperm.

Whether or not your guy was diagnosed with any specific problem, it is important to address his fertility because underlying, undiagnosed problems could exist that are not being caught.

Some causes of inadequate sperm production include hormone imbalances, post-testicular issues with plumping or ejaculation, trauma or accidents, varicocele, or dilated veins in the scrotum, undescended testis/testes, excessive xenoestrogen, which are environmental estrogen exposure; infectious disease of the epidydimis, a diseased endocrine (glandular) system affecting the hypothalamus, pituitary, thyroid, adrenals and the testes, resulting in low DHEA and testosterone levels, congenital abnormalities, urethral stricture, malnutrition, especially protein deficiency.

It can sometimes take two to three months to improve the quality of sperm, so you'll want to begin preparing as soon as possible.

Tests For Men
Here are some of the tests your husband/partner can request:

• Sperm analysis, including a sperm antibody test, which can determine sperm count, motility, morphology (shape), seminal fluid, volume of ejaculation, and pH level.

• A Hormone Analysis: Hormones include testosterone, follicle stimulating hormone, and lutinizeing hormone which are critical to sperm production. You may also want to have analyzed prolacin levels, thyroid stimulating hormone, sand ex-hormone binding globulin.

• Scrotal Doppler Ultrasound: measures the size of the testicle and look for blockages that involve transport of sperm out of the testicle.

• Transrectal Ultrasound: ultrasound technology is used to image the reproductive tract.

• A blood test to check for infections and hormone levels.

• A white blood cell count to detect infection, past infection, inflammation, low levels of inhibin B, or the compound alpha-glucosidase.

• Forward progression: this test measures the amount of forward movement in the sperm.

• Kruger morphology: if an abnormal morphology is found, this test allows the specialists to examine the sperm structure in great detail.

• Anti-sperm antibodies: this means the male has created an immunological response toward the sperm cells

• Sperm agglutination: sperm is examined to see whether there is any clumping together of the cells. Sperm agglutination can indicate the presence of sperm antibodies or bacterial infection.

• Viability: this test is performed if the sperm analysis shows that less than 30 percent of the sperm are motile. This test determines whether or not there is a presence of live sperm.

• Fructose: this test determines whether there is a blockage or no sperm at all being produced.

- An often overlooked cause of infertility in men is low-grade infection in the male urinary tract. Symptoms are often subtle and hard to diagnose, but they can include chills, fever, increased urination and intense burning during urination. Some physicians recommend culturing a semen sample to detect this mild infection.

• Cleanses

Here are some cleanses for men to consider before beginning infertility treatments.

- **A Parasite Cleanse:** Parasites can weaken sperm on a very hard-to-detect level. Health food stores carry 30-day parasite cleanses that can effectively remove parasites from the body.

- **Heavy Metal Cleanse:** Chemicals, pesticides and toxins in our environment have greatly impacted male fertility. Many men suffer from low-quality sperm because of these environmental toxins and chemicals. If possible, consider a heavy metal cleanse that can help remove these chemicals.

- **Liver Cleanse:** Just as detoxifying the liver is key to healing female infertility, it is equally important for men. Consider having your partner do a liver cleanse. The liver helps to filter toxins from the body, including excess hormones.

- **Candida-Yeast Cleanse:** can help rid the body of toxins.

- **Colon Hydrotherapy:** A colon cleanse can eradicate years of toxins in the large intestine, reducing the burden on the liver, pancreas, gall bladder and kidney.

• Holistic and Alternative Health Treatments to Consider

- **Acupuncture:** Acupuncture has been known to help men who have a low sperm count. It may be helpful for your partner to begin weekly or twice-weekly acupuncture treatments.

Make sure to let the acupuncturist know that you are looking to strengthen your husband's sperm Acupuncture points can help redirect Qi (energy) to key points in the body that assist in the smooth flow of blood to the penis and scrotum.

• Vitamins and Supplements

Here are some vitamins and supplements that can often help male infertility:

• **Vitamin C:** High-quality vitamin C supplements enhance sperm development. Some recommend 2,000 to 6,000 milligrams daily to prevent sperm from clumping or sticking together.

Foods that contain lots of Vitamin C include strawberries, citrus fruits, cherries, cantaloupe, broccoli, tomatoes, sweet peppers, mangos, kiwi, pineapple, grapes, peas, potatoes, parsley and spinach. Keep a bowl of these foods washed and easily available.

• **Zinc:** is very important to sperm quality because it increases testosterone levels, sperm count and sperm motility. Men should consider taking a zinc supplement or a high-quality multivitamin that contains zinc, as a zinc deficiency has been shown to cause or reduce male infertility. In addition to taking a supplement, foods high in zinc include oysters, organic meats, lean beef, turkey, lamb, herring, wheat germ, beans, sunflower and pumpkin seeds.

• **L-Arginine:** is an amino acid that enhances low sperm counts and poor motility. It is found in high amounts in the head of the sperm. Studies show that sperm and semen volume double with this amino acid.

Food sources of L-arginine include nuts, raisins, sesame seeds, brown rice, peanuts, almonds chocolate, meat and poultry.

• **A Multivitamin:** taken daily.

- **Vitamin E:** Studies have shown that Vitamin E increases sperm health and motility.

- **Folic acid:** Studies suggest that men with low levels of this key B vitamin have trouble producing healthy sperm. Folic acid reportedly improves sperm motility and sperm structure. Food sources include leafy greens, orange juice and spinach.

- **Korean Ginseng:** enhances testosterone and sperm levels.

- **Selenium:** should be taken as part of a quality multi-vitamin.

- **Coenzyme Q10:** increases energy production in the sperm and can increase motility and quality of sperm.

- **Omega-3:** acts as a hormone regulator.

- **Vitamin A:** helps enhance male hormones.

- **B-complex:** This vitamin is very important to male fertility. Vitamin B6 and B12 have been reported to improve sperm counts. Vitamin B12 can increase the quantity and quality of your guy's sperm. Foods that contain B vitamins include lamb, sardines and salmon.

- **Calcium-Magnesium:** aids Vitamin B absorption.

- **Vitamin A:** increases male hormones. Eat plenty of vegetables, fruit, oily fish and dark green leafy vegetables.

- **Royal Jelly:** can help optimize hormonal balance.

- **Manganese deficiency:** is known to result in testicular degeneration. Foods with manganese include: whole grains, green vegetables, carrots, broccoli, beans, nuts, pineapples, oats, rye and eggs.

• Things Your Guy Can Do To Improve His Fertility

• **Visit The Dentist:** Make sure your husband has his teeth cleaned, thus eliminating the possibility of infections in the gums or teeth.

• **Consider His Weight:** Too much or too little body fat can disrupt production of reproductive hormones, thus reducing sperm count. Try to help your husband/partner lose weight, especially scrotal fat, which can act like a warm blanket over the scrotum and elevate sperm temperatures, which in turn, kill and immobilize sperm. Excess fat around the waist is often associated with decreased male fertility.

• **Reduce Stress:** Encourage your husband/partner to take steps to reduce stress, as stress has been shown to negatively impact male reproductive hormones and lower testosterone.

• **Drink Lots of Water:** Make sure your partner is drinking plenty of high-quality, filtered water each day.

• **Touch, Touch and Touch Some More:** Stimulation increases hormones and improves fertility. Touch each other at length before intercourse to increase hormones, both his and yours.

• **Ejaculate Often:** Sex is good for sperm, because the less time spent in storage, the higher quality it will be and less DNA damage.

• **Enjoy More Sunshine:** Encourage your guy to get outside 10 to 15 minutes a day.

• **Balance The Body's Flora:** Eating a diet rich in nuts, seeds, fruits and vegetables can help encourage healthy sperm. Limit sugar, processed foods and encourage your guy to take a probiotic to improve digestive health and reduce inflammation. Reducing the amount of gluten consumed is also important.

• **Alkalize His Body With Greens:** Lots of healthy vegetables can help restore the acid-alkaline balance in the reproductive system to the proper sperm pH. A diet high in acid-producing foods such as meat, white flour, sugar, alcohol, coffee and soft drinks is to be avoided.

- **Nourish His Endocrine System:** The endocrine system is responsible for hormone production and secretions. Low sperm count or morphology is often caused by hormonal imbalance, and an over-stressed endocrine system.

• What Your Guy Should Avoid To Protect His Fertility

- **Keep It Loose:** Have your partner wear loose fitting boxer shorts, instead of tight underwear. Avoid boxers, briefs or bikinis.

No tight clothes around the genitals please.

- **Just Say No To Lubricants:** Avoid lubricants during sex. Lotions or lubricants can interfere with sperm motility.

- **Don't Let His Sperm Get Too Hot:** Heat can deter the healthy development of sperm. Genitals should be kept cool when possible. Lap top computers can increase scrotal temperature, which hurts sperm production.

Avoid hot tubs, saunas and Jacuzzis. Wear cotton boxer shorts rather than jockey shorts to keep sperm from overheating. Avoid long drives, and never let him put his cell phone in between his legs while driving. Avoid hot baths or overly long hot showers.

If your guy has a job that requires him to sit a lot each day, this could be causing high testicle heat. Encourage him to get up and walk every few hours.

Avoid heated car seats, electric blankets and heating pads that increase testicular temperatures—always remember sperm works better when it is cool!

If there is a chance that your partner is experiencing too much heat in his genital area, you may want to try artificially cooling his testicles with ice, a cold bath or shower. Always remember: Sperm counts are higher in the cold weather and in the morning.

• **Stop All Cigarette Smoking:** Smoking reduces sperm count and motility. It also increases the risk of genetic defects in an embryo. All smoking should be stopped.

• **No Marijuana:** Chemicals from marijuana have been reported to build up in the testicles and can cause impotence and a lower sperm count.

• **Take A Look At Prescription Drugs:** If your husband is on medication, you may want to evaluate if it is safe for him to take a break while you are trying to conceive. Some prescription drugs can negatively effect sperm count. This is a matter to be decided with a doctor's approval and notification, as some medications are absolutely necessary for various mental and physical health conditions.

• **Reduce Bicycling Activity:** Bicycling can raise scrotal temperature and critical arteries and nerves can be damaged by repeatedly banging the groin against the seat.

• **No Oral Sex:** Saliva can kill sperm. Avoid oral sex at this time.

• **No Extreme Exercise:** Extreme exercise can lower the sperm count.

• **Cut Down Or Reduce Alcohol:** Alcohol interferes with the secretion of testosterone and lowers sperm count. Alcohol can also depletes vitamins and minerals in the body and an overworked liver can cause a rise in estrogen

• **Stay Away From Water Bottles That Contain Bisphenol A (BPA):** Be aware of Bisphenol A (known as BPA) a hormone-disrupting chemical that is a common ingredient in water bottles, canned goods, and other products. Researchers have found that men with higher urine levels of BPA have decreased sperm concentration, decreased total sperm count, decreased sperm vitality and decreased sperm motility. BPA can also be found on cash register receipts and metal cans.

- **Avoid Soaps and Deodorants That Contain Phthalates:** Phthalates are another group of chemicals that have been shown to wreak havoc with reproductive health.

They are commonly found in vinyl flooring, detergents, soap, shampoo, deodorants, fragrances, hair spray, plastic bags, vinyl shower curtains, scented soaps, cleaners, garden hoses, and sex toys.

- **Be Aware of Chemicals In His Environment:** Other chemicals that are linked to decreased fertility include: Methoxychlor and Vinclozin, an insectide and fungicide, non-fermented soy products that contain hormone-like substances, and fluoride.

Avoid plastic containers for food storage, plastic bottles, wraps and utensils.

Be aware of office paper products whitened with chlorine. Use only non-bleached coffee filters, paper, napkins and toilet tissue to reduce dioxin exposure.

- **No Chlorine Products:** Avoid chlorinated tap water, chlorine bleach and other chlorinated products.

- **No Deodorants:** Avoid synthetic deodorants and use only organic products whenever possible.

- **Reduce Cell Phone Usage and Contact:** Cell phones can negatively impact the brain's pituitary output. Ask your guy to cut down on using his phone, and tell him not to carry it in his pocket. Try to encourage him to keep wireless items that transmit EMFs away from his body.

- **Reduce WIFI Usage:** Wifi signals contain EMFs that have been found to lower sperm count.

- **No anabolic steroids**

- **Some studies suggest anti-ulcer drugs decrease sperm count**

- **Avoid Cottonseed toxins hidden in food**

- Avoid pesticides

- Avoid growth hormones

- **Reduce or Eliminate If Possible Caffeine:** Excessive amounts of caffeine can impact sperm counts. Caffeine, found in tea, coffee, chocolate, cola, energy drinks, some medications, and stimulants to keep people awake, should be reduced or eliminated.

- **Reduce Contact With Lawn Care Products:** Stop using bug sprays, lawn sprays or pesticides to treat lawn and garden.

- **No More Microwaves:** Do not microwave food in plastic.

- **No Polyester:** Stop wearing polyester clothes.

• Fertility-Enhancing Foods for Men

Here are the foods your guy should eat to maximize his fertility.

- **Lots of Green Vegetables:** Green vegetables are needed to make your guy's body more alkaline. Juicing a glass of green juice each day is one way to ensure your husband has the greens he needs.

- **Spinach** is high in potassium, which improves sperm concentration.

- **Cauliflower** provides choline, that has been shown to improve sperm quality.

- **Add extra tomatoes to his salad**, as some studies have shown that the lycopene in tomatoes increase sperm count.

- **Red peppers, kiwi, lemons and strawberries** are all high in Vitamin C which has been shown to improve sperm count and motility.

- **Sardines** are rich in Omega 3's and a good source of Coenzyme Q10.

- **Avocado** has L-carnitine which promotes healthy sperm, can boost sperm motility and is packed with Vitamin E, Vitamin B6 and folic acid.

- **Pumpkin seeds** are high in zinc, loaded with omega-3 and should be a daily part of his diet.

- **Broccoli** is high in selenium

- **Wheat germ and almonds** are high in Vitamin E

- **Whole grains like oatmeal and brown rice**

- **Extra-virgin olive oil**

- **Oysters** contain a high level of zinc, which helps increase production of sperm and testosterone.

- **Brazil nuts** are rich in selenium, a mineral that boosts sperm production and mobility.

- **Walnuts** contains arginine, which increases semen volume and Omega-3s that improve blood flow to the penis.

- **Molasses**

- **Apricots**

- **Watermelon**

- **Sesame seeds**

- **Maca**

- **Spirulina**

- **Foods High In Antioxidants:** Sperm is damaged by free radicals and antioxidants can prevent cell damage. High antioxidant foods include: blueberries, blackberries, kale, garlic, Brussels sprouts, plums, red peppers, broccoli and red peppers.

- **Asparagus:** contain high amounts of Vitamin C, which prevents sperm from oxidizing and protects the cells of testes.

- **Bananas:** contain bromelain, that help increase stamina and boosts the body's ability to make sperm.

- **Wild fish**

- **Dark chocolate** contains L-Arginine, an amino acid related to the arginine in walnuts.

- **Garlic** contains allicin which increases blood flow to the genitals.

- **Pomegranate** contains an intense cocktail of antioxidants that can lower a chemical in the blood called malondialidehyde that destroys sperm.

- **Organic Free Range Meat:** Some nutritionists recommend eating organically-raised, free range meats, instead of conventional meat that contains hormones and antibiotics. Eat grass fed and organic cattle.

Conventionally raised cattle can sometimes contain high levels of hormones and antibiotics which can contribute to estrogen dominate conditions.

- **Free Range Organic Chicken:** Conventionally raised chicken is sometimes full of antibiotics and hormones which can negatively impact hormonal health.

- **Kiwi** fruit is high in zinc, which helps protect sperm from chromosomal and bacterial damage.

• Foods To Avoid or Eliminate

• Your partner should eliminate, or at least cut down, on alcohol, beer and wine while you are trying to get pregnant. Alcohol can lower sperm count, weaken sperm, and impede the secretion of testosterone. Studies have shown that alcohol can decrease sperm count for as much as three months after a big drinking fest.

• Encourage your partner to avoid sugar. Eating lots of sugar often results in hormone imbalances and robs the body of key nutrients.

• Cut down or avoid whenever possible white flour or gluten. If someone is sensitive to gluten, it can cause malabsorption of important nutrients, such as zinc, and increase inflammation throughout the body.

• Reduce or avoid foods with hydrogenated oil as much as possible.

• Reduce or avoid caffeine, which can reduce sperm count and motility. Caffeine is also detrimental to adrenal function, a gland key in productive hormones. The constant stress of caffeine can cause the body to focus on dealing with stress hormones, instead of reproductive hormones.

• Reduce or avoid animal products with a high fat content that contain hormones.

• No fried foods

• No hot sauce

• Avoid fried, charcoal-broiled or barbecued forms of cooking.

• Avoid soy. Soy is high in phyto estrogens, which can upset the hormonal balance in man. The estrogen-like compounds in soy can dramatically lower sperm counts. Texturized soy protein is in many meat substances used in fast food chains, and is also found in cereal, snack crackers and protein shakes.

• Avoid soda

• Stop drinking milk for now, since many dairy cows are fed estrogens to produce more milk. If you must drink milk, try to drink milk that is organic and not from estrogen-fed cows. Dairy that is not organic may contain hormones and antibiotics which can contribute to increased estrogen levels in the body. Keep dairy to a minimum.

• Avoid processed grains, GMO corn and corn products, and corn chips.

• Conditions To Have Checked

• Be sure your husband is aware of any food allergies he may have.

• Some cases of male infertility are linked to viruses. It would be helpful for your partner to do a parasite cleanse. Investigate whether your guy has an infection, which could be lowering his sperm count.

• Micro-organisms and bacteria may be the cause of fertility problems. Approximately 15% of cases of male factor infertility are reportedly caused by bacteria, parasites or viruses.

• Chlamydia

• Elevated prolactin levels

• Triglycerides: a sign of metabolic syndrome and insulin resistance

One More Thing:

• There is some research that suggests that sperm levels are highest in the morning, and this could be something to speak to your doctor about when scheduling IVFs and IUI's.

Chapter 3: How To Prepare For the Journey Through Infertility

• Prepare To Take Responsibility for Your Own Healing

This journey is your responsibility and yours alone. Your journey to motherhood is not the responsibility of your doctor, your husband, your mother, or your best friend.

You will ultimately fare better if you take responsibility for your infertility treatments, rather than hoping someone is going to come and pave the way for you or rescue you.

You are in charge and responsible for all the hard work your infertility treatments will demand and require.

Accepting the responsibility of finding a good doctor, showing up to all your appointments, and doing whatever it takes to heal your body, will empower you to make good choices, be organized, self-disciplined, and do whatever you can to improve your chances of conceiving the baby you so deserve.

You are the one that must go to the appointments, take the medications, change whatever needs to be changed and sacrifice whatever needs to be sacrificed, in the quest to have a baby. You are in charge. You make the choices. You ask the questions. You do the research. You explore your options. You ask to try another medication. You change doctors. You eat healthy. You show up on time for the appointments. The choices, the actions, are all up to you.

You want this baby, you need to understand you are the driver. You are not a child resting easily in the arms of your doctor or anyone else.

Relying on the word of any one doctor, or any one clinic, or any one person, is a big mistake. Starting right now, you need to take responsibility for your treatment--not hand it over to anyone or rely totally on anyone else.

Many women have made the mistake of letting the course of their treatment be dictated by one person--usually a medical professional--only to find out later that person had been on the wrong track.

By putting yourself firmly in the driver's seat, you will not be afraid to ask for things, push for more, change course when you see the need. You will not be tethered to a treatment that is not working for you. Nor will you be a victim to whatever some authority figure sees fit for you, especially if their pronouncement or decision isn't bringing you the desired results.

Stay in charge and realize that no one can run this race for you but you.

Taking responsibility does not mean blaming yourself, hating yourself, or beating yourself when you hit hard times and disappointments. It is not your fault when a cycle doesn't work out and you are not pregnant yet.

Taking responsibility means educating yourself, speaking up for yourself, advocating for yourself, believing in yourself. You need to understand and fully realize that you--and only you--are responsible and in charge of your infertility treatments and journey.

• Prepare to Work Hard

Once you accept the responsibility, it is important to understand that a lot of work may be required to beat infertility.

Infertility treatments require going to lots of appointments, and doing whatever you can to improve your health. This journey takes effort and push.

Accepting the hard work involved will make it easier, and hopefully empower you to do what is available to heal your infertility.

• Prepare To Talk Positively To Yourself Each Day

Starting now, you need to tell yourself every single day that your body can and will get pregnant and give birth.

Say right out loud that your body is healing from infertility, that it is only a temporary condition, and that you are capable, able and strong enough to have a baby.

Repeat over and over again that your body is ready, willing and able to receive and nurture a new life.

It is key that right from the start of this journey, you understand the importance of your self-talk. At this time, you must be your own best friend, your personal cheerleader, your own fertility coach, as you consciously choose to speak words of hope, health and healing to your body.

What you speak aloud and what you speak internally must be positive. No dire pronouncements. No words like, "I'll never get pregnant" or "this won't work out."

You must commit right now that you will speak to your body in a way that
encourages healing, confidence, success, and growth.

All the self-hating, blaming words must end now.

Stop the negative self-talk that the body listens to, and ultimately obeys, on an unconscious level.

Start talking to yourself and your body, both silently and aloud, about the success and healing you are soon going to experience. You need to tell your body that yes, you are going to have a baby. Yes, you are going to be a parent. Your self-talk needs to be affirm a good and beautiful outcome for your efforts.

Let your body know you love it and you have faith it will find a way to conceive, carry and give birth to a beautiful baby.

Let your ovaries, vagina, kidneys, adrenal glands and liver know that you love them and you believe in their power. Hug yourself, soothe yourself. Stop the voices in your head that call you weak, powerless, sickly, infertile.

Never ever say "this won't work."

When you are feeling down and you can sense that your internal whisperings are going to be negative, stop and envision how lovingly you would talk to a friend in this situation.

Just as you need to talk kindly to yourself, be aware of the words you use when speaking to others about your infertility. Even if you feel discouraged, NEVER EVER say out loud, "I doubt I will get pregnant" or "I don't think this will happen for me."
Repeat: even during difficult times, never let negative words that predict an unhappy outcome for your efforts escape from your lips.

• Prepare To Never, Never, Never Give Up

Get ready to persevere, persist, and try try again. You need to decide right now that you will jump over every hurdle, cross every river, take every risk, to reach your goal of becoming a parent.

From the start, you need to decide that giving up is not an option-- unless you come to a point that you've found peace with not having biological children and have found another alternative that feels like the right path to take.

Persevering means that you will stay with this until you reach your desired outcome.

A note here: If you decide to change your goal, from perhaps giving birth to a biological child to adopting a child, that is not giving up, but making a different, but wonderful, life choice.

Or if you decide having children is not a priority, that is fine too. Persevering is worth it if you desire the goal and quitting feels like the worst option.

• Prepare To Get Up Fast When You Are Knocked Down By the Word No

You are going to hear the word no sometimes. That is a reality infertility patients need to understand from the very beginning of this journey. Get ready for them and accept it.

If you know the punch is coming, it will still hurt, but maybe not as much as it would if it came unexpectedly and surprised you.

If at times you hear the word, 'no' such as 'no, you are not pregnant' consider the no's nothing more than a missed shot that is a part of this game—a ball that didn't make the hoop this time around and prepare to shoot again.

Prepare to hear many no's on the way to yes. You prepare, not because you are pessimistic or dismal, but so if a 'no' does come your way, it will not knock you down and break your heart so badly that you refuse to try again.

A 'no' should not surprise you, or trip you up, to the point that getting back up to try again feels impossible.

Disappointment and failure is an inherent part of this process. If you expect that disappointment is part of this game, you won't be shocked when something doesn't work out or the nurse calls with a no.

You just have to realize that the disappointments don't mean you are not going to someday arrive at your destination. It does mean, however, that you will need stamina and perseverance to stay in the infertility game.

But remember: one win in this game means a lifetime World Series status. In this tournament, you don't need ten wins to be a big winner-- you need only one.

You absolutely can't let a temporary loss that comes in the form of a "no" make you so sad that you stop trying.

There will be disappointments during your infertility journey that can make you so sad that they will threaten your ability to get up and try again. The grief and disappointment that can occur during infertility treatments is a threat to a women's ability to plow through the hard times. A person can feel so defeated by a cycle gone wrong that they choose to stop the game altogether and give up the fight. Prepare internally for those hard times, so if and when they do come, you are not knocked out of the game and can re-enter strong and ready to do whatever it takes to improve your chances of giving birth.

While you have every right to want to lock yourself in the house because your neighbor is suddenly pregnant with her fifth child and she chose you to complain to, you do not have the luxury of licking your wounds for too long. You need to be ready to get over it quickly and move on to the next cycle, the next medication, the next clinic, the next acupuncture appointment, the next whatever that is going to move you closer to giving birth to your baby.

You may be one of the lucky ones, and with a bit of medical intervention, wham, you're pregnant. It happens to some women this way. You could very well be one of them. I wish this for you--you certainly deserve it. But if not, it doesn't mean you are not going to get pregnant and have the babies of your dreams. It simply means that you must prepare not to get defeated by the nos.

When you try everything one month, and the nurse calls to say, "no, I'm-sorry- you are not pregnant" you have every right to despair, but then if you want to win and see your dream come true, you must muster your strength, schedule your appointments for the next cycle and try again.

When some cynical doctor tells you he or she doesn't think you can ever get pregnant, you ignore him or her, and get a new doctor who is willing to try a new medication or a new procedure and you try again. You don't get stuck on the negative words of anyone, even authority figures you may have great respect for.

You might hear lots of discouraging talk, read lots of bad statistics, hear lots of no's. You may have despairing moments--it is all part of this process. It is the person who perseveres through these rough times--who keeps making good choices and keeps trying new avenues--who has the best chance of reaching their goal despite the hurdles in the way.

I have a dear friend who underwent four IVFS before she got pregnant and gave birth to her beautiful son. One look at this boy, and you know he was worth it. Just keep in mind, however, what she went through: four IVFS, a few miscarriages, one ovary that wasn't working, and lots of people who said things like, "you did three IVFS. They didn't work. You only have one working ovary. Don't you think it is time to give up."

To continue, you have to accept as part of the process the defeats. The no's cannot be allowed to hold you hostage or push you permanently down into a hole of despair—even when it is your right to feel despair.

Remember: one no, 10 no's, 20 no's, do not have to mean defeat.

It only takes one yes in this game, amidst all the nos, to get you what you most want.

You, my strong mother warrior, are a fighter in the ring--you can take some brutal punches and even flat-out knock downs, and still come out a winner.

Remember: your chances of winning increase when you refuse to stay down no matter how devastating the punch.

The more you try, the higher the odds are in your favor. Wallowing too long can leave you stuck, and you could miss key chances to get pregnant. So cry. Scream. Wail. Just don't stay down long. Get up. Try again. Move on. Prepare for the no's so when they happen, you'll be ready.

• Prepare to Put Certain Parts of Your Life on Hold

Infertility requires a certain amount of sacrifice. Certain aspects of your life will have to put on hold. Getting pregnant and healing from infertility requires that you make this a priority in your life. It may mean that some of your goals will have to be put on hold, routines will have to be changed, so that all your resources and focus can be on having a baby. You may have to use extra money for treatments that you normally would have used for other things. You might have to put certain house renovations on hold.

You might not be able to commit to as many social functions. You might have to scale back on your work, or use all your vacation time or sick time on infertility treatments. You may need to set aside time at night to prepare healthy foods, instead of watching TV. You might have to be at the clinic early in the morning for blood work, maybe a lot earlier than you used to being out. Sometimes, you may have to change your entire work schedule.

Getting your body ready for conception may mean giving up things and putting in place other things. It may mean a change in lifestyle, a change in eating habits, a change in routine, a change in how you spend your money, a change in where you spend your time, where you vacation, and how you live your life on many levels. These sacrifices will eventually not seem so bad, but preparing for them right from the start will be helpful, so you are not surprised or thrown off course when they happen.

Sacrifice requires keeping your eye on the outcome rather than on the deprivation of the moment.

Sacrifice requires being flexible, and understanding that eventually, you can get back to your normal life and routines, but not right now--right now, your goal of getting pregnant has to take precedence.

Healing from your infertility needs to be a high priority in your life. You can't do infertility treatments and expect to do 1,000 other things at the same time.

When I realized I was in need of some serious healing, any extra money I had went to alternative holistic treatments that complimented my regular healing. I committed to acupuncture weekly. It costs me $40 a treatment. To many of you, that may not seem like a lot of money, but it was enough to mean I couldn't enjoy some small pleasures I once enjoyed, especially when I went a few times a week.

 I don't know what sacrifices you will have to make, what money you'll have to spend, what time you will need to put aside.

For me, infertility treatments meant no new clothes, no wild romps of eating anything I wanted. All extra money went to alternative holistic health treatments. Things like new items for the house became distant memories from the past.

We even had a friend live in our basement who paid $400 a month in rent--most of that extra money went towards alternative health treatments to aid in my body's healing.

Expect that, for awhile, certain parts of your life will be put on hold, so that you can give 100 percent of your energy, time and resources to getting pregnant.

• Prepare to Say Goodbye to Guilt, Shame and Self-Blame

Infertility is not a weakness, a curse, or a sin. Infertility is not something you should feel guilty about.

It is not your fault and it certainly doesn't mean you are not meant to be a mother.

Infertility is a temporary physical condition that can be treated and healed. Millions of women once diagnosed with infertility went on to heal and give birth to their babies.

Should a person with a bad cold feel guilty because their nose is running? Doesn't a person with a cold take Vitamin C and rest, knowing that with some orange juice and chicken soup, their nose will eventually stop running and they will return to living without a cold?

Is a person with cancer somehow to blame for the cancer? No, the body sometimes gets on the wrong track, and whether it is a runny nose, an arthritic knee, cancer or acne, we should never blame ourselves for the times when the body goes awry. We are not physically perfect, nor should we expect ourselves to be.

What we are, and what we can expect from ourselves, is the capacity to heal and renew from temporary physical conditions.

Instead of guilt and shame, we need to forgive our body, love our body, be kind and good to our body, and work slowly and lovingly towards healing our body. Illness is in no way a reason to engage in self-hatred.

The body cannot be beaten and shamed back into health. It can, however, be loved and soothed back to a healthy state.

Wipe away right now any archaic ideas that you are evil, flawed, or cursed because you are having trouble getting pregnant.

You are not a bad person because you have a physical problem with conception.

You are in simply a temporary state of infertility that can be healed.

Infertility is a malfunction of the body, just like any illness, and it is no reason to beat yourself up.

Does infertility make you less of a woman? No, no and no. No self-hate allowed. No needless shame or guilt is warranted. You need now to love yourself as much as possible.

What is there to be ashamed of? What is there to feel guilty about?

Infertility is not a statement about your character, your worth, your power as a woman, your ability to mother, your maternal calling, your right to be a mother, your childhood, your family history, your ability to mother, or anything else.

Infertility is the result of the body straying down an unhealthy track—a track, however, that you can lovingly lead your body away from so that you can ultimately get back on a healthy, vibrant, blooming and yes, fertile track.

Say a goodbye to emotions like guilt and self-hatred because there is no validity to them.

• Prepare to Hear Some Negative Comments About Infertility Even from the People You Love

Realize and accept right from the start that sometimes you will hear negative comments about your infertility, even from close friends and family.

Not everyone you love will support or understand what you are going through. Some of your dearest and closest friends and relatives may not understand or approve of your pursuing infertility treatments. Others may think it odd that you are having trouble getting pregnant, attributing the problem to something that is "all in your mind." Some may wonder why you want children so badly, labeling you as 'obsessive' or even 'imbalanced.'

Some people may feel it is morally wrong to get medical help to have a baby. Some may not be able to understand at all why you are having trouble getting pregnant. They may blame you and say you are too uptight, anxious or nervous.

Other people might feel uncomfortable seeing someone ardently pursuing something that isn't coming naturally. These are the type of people who may desperately want pancakes for breakfast, but if life serves them up scrambled eggs, they will say thank you, eat them, and never dare to ask for pancakes again. Some people take what they are given, and don't rock the boat by going after what doesn't come naturally or easily.

By pursuing infertility treatments, you are rocking the boat and saying that you are not willing to accept what life has served you.

You want a baby, and if it doesn't come naturally, well, then you will do whatever modern medicine has at its disposal to make this baby come alive.

That freaks some people out--and you need to prepare and know that, so you can get ready for some criticism and disapproval. You need to carefully select whom you will tell about your infertility treatments, and who you share information with.

There are some people who already have children, and maybe all they dream about is a quiet weekend away without the hard work of caring for kids. So to them, they really don't get what your intense longing is all about. They've sadly lost sight of the immense beauty and gift children are, and because they have lost sight, they can't imagine what the big deal is and why you seem so determined to have a baby. They may even try to convince you to let this go and stay childless. Beware of these cynics, who may simply be just exhausted parents in disguise or parents who have lost the ability to see the joy in raising kids.

Others may not see you as "the mother type" because they can't imagine you in a role they haven't seen you in yet. Ignore them. They obviously don't know who you really are and what you are capable of.

If they can't see your maternal abilities, that is their lack of understanding. These are the same people who will someday go on and on about what a great mother you are.

There are a host of other discouraging, negative comments people may send your way. To some older friends and relatives, the whole "science-making-a-baby-thing" can seem weird, odd, freakish and scary.

Don't let all these negative comments in.

Screen carefully who you let be part of this process. Only let in friends and family who are positive, and who can ultimately see a good result for you. People who say things like, "Maybe God doesn't want you to have a baby" need to be shut out during this time. Since when did they get the right to speak for God? Don't talk to negative people about your dream of having a child.

Try not to be angry at these type of comments--forgive those you love, but don't let your infertility become a topic of conversation with them.

If you are prepared for the negative comments, they will not throw you off course so easily or make you limp at the 'surprise attacks.' Instead, you will be cautious and aware of who you talk to about infertility. You'll also understand that nothing they say or feel about this matters. You'll realize that whatever negative shots are thrown your way come from ignorance, fear, misunderstanding or just plain stupidity. Don't let it get to you. Don't let the comments penetrate. Shake them off and keep walking towards your heart's true desire.

• Prepare To Get Organized

Getting organized is an important part of this journey. Purchase a date book or a blackberry where you can keep track of all your appointments.

Keep a notebook, preferably with pockets, where you can jot down any and all information that might help you with your treatments.
Helpful ideas, information from holistic practitioners, doctors and nurses, can all be stored in this notebook.

The more organized you are, the smoother this whole process will go.

What helped me was a daily calendar at-a-glance appointment book where I kept all phone numbers and appointments related to my infertility treatments.

I also had a big green notebook where I kept all information I gathered from books, magazine articles, television specials, on topics related to infertility, such as infertility medications, foods to help heal infertility. Anything I read or heard that might be of help to me all went into that notebook. Having all my information in one place helped me follow-up on things I learned.

Infertility treatments can be a bit like starting a new job: a lot is expected and there is little time to adjust.

You may need to organize what you will eat each day--no more 'I-have-nothing-in-the-house-so-sugar/fast food/low quality food/ will have to due.'

Any vitamins or herbs you will be taking need also to be organized. If you are doing several cleanses in preparation of fertility treatments, you'll need to organize these also.

In addition to keeping track and being on time for all your appointments with the infertility clinic, you'll also need to keep track of any appointments with alternative practitioners, such as chiropractors or acupuncturists.

If you are also planning to add some stress-relieving type of exercises into your daily routine, you'll also need to do some time management and scheduling to make this happen.

You'll also need to organize foods, snacks and containers for these items, so that you always have on hand healthy foods, instead of being forced to eat junk food or fast foods, because you are starving and nothing is available. That might also mean preparing foods at night for the next day, washing fruits or vegetables and putting them in bags, or cooking several healthy meals ahead of time and freezing them.

When I began to seriously understand the role I needed to play in my own healing, I had to schedule time for light swimming, time to prepare healthy foods the night before work and acupuncture appointments.

Being well-organized will also help you when you feel emotionally shaky and unsure of your next step. Knowing what you need to do tomorrow can help keep you on track moving forward towards your goal.

• Prepare to Switch Gears--and Switch Gears Often

Successfully coping with infertility can sometimes mean knowing when it is time to switch gears and try something new.

Switching gears can mean knowing when it is time to change doctors, try a different medication, or incorporate some holistic healing into your treatments.

Infertility treatments require the ability to shift gears and change tracks when the one you are on isn't working. It requires bending, twisting and contorting as the path unfolds. Being prepared to switch gears means being flexible and welcoming change when need is needed. It means trying new ways of healing when they are presented to you. It means not clinging to a certain doctor or a certain medication that isn't working.

This journey is not always Step A to Step B, it is sometimes Step A to Step N to Step Z back to Step C. Get your dancing shoes on and be ready for the trapeze act that will sometimes be required of you.

Don't stay stuck thinking there is only one way to reach your goal--if that path is not working, switch gears and be ready to go down a new path if you need to.

• Prepare To Tap Into Your Power

To endure some of the challenges of infertility, you need to tap into your power.

While you cannot control or determine the outcome of your fertility journey, you do have some measure of power. You have the power to make choices, power to persevere, power to pray to God, power to believe against all odds, power to think positively, power to phone a friend who is positive and encouraging, power to read a book or listen to music that inspires, power to exercise, power to communicate, power to connect to nature, power to eat healthy foods, power to get up the next day, power to walk forward, power to sing, power to dance--power to envision ourselves in a life with the children we most desire.

Get ready to tap into all the power that is yours, that God has given all humans, and that can help you as you strive towards this goal.

You have power over what you eat, what you drink, and what you say out loud and to yourself.

You have the power to endure pain when you have to. You may have to endure shots twice a day for several weeks, and you may have to do this even if you think right now you could never endure shots. I am the biggest chicken on the planet--a person who can tolerate very little pain--and after awhile, the shots seemed like no big deal to me. If I can do it, you can too. Trust me on this one. You are have more power than you realize. You will be amazed at the power within you as you walk through infertility. Get ready to embrace it.

• Prepare For The Hard times By Creating Happiness Zones in Your Life

You need from the very start of your infertility journey to create happiness zones that will give you some comfort and joy when the going gets tough.

A happiness zone is anything that nudges you gently over to a road of happiness, and shields you, even for a few minutes, from feelings of sadness, anxiety, anger and nervousness. A happiness zone can be a place you love to visit, time spent with a person who always leaves you feeling happy, a favorite picture, a game, hobby or a pet.

The more happiness zones you create in your life, the easier the hard times will be to endure. A happiness zone can be a weekly date with a friend, a singing or acting class, a knitting group, a book club, buying yourself flowers every Tuesday, taking yourself to a weekly picnic, or buying a fish tank, a cat or a plant.

Set up routines so you have pleasant experiences to look forward to each week. Is there a beautiful park nearby that you can take a walk at once a week? A place in your yard you can sit 15 minutes a day and enjoy the sunshine?

Have videos, music and books readily available that make you laugh and feel positive. Surround yourself with music that transport you back to happy times in your life.

Ask yourself: what makes me happy? Include these in your life more often! What can you do to make breakfast more enjoyable? Your drive to work? Your lunch hour or break time? Evenings at home? Saturday mornings?

Break it down by the hour if you have to—what would elevate your feelings of joy? It can be anything, from taking out your collection of childhood teddy bears and displaying them in the living room, to doing karaoke once a week with a new group of friends, to reading a chapter of the Bible daily.

Think about what made you happy when you were a child, a teenager and a young adult. Get ready to tap into the most ancient parts of yourself and start including those long-forgotten activities in your life.

In whatever ways you can, add fun and comfort to your home, your routines, and your life. These will lift you up as you walk this road.

• Prepare to Research the Subject of Infertility

Take the time to research and learn about the reasons why you may be having trouble getting pregnant. Visit the library and bookstore.

Google infertility. Phone holistic and alternative practitioners and have a chat. Ask questions. Read blogs on infertility. Exchange ideas with others who have successfully beaten infertility. Investigate what new medications and research is out there. You never know what nugget of information will turn be the one to turn the key to your body's healing.

• Prepare to Banish the 'No-You-Don't-Deserve-That Monster' Who May Lurk In Your Subconscious

Inside many of us, there lives a little no monster who is always telling us 'no'.

The little no-monster wants to punish and deny us.

The little no-monster will say, 'no, you can't have that!' 'no you can't do that!' 'no you don't deserve that!' 'no someone like you will never get that!'

If you are going to harness all your power to make a baby, you need to set the 'no-monster' straight right from the beginning, and let it know 'yes, I can have a baby' 'yes, I deserve a baby' 'yes, I am capable of giving birth.'

Tell the no-monster 'yes I can get pregnant', 'yes my body is strong enough to conceive a child and hold it safely for nine months', 'yes someone like me will have a baby' 'yes, I deserve this to work out.'

The no-monster will remind you of all the times in your life you tried and failed. It will remind you of all the times you really, really wanted something and you failed to get it. It will remind you of all the things you didn't achieve and all the people who hurt you. It will say over and over again that you are not the kind of person who ever gets what you want. It will tell you that you are a failure. It will tell you that woman with your type of personality/childhood/family history/experiences/ can't do this.

You need to tell the no-monster to SHUT UP AND GO AWAY!

You need to squash that voice, argue it away, and put your inner yes master to work.

Because inside you also lives a 'yes master.' The 'yes master' believes in you and knows you can win. This 'yes master' knows very well that you are very capable of having a baby.

Allow this 'yes master' to scream right out loud that yes, you deserve a baby. Yes, you will get what you want. Yes, you can achieve what you set out to achieve. The yes-master will remind you of all those times in your life when you worked hard and achieved your goal.

It will remind you that miracles happen everyday, and people who never imagined they could get pregnant somehow end up having beautiful babies.

It will remind you that although your road may be long and hard, you can still reach your destination. The 'yes master' will encourage you to never give up. It will help you tap into the strong, courageous part of you who is able to step up to the plate and do whatever it takes to win.

Let the 'yes-master' be your friend through this ordeal, and tell the 'no-monster' to shove off.

• Prepare to receive

Becoming pregnant is, in part, an act of receiving. Being open to conceiving a baby is the act of receiving a precious gift—a gift you very much deserve.

So starting now, get yourself in the habit of receiving.
Make receiving something you feel very comfortable with. Buy yourself small gifts every week, so that receiving becomes something you get used to.

Write down all the good things you've received in your life, things you willingly allowed yourself to receive, things that came to you just because you are a human and good things can sometimes flow to us if we allow ourselves to receive it.

Think of all the things you easily and freely receive in your life, such as air, gravity, sunshine, and a womb where your child can grow.

Wrap small presents and give them to yourself as a reminder that you, as a human being on this earth, have a right to receive good things.

Remember: you don't need to be perfect to receive good things.

You can be flawed, imperfect, and still be worthy of receiving good things.

Sometimes you will receive good things just because.

Sometimes you will receive good things because you worked hard for them.

Sit outside and allow yourself to receive the warmth of the sun. Sit under a tree and let yourself receive its cooling shade. Sit by the ocean and let yourself receive the calming sound of the waves.

Each week, take note of all the wonderful things you received that week--from a text that brightened your day, to a hug or kiss, to a good night's sleep, to a glimpse of something unexpected that just made you happy.

Let the emotion and experience of receiving begin to feel natural to you.

• Prepare to Change the Way You Care for your Body

Healing from infertility requires taking care of your body in a new way that you may have never done before. You may need to entirely change the way you eat, cook and experience food in your life. You may have to change your sleep schedule, exercise routines, and how you use food to cope with emotions and during times of fun and celebration.

You may have to pay closer attention to what you put on your skin, and around your body and in your environment, which can then enter your body. You may have to spend a lot more time preparing foods then you did in the past.

The upside is, not only will you be taking steps to heal your infertility, but you most likely will also start feeling healthier in every other way too.

• Prepare As If You Were A Professional Runner Training For A Race

While going through infertility, consider yourself a runner training for a race. Professional runners are aware that there are many obstacles that can come up during a race and they prepare ahead of time for them.

Successful runners develop the trait of resilience, which gives them the power to bounce back from setbacks. They acknowledge the setback, but quickly move past it so they can focus on the goal ahead.

They know the importance of developing mental toughness and strength so they can continue running, regardless of the conditions, distractions, and emotions they experience during a race.

A successful runner develops the ability to keep moving forward towards their goal, even when there are no immediate signs of winning or even being closer to the finish line. They develop an inner voice that says, 'I can do this. I have the resources inside of me to succeed.' They keep running towards their goal, even when the finish line seems impossible to reach. Some runners write positive sayings on their arms or water bottles so they have a motivational thought to carry them through. Some runners keep themselves going by visualizing how it will feel to get to the finish line and win the race.

While going through your infertility treatments, you plan ahead and prepare a strategy to follow even during the rough times. You develop a mental toughness, so you can bounce back from disappointment, whether or not anyone is cheering you on or believes you can win. You follow your plan of action, even when your goal seems elusive or faraway. You keep listening to that positive inner voice that says: 'yes, you can get pregnant' even when the finish line is nowhere in sight.

• Prepare To Be Self-Disciplined

Infertility treatments require a lot of self-discipline.

It takes self-discipline not to delve into a box of donuts when you are stressed.

It takes self-discipline to get to the clinic for blood work and ultrasound at 6 a.m.

It takes self-discipline to go to bed early.

It takes self-discipline to keep going to a myofascial release expert or a chiropractor week after week.

It takes self-discipline to remember to buy some walnuts and pumpkin seeds, put them in snack bags and bring them to work to eat during break, instead of grabbing something fast from the vending machine. It takes self-discipline to walk each morning to relieve stress.

Self-discipline means following through on what you start. Self-discipline means getting to your appointments on time. Self-discipline means continuing with treatments and foods that can heal you—even when they are inconvenient and boring. Being self-disciplined will help you stay consistent. It will help you say no when you want to say yes. Or say yes when you wish you could say no.

• Prepare To Connect To Your Body

Stop hating your curves, dreading your 'time of the month' and disliking the shape and size of your breasts. No, they are NOT too big/too small/too whatever. They are just perfect.

Stop hating the smells that come from your vagina or underarms.

Stop. Just stop.

Its time to start embracing your womanly, feminine body.

This includes your menstrual cycle, your pubic hair, your shapely (or not so shapely) backside.

Start honoring your period. No bad mouthing it, please. It is part of the birth cycle. Stop denying it and suppressing it. Love it and appreciate it.

Your body, in all its amazing womanliness, is trying to do its best for you. Say thank you to it. Give it a big hug. Show some gratitude.

Chapter 4: Emotions That Can Come From Suffering With Infertility

There are very difficult emotions that being an infertility patient will bring up within you.

Yes, you have every right to feel rage, jealousy, anger, resentment, fear and intense sadness. Infertility is hell. Pure and simple.

You have been through a lot.

You have a right to have a baby, and none of this is fair.

Having your life plan delayed can be frustrating and maddening.

It is not fair in any way that you should have to wait so long and suffer so much for something that is your natural birthright.

Being a mother may be something you drept of and wanted since you were a little girl. When it doesn't happen the way you once thought it would happen, you can feel devastated. Completely alone. Cast away on an island you never wanted to. Isolated from the life you imagined you would have.

Then, there are the daily injections, early morning ultrasounds, and month-to-month cycles that don't always work out, that can leave you angry, emotionally exhausted, grief-stricken and jealous.

Sometimes, you don't want to talk about it. You definitely don't want to be lectured about it. And you certainly don't want to hear one more stupid, insensitive person make a comment like 'just relax and it will happen.'

So you stay silent. Friends and family have no idea of the dark pit infertility patients sometimes end up in.

Going to social events can be painful, especially when they center around celebrations involving pregnancy, birth and children.

Here are a few ways to cope with some of the feelings and emotions that accompany infertility treatments:

Anger: Infertility is hell (I said it before and I will say it again) and if you feel angry about the whole thing, you have every right to feel that way. We feel angry when we are frustrated and unable to get what we want.

Anger is an emotion that is often a combination of feeling powerless, afraid and hurt.

Anger sometimes appears in the form of resentment, irritability, rage, animosity, and bitterness.

In Chinese medicine it is believed that anger affects the liver, which is a key organ in infertility. The more you release the toxins in your liver, the less your body will be able to hold onto anger.

There are also alternative/holistic therapies that can help release anger, such as craniosacral/myofascial therapy, acupuncture, and homeopathy. Massage and trauma release can also help release anger. Swimming can be a safe way to release anger. I started swimming when I began infertility treatments, and once found myself sobbing after a very intense swim. I didn't know why I was crying, but I sensed my body was releasing pent-up anger.

Spending time in nature, sitting by the ocean, are also ways to release anger.

When you begin to feel anger, try to do one thing that gives you a feeling of control in your life, such as juicing a green drink, saying a positive affirmation, or going to an acupuncture appointment. Close your eyes and picture the part of you that is angry and ask that part of you: what can I give you right now that will help you feel better?

Let your inner child know you will help her have the baby she so desires. Comfort her. Ask her: what is it you want honey? Then listen closely for the answers.

Remember: anger is a secondary emotion. There is something you feel before you feel angry. Try to identify what emotions you feel before you reach anger.

When you begin to feel angry, say: 'I am powerful. I am powerful and able to get what I want.'

Do something creative that gives your anger a chance leave your body and take another form outside of yourself.

Anger does not have to trap you into a helpless state that leaves your body stressed. Acknowledge it, give yourself something that it needs, and release it when you can.

Jealousy: Jealousy is an emotion everyone feels at one time or another, regardless of our circumstances and situations in life. We all feel jealous when we see someone with something we desperately want, but don't have. It is easy to feel jealous of women who have children. Don't feel guilty about experiencing this emotion. Jealousy often comes from a perceived scarcity in an area of your life. So rather than seeing other people's babies as a slap in the face, begin to see it as a cue that 'if it is possible for them, it is possible for me.'

The next time you see a mother with her children and you feel jealous, say to yourself: if it could happen to her, it could happen to me.

Think of it this way: her success today mirrors the potential for your success tomorrow.

When you hear of a baby shower or find out a friend is pregnant, it means that pregnancy and birth are conditions possible in our world— possible for them and possible for you.

Realize that just because you don't have something today doesn't mean you won't have it tomorrow.

Try, (I know how hard this is) to keep a vision of a tomorrow where you have the babies you deserve.

Repeat: 'There is enough to go around.' 'There is enough for everybody.' 'I too can have what I want.' 'I will have a baby too.'

When you see a baby, repeat the words: 'babies are born, babies are here, babies are everywhere, and my baby is coming too.' Or: 'this just proves that babies are always coming and my baby is coming too.'

Feeling robbed and jealous are not emotions that just disappear overnight. Nor should you feel guilty when you experience them. Just keep reminding yourself that every baby you see is a reminder that babies are born everyday—and one of these days it could very well be your baby that is born! Keep a note on your refrigerator that says: "There is enough for everybody! There is enough for me! Lots of women have babies and I will have one too!"

Frustration: Frustration is a common emotion for those coping with infertility. It is frustrating to want something very badly and not be able to get it.

Frustration is an emotion linked to feeling helpless and powerless, a combination of feeling disappointed and angry. So taking some type of action, such as doing something new to heal your body, can be a remedy for this emotion. When you take action, you are reminding yourself that you are not powerless.

Remind yourself each day that you are not helpless, you are not powerless, and that your body is capable and able to heal if given the right tools.

For me, prayer gave me a feeling of power and trust in God that I needed when my own efforts felt blocked or thwarted.

When I was frustrated, I would write a list of what I was going to do the next day to help my body heal from infertility. Making that list gave me a sense of power because—I was doing something to help myself heal from infertility.

I was showing myself that I could find solutions to my problems and that with the right steps, things could work out for me.

Taking action and responsibility is what will help alleviate feelings of frustration.

Fear: Fear is an emotion that sometimes accompanies infertility. You may fear never getting pregnant or you may fear some of the procedures and tests you have to go through.

According to Chinese medicine, excessive or prolonged fear drains the kidneys and suppresses Qi energy in the body. Fear is an emotion that can wreak havoc with your hormones.

Fear is an emotion that is caused by the belief that something is dangerous, likely to cause us pain or is a threat. To cope with fear, name it, face it and acknowledge it. Go within and write down your fears concerning infertility: do you fear not getting what you want? Or getting what you want? Once you name your fear, you then can begin to find ways to calm your nervous system and let it know you are safe.

Remember: never let the fear of striking out keep you from playing the game.

Sadness or Grief: Feeling grief-stricken and extremely sad are normal emotions that infertility patients often experience. Never feel ashamed or weak because of your sadness. You have a right to it. Sometimes, you just have to give yourself permission to feel sad, while at the same time, do whatever you can to keep the endorphins or "happy chemicals" in your body moving.

Chapter 5: Coping With The Ups and Downs of Infertility Treatments

How do you not go crazy when you run into an old friend who has three beautiful kids and just announced she is happily pregnant with her fourth?

How do you keep going, when the shots, the appointments, the painful tests, seem never ending?

How do you persevere when the nurse calls again with another, 'no, I'm sorry' message.

Sometimes, not being able to get pregnant is nothing short of torture, anguish, a raw clawing frustration, because what is natural is not coming naturally.

There were times during my infertility treatments when I was hysterical, depressed, unable to be consoled.

This is no easy time and no easy task.

There will be times when you will rightly feel very angry, frustrated and even downright hopeless. My guess is that you are a lot stronger than you think you are, but feelings are feelings and sometimes they are just there and can't be ignored.

Here's what five years of infertility treatments taught me about coping with the ups and downs that accompany this difficult and trying process.

• Accept the Fact That Infertility Is Sometimes Going To Be Heartbreaking

Yes, enduring infertility is hard. Very very hard. Wicked hard (if I dare flashback to my 1980s youth) Once you accept that is hard, you can go from there. This is not an easy road, but you are inherently strong enough and capable enough to handle the difficulty.

Once you accept the difficulty of this process, you won't be surprised at the work and perseverance sometimes needed to get through this.

Accepting that it will be hard means you will accept the work, and have the patience and perseverance to get through it.

And, most importantly, you won't be shocked when you hit some very hard bumps in the road.

• Accept That Some Days You Are Just Going To Fall Apart

There are going to be days when it all gets too much. The unfairness of what you are going through, the longing for a child that continues to be unfulfilled, the raw pain of seeing a world filled with pregnant women and babies, and you somehow denied that joy, will all get too much. When that happens, you might collapse into bed, cry uncontrollably, rage at your husband, flip out at the next friend who tells you to just relax. You won't always behave appropriately, you might do unproductive things. Sometimes you might just feel like the pain of it all is going to kill you.

Knowing ahead of time that this might happen won't relieve you of the pain, but it might help you remember that thousands of women who experienced infertility also have had bad days like this—and thousands of them now have children. Eventually, many of them got pregnant and gave birth, despite heartbreaking disappointments.

That lady you walked by in the supermarket with the adorable kids who made your heart ache? She very well could have been an infertility patient once upon a time.

Know this: you may be crying hysterically today because you are not pregnant, and a year or two from now, you might be spending your day taking care of your sweet baby.

• In Your Darkest Moments, Remember What Choices Are Still Available to You

During the moments when you feel you can't take anymore, ask yourself this question: what is one thing I can do today that will move me one step closer to my goal?

You got a call and the news was bad: no, you are not pregnant. In that moment of complete disappointment, stop and ask yourself: what is one positive action I can do right now to help me get one step closer to having a baby? Before you fall apart, before you start crying, ask yourself this one question and immediately take a step towards this positive action.

• Never Forget the Link Between the Choices You Make and the Consequences That Follow

It is easy to feel helpless during infertility treatments. It is easy to feel like you have no control over the outcome, and to some degree, that is true. However, you do have choices that are under your control.

Everyday, you can make choices that can either empower your body or debilitate your body. While you cannot guarantee the outcome of your infertility journey, you can improve your chances by making good choices. You can choose to consume less sugar and caffeine, and as a result, your health could slightly improve. Choose to walk 15 minutes a day, and you may lose weight, which in turns helps balance your hormones.

• Take Control Of What You Can Control

To cope with all the things that happen during infertility that are out of your control, learn to take control of what you can control. You have control over what enters your mouth and what you put on our skin. You have control over what type of water you drink, what types of cleaning chemicals you use in your home and yard, and what types of holistic healing you bring into your life. During your moments of despair, grab hold of what is still under your control and do the best, most positive, healing action available to you. What you can control, control well.

• Just Say No To Denial

To beat infertility, you have to face head on the problems you are experiencing. During treatments, don't allow yourself to go into denial if that will inhibit your ability to make choices that will help heal your body. Do you have the right doctor—one who is proactive, open to suggestions and ready to try different medications? Or are you ignoring that nagging feeling that your doctor is not on the right track with your treatments? Have you been on the same medication for a long time and it is not working? Come on, be truthful, look straight at it, no more hiding the truth from yourself. Is there a condition your body is suffering from that you are not paying attention to, such as exhausted adrenal glands, a parasitic infestation, a lack of sunlight or sleep, or chemicals in your system that need to be released? Face it, name it, look straight at it, and then work to fix it. Denial is not your friend in beating infertility.

• Make it Easy To Hope By Physically Showing Your Complete Belief That You Will Someday Have a Baby

It is important that you physically showcase and manifest in some way your complete and utter belief that you will have a baby.

One summer, I was recovering from a very painful laparoscopy and feeling incredibly broken over not being pregnant.

While out shopping, my best friend Leah suggested I buy a photo album titled: "Summer Memories with Baby" that we saw.

Leah said, "Next summer, you'll be putting pictures of your baby in it."

I wasn't feeling at all hopeful, but I listened to Leah and bought the album. From the very first night that it sat on my nightstand, it gave me hope that yes, somehow, pictures of my baby would actually fill this album someday.

Buying it was an act of courage and faith.

Leah turned out to be right: the next summer, I had pictures of my new baby to put in the album. When I was feeling defeated, Leah pointed me towards a way to give myself what I needed: a physical, tangible symbol that my dream of having a baby would come true.

To this day, this album sits on my nightstand, a physical symbol of hope at a time when hope was very hard for me to feel.

Put some physical manifestations of hope around you, i.e. a stuffed animal you will give your child, a photo album that says baby's first year, a toy.

By doing this, you will be moving past your present reality into a new reality--a reality where you absolutely know and believe that your baby is on the way to you. Thank you Leah.

I hung a poster in my kitchen entitled "Relax...God is in Charge." Reading this poster always gave me a sweet, calming sense of peace. If there are sayings that give you feelings of hope, joy and peace, put them in places where you can read them daily and let your body experience the positive force of these words. Put symbols, pictures, quotes in your everyday life that make it easy for your mind to float over to the realm of hope.

• Listen To Your Body

Ssh, listen. What is your body trying to tell you? During infertility treatments, it is important that you start listening for the subtle and sometimes not-so-subtle messages your body is trying to send you.

Listen to that inner voice that knows what your body needs to heal. Don't shut this voice up--it may be of great help to you.

If suddenly you get the urge that your body needs a certain food or treatment, honor that inclination. You know more than you consciously realize about what your body needs to get pregnant.
Keep a journal where you ask your body questions like: why are you having trouble getting pregnant? What can I do to help you get pregnant? and let your deep subconscious speak and reveal what it needs.

• Keep Reminders in Your Home of the Times When Seemingly Impossible Dreams Came True and You Got What You Really Wanted

Hang diplomas and awards from school. Frame letters and cards from family and friends. Call it: My Wall of Happy Ever After or The Wall That Proves Dreams Come True.

Display achievements in your life that resulted from a lot of hard work, along good things that came for no reason at all. Display photos of a wonderful vacation, a picture of the first house or car you ever bought, a gift from a friend, your wedding photos, a love letter, a seashell--anything that reminds you of times in your life when dreams you worried were not attainable came true. Look at these reminders often. Write the story of how you met your true love, found your lovable dog, or got to experience something you never thought you were going to be able to experience.

• Memo To You: You Are Not A Victim

While you are being treated for infertility, remind yourself that you are not a victim.

A victim has no choices. A victim cannot change their situation. A victim is forever stuck with the same problem. A victim has to rely on someone to save them. A victim is passive. A victim is without hope.

You, on the other hand, can do things to change your situation.

You can...

--Ask your doctor questions, change doctors if your doctor is not aggressive enough or fails to listen to you or doesn't try every possible procedure and every possible medication to get you pregnant.

--Try a new medicine or research medicines and ask to be put on a different medicine than one you are on that is not working.

--Request every test available.

--Eliminate white flour products and trans fats from your diet.

--Eat lots of romaine lettuce, spinach, chicory, and other good-for-you green vegetables.

--Go to your primary care doctor or allergist and request tests to determine if you have any food allergies that are weakening your body. Armed with this information, you can stop all foods that are not promoting your body's optimum health.

--Do a parasite cleanse and get unwanted parasites out of your system.

--Do a yeast cleanse and balance the flora in your system.

--Do a liver cleanse and rid your liver of toxins.

--Have your thyroid checked.

--Get several colon cleanses that will release toxins and help improve your elimination

--Start walking, singing, deep breathing, gardening and drawing, to release stress.

--Find an acupuncturist who understands infertility and begin weekly, twice or three times weekly treatments to strengthen your chi, or life energy.

--Keep a journal and express and release negative feelings.

--Pray. Then pray again. Then pray some more.

--Talk to people who are positive, supportive and believe in your ability to have a baby.

--Listen to healing music or music with positive messages.

--Paint the walls in your home beautiful colors that make you happy.

--Stop watching TV programs that are frightening or upsetting and instead start watching shows that make you laugh.

--Avoid situations that drain your energy.

--Visualize the day your baby is born.

-- Speak about your journey to having a baby with confidence, optimism, and total belief.

--Get rid of the doctor who doesn't act fast enough, aggressive enough, or just keeps telling you to relax.

--Find a doctor who answers all your questions, listens to your ideas and suggestions and who is aggressive in their treatment.

--Choose an infertility clinic with a fantastic success record.

--Go to a top notch chiropractor and get your spine aligned, and wear good walking shoes that doesn't throw your spine and hips out of alignment.

-- Find a myofascial release specialist who specializes in trauma release to help you let go of emotional blocks or trauma in your body.

- **Remind Yourself That Your Infertility is Temporary**

When you are having a bad week, remind yourself that infertility is not a permanent condition. Remind yourself that infertility is a temporary condition. Temporary, temporary, temporary. Put that word right in your head: temporary. Infertility is temporary. Temporary.

From day one, start looking at infertility as a temporary condition. Infertility is not and should not be considered a permanent condition. Start seeing your body as capable of healing from infertility. Stop viewing this as a permanent condition that your body can't escape from.

If you were suffering with a toothache, would you imagine yourself permanently having this toothache or would you think: 'I have a toothache, I'm going to go to the dentist and be treated for it, and it will be gone'.

See your body in a state of positive change heading towards conception and pregnancy—with infertility as only a temporary stage you are passing through.

Even if you are officially diagnosed with 'unexplained infertility', it is only a temporary label explaining what your body is experiencing at this moment.

It is not a lifetime sentence.

The human body changes minute to minute, based on factors like, what we eat, what forms of healing we allow ourselves to experience, the environment we put ourselves in and elements we use to connect physically and emotionally to our healthiest self.

Our body is always in the midst of change and always capable of change. A woman weighing 200 pounds is labeled "grossly obese' by her doctor, but if she begins exercising and eating nutritious food, a year later, that label is no longer applicable because she made different choices that changed the state of her body. Consider your body as the composite of many ingredients that result in a recipe, which is the state of your health. If you change the ingredients, you change the recipe.

Your body has the power to heal and change from an ill and infertile state to a fertile healthy state.

• Keep the 'Happy Chemicals' In Your Brain Flowing

Work hard to make sure the 'happy' chemicals in your brain are working at their maximum capacity. Infertility can be devastating to your emotional self, so try to counteract it by revving up the happy-chemicals your brain. Exercise gently, eat lots of green vegetables, get lots of sleep, reduce your coffee intake and take extra folic acid.

Research has shown that embracing a positive new goal stimulates the release of dopamine, believing in yourself triggers serotonin. Putting yourself around people you trust releases oxytocin. Sniffing vanilla and lavender releases endorphins. Knitting or sewing can give you feelings similar to meditation. To enhance your positive experiences, write them down.

• Remind Yourself Of What Helped You Cope with Challenging Times in the Past

What kept you emotionally strong and able to cope during hard times in your past? What helped pull you back from despair?

When you were sad, where did you seek comfort and find relief?

How did you keep yourself motivated and forward-moving during the rough patches in your life?

Spend some time recalling how you dealt with challenging situations in the past, and be prepared to tap back into these sources of strength.

For me, what helped me to cope was my reliance on God. God has always My faith reminded me that God can help us conquer even the most impossible situations. I often reminded myself that God could give me strength to do anything, even when in my own human strength, it did not feel possible. I often thought to myself: if God could open the Red Sea, or shut the mouths of lions, or save three young boys from a fiery furnace, then this is very possible for me. Now ask yourself: what helped me cope in the past that I can tap back into when I need it?

• When You Are Going Through A Rough Patch in Infertility Treatments, Turn It Into A Happy-Ever-After Story

When you are going through a particularly rough time, write a story about the challenges you are facing, but write into your story a happy ending with you giving birth to a child. Project yourself into a future where you finally get pregnant and have the baby you dream of. When you endure a cycle that is grueling, sit down and write about it—just make sure to add the happiest outcome you can imagine. Don't worry if the story is well-written, grammatically correct, or even makes sense— as long as you write a happy ending to it.

• Switch It Up

Switch it up: you are not a woman without a baby—you are a woman preparing to be a mother. If anyone asks if you are pregnant, don't say no, instead tell them you are are 'prematernal.'

You are not a infertility patient—you are a mother preparing her body to incubate her baby who is coming soon.

You are not a woman who didn't get pregnant this month—you are a woman whose child is going to be born 10, 11, 12 months from now.

Instead of calling yourself 'infertile' call yourself pre-pregnant.

• Believe and Act With Complete Confidence In A Positive Future

Write letters to your future child, start planning a Disney vacation for five years in the future. Act as if the arrival of your child is inevitable.

• Adopt a 'Next, Next, Next' Attitude

I once had a wise friend tell me that in to succeed, you can't let yourself get stuck when you have a goal. When things go wrong, instead of wasting time wallowing think: next, next, next. When things are difficult, take the next action, make the next choice, do the next right thing.

If your doctor tells you there is no hope, get another doctor. Next.

If the medication you have been taking doesn't seem to be working, ask to try another medication. Next.

The nurse called and told you your cycle didn't work out. You reschedule for your next cycle. Next.

If what you are doing doesn't seem to be working, start doing some research and try something new. Next.

Don't get stuck no matter what. Take a next-next-next approach and keep going.

• Develop a Strategy

Military commanders do not enter a war without a clear strategy. When you are fighting something, you need a strategy to beat your opponent and win. That means understanding who your enemy is and what is needed to defeat it.

It means knowing your strengths and weaknesses, what obstacles might come in your way, and how you will overcome these obstacles.

During my infertility, I spent a lot of time researching how the body works, and what can set the body on a wrong track. I began to understand the "enemies" of my fertility, or the places where my body was weak and needed help.

You need a strategy for how you will eat, how you will give your body the amount of sleep, water and sunshine it needs, how you will release your stress and trauma, and how you will maximize the strength and health of every organ in your body.

Having a strategy with a clear path and a series of steps can help keep you on the right track, even during the rough times.

• Every Night, Ask Yourself: What Is One thing I Can Do Tomorrow to Improve My Chances of Having a Baby?

Make a list each night before bed of what you can do the next day to move you one step closer to getting pregnant. Note what you have to prepare that night so you can accomplish your goals the next day. When you wake up, look at your list from the night before and get to work. Use this list as a guide for how you are going to stay on track that day. For example, can you have green tea on hand for the drive into work, instead of the big coffee you used to start your day with?

• Don't Give Any Medical Professional Too Much Power When it Comes To Your Treatment

Always get a second opinion. Remind yourself that doctors are not always right. Just because one doctor is discouraging or sees no hope for you doesn't mean you have to take their diagnosis as a final statement on your fertility. Just because one medical professional sees your situation a certain way doesn't mean it is the only truth or your condition. Get a second, third, or a fourth opinion.

Once, I had a very well-respected doctor, named as the best infertility doctor in New England, tell me that my eggs were "bottom of the barrel" and it was unlikely I would ever get pregnant again, and that I should consider using an egg donor if I wanted a second child.

For a few minutes, her words totally knocked me down and out. I felt broken, shrunken, put in my place, defeated. I wanted a child with my own eggs, thank you! Not that it isn't a great option for many, but for me at that time, it wasn't something I was comfortable with or willing to do. On the way home from that hope-shrinking, earth-shattering encounter, I stopped at a natural food market and started looking through books. I guess without knowing it, I was searching for some glimmer of hope.

I found a second wind in a book written by Christine Northrup. In it, she wrote about how in other cultures, women in their 40s become pregnant without a lot of problems, and that some of the infertility problems in our culture could be because of our cultural attitudes toward aging. This information gave me some of hope I needed at that moment.

When I got home, I was still feeling really shaken up, so I phoned my mother. Thank God for my mother, who immediately told me to get rid of that doctor and get another one! My mother was absolutely right. During my meeting with this doctor, she had refused to answer any of my questions from a list I sent her weeks before our meeting, refused to consider trying another medication, (which my next doctor did try and it worked) and seemed more concerned with not being bothered with too many questions, than really helping me get pregnant.

The doctor I chose next was a wonderful man, who listened to me, took the time to answer all 21 of my questions, and agreed with me that it was time to try a more aggressive medication. He even had selected the same medication I had requested my other doctor try with me. I wonder now: why didn't that other doctor want to try me on a new medication? Why did she refuse to even consider it?

Was she afraid that if I didn't get pregnant, her success rate would drop, and her ranking as the best infertility doctor in the area would be threatened? Did she advocate egg donation because she thought it would up my chances of becoming pregnant—and, in turn, make her statistics look better? Was there some financial or professional benefit to her if I went with her suggestion, rather than to continue trying with my own eggs? Was I simply a pain-in-the-butt patient she wanted to get rid of because I was too intense, showed too much emotion, worked her nurses too hard, and asked too many questions?

Whatever her motive, she almost stopped my son from being born. If I was willing to keep trying, why did she want to persuade me not to try? Was she really thinking of my best interests? Nope. And that is why you can never take one doctor's pronouncement as some type of irrefutable gospel. Please, don't get sucked in just because some magazine names a doctor as one of the best in the region—they may be doing things to falsely up their statistics or hiring a publicist to market and promote themselves to the media behind the scenes. Or maybe they simply bought an ad in the magazine to garner this rank.

Please don't be deceived because your doctor is loved by everyone you know—if they are giving up on you and you do not want to give up—go find a doctor willing to fight for you and your future child. My doctor was extremely popular, which shows that you have to judge a doctor on what they are doing for you, not for everyone else.

The next doctor I had, who worked in the very same clinic, was completely different--proving that there are doctors who respect their patients and who are willing to go the extra mile.

I wonder now what would have happened if my mother hadn't given me such good advice to get rid of this doctor? What if I had been a more compliant personality and I believed the good doctor, deeming her to be an expert that "knows better"? Well, today I would not have my son.

My gorgeous beautiful son from my own bottom-of-the-barrel eggs.

Someday, I'm going to send this doctor a picture of my beautiful son, and in blazing letters across the picture I am going to write: "THIS IS WHAT BOTTOM OF THE BARREL LOOKS LIKE."

So don't listen. Shut those bad guys up. Dump them. Move on to someone who believes in you.

If a doctor tells you to give up hope, thank them kindly and find a new doctor who is willing to investigate your particular condition and get to the root of the problem. Ultimately, you have to be your own advocate. There is no one in this world who is going to fight for your child to come alive like you can.

Make God your partner in this fight--not any one doctor or medical professional. This doctor seemed so nice when I first met her, but ultimately she could have stolen my son's right to life away.

• **Understand That In Many Ways, This Journey Is One You Are Sometimes Going To Take Alone**

Infertility can sometimes be a very lonely experience. Family and friends who love you dearly may not always be able to understand the depth of your pain.

Even your husband may not always understand your drive to have a baby. He might not always have the patience infertility demands. He will not always say and do the right thing.

While my husband wanted children as badly as I did, he sometimes lost patience with me and the whole process. Sometimes he thought I was too obsessive. Many times, I trudged on alone, because he was too tired and too angry to really be beside me through the ordeal. Other times, he was my knight in shining armor. We got along a lot better when I realized there were times I had to rely on myself and God, and not anyone else.

• Find Places Where You Can Safely Pour Out Your Grief

Infertility can bring up a lot of grief, especially when things don't go right or are taking longer than you wish. You need places and people where you can pour out your grief in a safe, non-destructive way--not in a way that paralyzes or cripples you.

Do you have a friend who can listen to your intense grief and not lecture, criticize or try to get you to give up?

Do you have a family member who is kind and can listen to your most intense feelings of anger, jealousy and grief, and not make you feel silly for your emotions?

It is important that when you need it, you have a friend, a family member, or a group where you can voice your feelings without feeling judged.

This is not the time to confide in people who are downers on the subject of fertility, or somehow think it is okay to pop your balloon of hope. Surround yourself with people who believe in your body's ability to heal and who can see a positive outcome for your efforts. Whether it is a friend at work who also went through infertility, a blogger, or your Mom, talk, vent, cry, brainstorm with those who are positive and who can give you a sense of 'I'm here for you' at this time.

Stay away from anyone who is negative or will say and do things that will rob you of your optimism or power.

Avoid those who find it hard to empower anyone except themselves. Don't share your sadness with those who might underhandedly steal your ability to see this all working out.

Confide in people who will be positive and upbeat about your getting pregnant.

I was fortunate enough to have a few people like that in my life.

My mother, for one, was my greatest cheerleader and helper. She always told me she knew I could get pregnant and have a baby.

Leah, my dear sweet Leah, who also was my greatest cheerleader (you can have more than one).

Judy, my dear sweet Judy, who one day at work out of the blue looked at me and said, "I can see you with a little girl with cork screw curls." How did she know I would end up having a daughter with beautiful curls?

Or Peter, my dear beloved friend, that I phoned late one night when I was in despair, who declared without hesitation that I would get pregnant.

There were others too, but I will never forget the words of people who believed in a happy ending for me, when I could barely believe myself.

I cherish those friends and family members who said words that gave me hope instead of crushing my dream.

Beware of therapists or counselors who want to beat you down with "realism." At the infertility clinic I went to, there was a counselor who was like sheer poison to patients like me. In my darkest times, she said the most negative words to me and I have no idea why.

When you undergo infertility treatments, you need words of hope.

Your body needs to be told over and over and over again that it is strong enough, healthy enough, and capable of getting pregnant.

If you have a family member or friend who tends to be negative about the whole process, you need to ask them to please stop doing this. Once someone told me they thought God didn't want me to have children. I asked her to never, never say that to me again. Her words were stealing my hope, and I was feeling doubtful enough already. My body couldn't afford to listen to such negative predictions even for a minute.

You need to find people willing to hear your pain, see your tears, hear your screams of anger, and still say, "I think you will have a baby."

Understand that there are people in this world who, due to their own disappointing experiences, don't really believe people can do much to change their bad situations. They see going after a dream as a waste of time. Or maybe they are just jealous and unable to really wish good for anyone but themselves. They slyly discourage you, because they want to be the only one with a happy-ever-after story.

Others don't understand the power of choice, perseverance, and will.

They just don't get that today's no can be tomorrow's yes.

Some people have tried for dreams that never came true. They think they are doing you a favor by dousing you with realism, so you won't get disappointed. They are, of course, completely wrong.

Bottom line: confide only in positive, helpful, hopeful, people who aren't too afraid or too jealous or too sad themselves to see you have a win.

• **Understand the Power That Lies In Your Passionate Desire for Children**

To endure all that is going to be asked of you, you need a mighty big motivator—and wanting a child passionately can be the motivation you need to get through this.

Your intense desire to be a mother will help you override the physical and emotional pain of infertility treatments. Your passionately wanting a child is an asset, not a liability.

When the yearning and longing for a child feels intense and painful, remind yourself that it is this yearning and longing that will help see you through to your goal. Feel the pride in knowing that your desire to love another human is that big, that consuming, that deep, and something you should respect yourself for.

• Be Patient

When you are having trouble coping, remind yourself that getting healthy and restoring your fertility takes patience.

The body doesn't heal overnight.

Once, after six months of weekly acupuncture treatments, I asked my acupuncturist if I was getting healthier. I expected glowing remarks about how all my effort was paying off. Instead, he answered, "A bit. You are still very weak." What? After all I had done? I was pretty discouraged. I thought I was going to hear about all the progress I was making, but despite this not-so-encouraging diagnosis, I kept going to acupuncture weekly.

I had to be patient, whether I liked it or not. In time, I grew to understand that my body was changing and healing with every appointment, even if it was ever-so- slightly, and that continued effort would eventually see my body to a different and better place.

If you are making good choices for your body, keep on making these good choices. Eventually they will pay off, even if it takes all your patience to keep on track for the long haul.

• Take Your Power, Acknowledge Your Power, Harness Your Power, Utilize Your Power

Never for a minute take a fatalistic approach to infertility.

You can't control the outcome of your infertility treatments. Nor are you at fault if this doesn't work out, but you do have some power
in this situation.

Not total power. Not complete power, but you do have some power.

You have the power to pray. You have the power to stop letting foods, chemicals, toxic substances into your body that could weaken you. You have the power to believe in yourself. You have the power to eat well.

You have power over how you use your words, and whether or not you will speak with positive belief or negative dread.

While you are not all powerful in this process, neither are you entirely helpless and powerless either. Whatever measure of power you have, grab hold of it and be aware of it.

• During the Hard Times, Remember To Conjure Up Some Good Old-Fashioned Persistence

Remember the old saying: if at first you don't succeed, try, try again. This basic, bottom line way of thinking might mean the difference between having a baby and never having one.

Let yourself persist. Throw yourself over the bar and persevere, persevere, persevere. Don't see a no this month as a no forever. A no today does not mean a no tomorrow. I have a neighbor who did four IVFs—four! She was almost 45 years old, had only one working ovary and she miscarried a few times.

She had every reason to give up after three IVFS--but she didn't! Something inside her--call it faith, the ability to persevere, the ability to mourn the disappointments and heartbreaks and allow herself another try--and she continued on to number four.

Well, attempt number four turned out to be her winning try and she gave birth to a beautiful, healthy, lovely baby boy.

No one is going to lie and say persevering is easy. After you've had a few hard disappointments, it is hard to continue. But giving up can ultimately be the most disappointing turn of events of all.

Keep trying if you can. Don't listen to people who try to make you quit.

Here's the thing: to persevere in the face of defeat, you need to call upon the strongest parts of yourself. For me, that was my faith in God.

If God didn't give me the privilege of prayer, I would not have been able to endure month after month of 'no, you are not pregnant.'

Along with prayer, I tapped into the willpower inside me. I am passionate and very clear about the vision I have for my life. When I am 80 years old, more than anything in this world, I want my children beside me and I want to have had the experience of raising a family. That vision of my future kept me going.

If I had let the many disappointments I experienced during infertility weaken my vision, I would have never attained my goal of having children, but instead I would have been frozen by the disappointments into a life I didn't want.

Unless you give up in peace, and are moving on to another purpose, you could possibly stay stuck in the yearning.

To get my two children, I underwent a total of 15 IUI cycles, three IVF cycles and four operations. Was it worth it? Yes. Without a doubt. As hard, long, tedious, excruciating, insanity-making and crazy-making as it was, it was worth it.

After I had an operation for what they thought was fibroids, incorrectly diagnosed by that renowed doctor I spoke of earlier who called my eggs bottom of the barrel, I was asked to do the balloon test--a nasty test where they inflate a balloon into your vagina. I hated doing this test and was angry that they requested it after just having undergone a painful operation that was a result of a misdiagnosis.

I did it anyways. Why? Because I had to. Because they wanted me to. Because I knew that to ultimately get what I want I had to conform to the requirements of the clinic. So I persevered.

Keep trying. Go for one more cycle. Don't listen to all the people who tell you to quit, that because it didn't work this month or this year or even for the past few years that obviously it is never going to work.
Ignore the people who say, "Can't you see that maybe you are not meant to…? Haven't you already tried this and that?" Shut them out of your brain.

One more time--and it may be the time your body is ready to be pregnant and deliver a baby. Do one more thing. Call one more person. Try another clinic. Persist, persist, persist. Bang on every door.

Read every book on health available, because one of those books may hold the answer for you. Get another physical and have your body checked completely. Do it again and again if you have to. Don't be afraid to stomp your feet and scream, "I WANT A BABY AND I'M NOT GOING TO STOP UNTIL I HAVE ONE."

However, if you've come to a point where infertility is just too emotionally painful and you cannot hear one more no, consider the alternatives. Adoption is also having a real baby of your own, a beautiful option, and not one that precludes you from continuing to try for a biological child someday.

At one point, I made a pact with myself that if I wasn't pregnant by a certain time, I was going to start the adoption process, while continuing infertility treatments. I knew I was yearning and ready to love a baby, and if I was blessed with an adopted baby, that would be a grand and wonderful privilege.

Not to say I gave up my dream of a biological child, but I realized that emotionally I needed to give myself options if I was going to mentally be able to continue infertility treatments. I realized, from watching friends who had the privilege of adopting children, that a child is a child is a child, and a child's laughter is a child's laughter, and reading to a child before bed at night is reading to a child before bed at night, and making someone else's life happier and better is a grand purpose and mission, regardless of whether or not that child shares your DNA.

But if adoption is not something you feel ready to consider, don't give up trying to give birth to a baby. You might be inches away from your dream and not even know it.

Sometimes it is that one-more-try that can bring results.

For example, before I got pregnant with my son, I was on the verge of giving up. I had suffered a lot of disappointments and cycles that didn't work out. I had an operation for what they thought was fibroids. Then, I tried a second IVF, which didn't work out. At that point, my doctor told me to pretty much give up. But it was that one more try where I finally found success.

• Make The Process Of Infertility Treatments As Pleasurable As Possible

When I first learned that I would have to take shots every night to prepare for an IVF, I didn't think I was going to be able to handle it. But then I stumbled onto something that made the whole process easier and lighter: I had recently got a beautiful book of recipes from bed and breakfast inns. It was a sweet, pretty, cozy book, with recipes for things like blueberry muffins, apple butter and raspberry jam. I found that if I read a recipe from this book, while my husband gave me my shots, the whole thing was a lot more bearable.

This lovely book had a beautiful white and blue cover. Just looking it would calm me down.

So instead of looking at the needle about to be jabbed in my leg, I put my eyes on this romantic little cookbook, and I was whisked away to quaint inns across the country, visions of blueberry this-or-that dancing in my head.

You, also, can find ways to make the most difficult moments in your treatment bearable.

Listen to great music while driving to the infertility clinic.

Get to know the nurses and other medical staff at the clinic, and bring them flowers occasionally--brightening up their day can give you a boost too.

• Stop The 'I Should Have' or 'I Shouldn't Have' Talk

Infertility is not your fault. Stop blaming yourself, with thoughts like, 'I should have had children sooner' or 'I shouldn't have done this or that.' This is not your fault. For some reason, infertility seems to be an illness where women like to blame themselves.

• Harness the Power of Positive Words When The Nurse Calls With Disappointing News

You need to be aware of the self-talk that occurs within you when a cycle doesn't work out. When you hear a 'no', do you say to yourself, 'this will never work out for me.'

Be very watchful of the words you use, especially when you hit a bump in the road. Your body listens to the conversations you have with yourself and it follows suit.

If you say things like, "I probably won't ever get pregnant" well, if you have an obedient body, it might just live up (or down) to your expectations.

After you get off the phone with a nurse who has devastating news, before you start crying, repeat these words: tomorrow it will all work out for me, tomorrow it will all work out for me, tomorrow it will all work out for me.

Use your words to propel you towards what you want.

Let words come out of your mouth that will help create a positive, healthy vibration within you.

Even in your most difficult moments, speak of getting pregnant as if it already happened. Let your words stamp on you a definite 'yes, my body will physically manifest a baby soon.'

If a cycle didn't work out, say to yourself: my body is getting more and more fertile every day. Or 'my baby is on their way to me.'

Never let yourself say words that carry a defeated, sad prediction for yourself.

Keep repeating, "I will get pregnant and have a baby...I will get pregnant and have a baby...I will get pregnant and have a baby" regardless of how disappointed and sad you are feeling.

• Coping With the Unfairness of It All

Is it fair that you should have to suffer with infertility, when other women seem to get pregnant without barely trying? Is it fair that you are invited to yet another baby shower for the lady down the street who already has two adorable kids? No, it isn't fair at all. Do you have a right to feel sorry for yourself? Yes, you definitely do.

But just because something is not fair doesn't mean that ultimately you can't get what came easily to someone else. Maybe your road is harder and longer than some other women, but you can reach the same destination as much as a person who got pregnant without trying.

• Give Yourself A Break and Get Away

If you are feeling overwhelmed, consider a vacation, a day trip or a weekend away. It could be something simple, like a visit to a lake less than an hour from your house, a trip to the beach, an afternoon at a local park or museum. A change in environment can sometimes give you the break you need.

After a key IUI, I spent a week at the beach with my parents at a rented cottage at a relatively inexpensive beach only 35 minutes from my house. I didn't need an island getaway to benefit from the healing power of sun, sand and ocean. I took this time off during a busy time of year at work, but I knew that in the long run, being at the beach would help me conceive my child. It was my ninth IUI, I was very discouraged, so drastic action was needed.

Well, I did the IUI on a Saturday morning and then spent the rest of the week at the beach, doing nothing but sitting in the sun and swimming lightly in the ocean. Sometimes the body needs rest, sunshine, and a place to feel at ease. I felt more relaxed that week than I had in years. I made sure to set my vacation up in a way that no pressure or stress would be involved in my vacation. No heavy traveling was required, or getting adjusted to an unfamiliar place. Wouldn't you know it--I conceived my beautiful daughter during that IUI!

Take some time to discover places within a 30 minute drive that can give you that same feeling of rest, peace, and escape. A change of environment might be exactly what you need.

- **Take Daily Mini-Vacations**

Maybe you can't get away on a vacation right now—but you can enjoy daily mini-vacations. Start by listing three places within 15 minutes of your home that you can enjoy on a daily or weekly basis.

Some examples include:

a favorite park
a walking trail
a relaxing bookstore
a fun and interesting store
a friend's home where you feel loved and accepted
a home of a wonderful relative
a place of worship
a restaurant within your budget
a bowling alley
a coffeehouse
a farm or farmstand
a lake
a pond
a walking trail
a college campus
a pool
a library

a newspaper stand
an animal rescue center (lots of little kittens put a smile on my face!)
an outdoor garden
a museum with outdoor benches

• Read and Flood your Mind with Hopeful, Positive, Miracle Stories

Go to a bookstore or library and find hopeful, inspirational stories that lift your spirits. Read uplifting passages from the Bible. Read the life stories of people who overcame almost impossible adversities. Read stories in the Bible of people like Hannah and Sarah. There is a lot of information out there that is negative, discouraging and cynical. Avoid this information at all costs.

Avoid reading information on infertility that is loaded with discouraging statistics. Avoid any form of disaster reading. Refuse to take in information that sours your spirit and leaves you feeling hopeless. If ever in your life there was a time to feed yourself as much optimism and hope as possible, it is now.

Read personal growth books that uplift, encourage, and bring you to a place of joy. I typed up passages from the Bible and positive messages from various books and I read them daily.

• Press Your Happy Buttons—A lot!!

To keep going, you need to press your 'happy buttons' as often as possible.

A happy button can be rereading a much loved book, hanging a picture in your home that brings you joy, or enjoying a dinner out at a restaurant you love.

You need to pursue putting your body into a state of
joy as much as possible--because it is in this state that healing and conception has a better chance of taking place.

• Don't Listen To Anyone Who Blames You For Your Infertility

If someone tries to criticize you or blame you for your infertility, walk away, ignore them, refuse to listen. If someone says: 'you are just too uptight' or you are having trouble getting pregnant because you are…" Say: thanks, but no thanks. Here's an alert: millions of women who are uptight, nervous and stressed get pregnant every day.

Fertility is a complicated medical condition and no one is to blame. The body sometimes does what it is suppose to do and sometimes it doesn't. But…(and here's the but)…just because the body isn't doing what it is suppose to do today doesn't mean it won't make a switch and do exactly what it is suppose to do tomorrow.

So tell any well-meaning, but oh-so-annoying-people, that IT IS NOT YOUR FAULT and walk away. You don't have time to listen to this garbage.

• Treat and Alleviate Depression

Doctors have found that infertile women can boost their odds of getting pregnant by alleviating their depression. However, the catch-22 is: being infertile can cause depression, so how do you treat depression while battling infertility that can cause depression?

• Increase your intake of folic acid. Researchers have found that blood levels among those with depression had much lower levels of folate (folic acid).

• Take a high-quality B-complex. The B vitamins have been shown to help reduce depression.

• Find out if you have an iron deficiency. Depression is often a symptom of chronic iron deficiency.

• Take a high-quality calcium/magnesium supplement.

- Lack of the mineral zinc is linked to depression. Low levels of zinc in the body have been shown to result in paranoia and fearfulness.

- Include omega-3s and foods rich in omega-3s in your diet more often.

- Increase your social support. Join a support group, a neighborhood book club, or attend a weekly meeting with those you have something in common with. Positive social support can do much to alleviate depression.

- Learn how to deep breath.

- Try to include in your daily schedule time with supportive people, friends and family; a mild form of exercise, time outdoors, and time helping others in some way, such as writing a card to a sick friend, sewing a blanket for a children's hospital, or dropping off some baked goods for a friend.

- Restructure how you talk to yourself—remember: positive words, positive words, positive words.
You deserve an internal best friend who speaks kindly to you, not an internal enemy that is always badgering you.

- Keep your blood sugar levels stable by eating several times a day and avoid white flour and sugary foods.

- Tell yourself 'I love you" several times a day. Whenever you start to feel sad or hopeless, say, "I love you" to yourself.

Chapter 6: The People In Your Journey and Some of the Rude Comments You May Hear Along the Way

This is not to be misinterpreted as an exercise in dumping family or friends, because people are not perfect and we should not expect them to be, and there are people in our lives, as unpleasant as they may be, that we simply need to forgive, stay connected to and be around. Despite their flaws, we owe them something. That being said, as you walk this journey, you need to be ready for some of the stupid, rude and totally insensitive comments you are going to hear. Sometimes, people you love will say really dumb things. Other times, it could be a stranger who zaps you with a statement that leaves you breathless and feeling punched in the gut.

Here are a few of the stupid, rude, thoughtless and COMPLETELY FALSE comments you may have to deal with, and how best to respond:

- **"Maybe you weren't meant to have a baby":** Yes, you were meant to have a baby. Yes, you were. Millions of women have babies whether they want them or not, whether they will be good mothers or not, so why shouldn't you have a baby? In fact, there is NOT ONE REASON IN THIS UNIVERSE why you should not have a baby.

This person is either jealous of you or just likes to pop the balloon of hope. People who mouth off a comment like this mistakenly feel they have some sort of moral authority. Ignore them. They are wrong. Completely and utterly wrong.

- **"Aren't you a little too old to be trying for a baby?"**

Whoever got the idea that a young mother is better than an older mother has not seen the millions of mothers in their 40s and even 50s who mother with great patience, love, insight, wisdom and kindness.

This person obviously doesn't understand that with age comes maturity and wisdom.

Someone who makes a comment like this may be focusing on the energy level of children, forgetting that even most 25 year old mothers are not out playing baseball with their kids everyday.

Whoever throws out a comment about age is ignorant of the fact that a woman of any age who is ready and able to love a child, and who is brave and strong enough to endure infertility, is more prepared, capable and ready to mother than almost anyone.

A good mother is a good mother, whether she is 21, 31, 41, 51 or beyond.

- **"Why don't you just adopt?"**

A person who says this perhaps does not understand or is not sensitive to the desire to have biological children.

Maybe they don't have children, so to them, what difference does it make how you get a child. Or they have children and it came so easily and naturally, that they don't see it as a privilege or any big deal.

The comment wreaks of ignorance and lack of judgment.

Here's the thing: adoption is a wonderful opportunity for those who are ready and willing to embrace it. However, if this is not the path you desire, DO NOT FEEL GUILTY!!!!! You have every right to a biological child, and even if your desire for a biological child isn't coming easily— IT DOESN'T MEAN YOU WON'T HAVE ONE EVENTUALLY. This type of comment throws guilt in a direction it should not be thrown. Adoption is something that a person should do only if they passionately want to, not because they feel guilted into doing it. You have a right to want a biological child, and a right to take advantage of whatever is medically available to make that happen. No one has the right to make you feel guilty about this, and or rob you of a natural right.

- **"Don't worry! Just relax and it will happen"**

This comment often comes with all the best intentions. Perhaps this person feels sympathy for you, but doesn't know what to say to express themselves. Maybe they don't know much about infertility and are not educated on how the reproductive system works. Maybe they want to comfort you, and this is their attempt to do so. Maybe they mistakenly believe that by saying this, you will relax a bit and get pregnant.

When you get this type of advice, you need to remember that millions of women get pregnant every day under all kinds of conditions, including stress, war, famine and other horrific environments that are definitely not relaxing.
It is very unlikely that as you go through infertility you are always going to feel blissed-out and relaxed—and for that, you should not feel guilty.

- **"Maybe its for the best. Maybe you couldn't handle it"**

 This comment often comes from either someone who has children and really doesn't enjoy being a mother, and deep down feels they were handed something they couldn't handle, or the person is the competitive type who likes to one-up others and takes odd pleasure in put downs.

When you get this type of comment, remind yourself that you are going to be a great mother. Just because no one has seen you in action yet, doesn't mean you are not going to be the best mother around.

Your friends and family have not seen your maternal side in action yet. Maybe at this point, they are unable to envision the mother you are going to be. Maybe they are so focused on lifestyle choices, personality traits, and attitudes that serve you well now that they can't see the maternal potential inside you. But just wait—someday they will stand back in awe at the amazing mother you are.

If you desire to love a child, then you will find ways to raise your child in safety and love, whether you have any experience caring for a child or not.

If someone doesn't see your potential to do that, well, they are clueless as to who you really are.

Hold tight to the vision you have of yourself as a mother regardless of how others see you—other people can often only see what is right in front of their eyes and do not have the insight to see the maternal flower inside of you waiting and ready to bloom.

• "Having children at your age is risky. They might be born with a disability or special need"

This comment most likely comes from a person who likely always sees the glass half full, lives their life in fear, and does not embrace risk. They also like spreading their gloom around, perhaps because they see trouble lurking around the corner, instead of opportunity and hope.

Here's a little thing someone who makes a comment like this doesn't realize: any child can be born with a disability and age doesn't have as much to do with it as we like to think. Having a child at any age, even for teenagers, comes with some risks. Good prenatal care and nutrition can do much to eliminate the risks. Be brave and step forward, and don't let those who lack courage stop you.

Their warnings are not warnings that will protect you in any way. In fact, their warnings are actually vicious thieves who could rob you of what you want most. Feel sorry for anyone who says this to you: life is probably a bit too scary for them to ever enjoy.

• "I'm the opposite. All my husband had to do is walk by me and I got pregnant"

Wow, this person really likes to feel better than others and gets a real kick out of a chance to self-promote how great they are. Tisk, tisk, tisk, didn't their mother teach them better than this?

Maybe you should just congratulate them and say something like, 'wow, you are so much better than me. I wish I was like you" because bottom line is that is exactly what they want to hear.

Just remember: some women get pregnant easily and some don't—and someday, when you are snuggling with your beautiful baby, it won't really matter how you got to your moment and how they got to their moments, because you will be enjoying the same prize.

It isn't fair, of course, that their road may have been a lot easier than yours—but ultimately, you can have exactly what they have and more. Plus, you'll always have your good manners that they obviously lack.

- **'Maybe God doesn't want you to have a baby'**

In my opinion, whoever dares say this to you is stepping on sacred ground. Ask them: when did God give you the right to speak for Him? Since when do they get to speak God's intentions for you? According to the Bible, God loves us and wants great things for us. God is love—and love never denies, but gives. This person really has no understanding of God's true personality. Perhaps they should sit down and read the Bible closely. God is complete goodness and love—not some punishing father ready to deny us. If they see God this way, perhaps they need to get to know Him better. It is rude, presumptuous and ignorant to speak for God or to assume that a physical condition like infertility is the result of God's withholding something from one of His earthly children.

Would they say to a person with cancer, "this is God's will for you." Probably not—because we look at other diseases as physical problems that deserve treatment. So why is infertility a disease that is viewed differently?

Ignore this person and remind yourself of the scripture at 1 John 4:8, "God is love" and spend some time thinking about how someone who is pure love gives and provides, not takes away and denies.

If this statement is ever thrown at you, immediately begin repeating: God is love, God is love, God is love, over and over again.

- **"Didn't you try this before and it didn't work out?"**

 Yup, and trying again is what winners do so they ultimately get what they want. A person who might not like to repeat their efforts without immediate reward—also known as lazy—might come up with this one. Again, ignore and move on. They don't know what they are talking about.

- **"I went through infertility treatments and they didn't work"**

 Of course, sympathize and feel badly for this person, but remember: their journey doesn't have to be your journey. Their experience doesn't have to be your experience. Their outcome is not going to be your outcome. Just because it hasn't worked out for them yet doesn't mean it isn't going to work out for you. Different people, different choices, different results. They are not hopeless and either are you.

Whether or not they ever have a baby doesn't mean you do not have the right to get the children you want. Don't bother arguing with that person or trying to convince them that your path will be different than theirs. Be kind and walk away. New treatments, new medications, and new ways of healing from infertility are being offered everyday.

And remember: you have every right to have this work out—even it didn't work out for someone else.

- **"Aren't infertility treatments dangerous? I hear the medications can cause this or that"**

Well, doesn't everything have a little bit of danger in it? It takes courage and the ability to risk-take to go after anything in this world. If you want a baby, than any obstacle is worth climbing over to get it. Danger/smanger/ignore and move on.

- **"If I were you, I wouldn't get so worked up about this"**

Well, obviously, they are not you. Maybe this person never really wanted anything that badly. Or maybe they are just super insensitive to other people's pain. Whatever the reason for such a comment, it shows a lack of insight—infertility is very much a reason to be worked up. This passion will also make you a great mother someday.

- **"You've already been through so much. If I were you, I'd give up"**

Well, I'll say it again--they are not you—you are stronger, braver and able to walk through fire to get what you want.

Maybe they just don't have the guts you have. Maybe they already have what they want, or they don't want anything that badly, that seeing you make so much effort is unnerving to them. Don't listen. Be proud that you can continue on despite the difficulty involved.

Chapter 7: A Note About Husbands and How To Not Let Infertility Ruin Your Marriage

Here are my thoughts about husbands:

Infertility can be rough on a marriage.

From the day you start infertility treatments, it will be best if you let go of the idea that your husband will always be able to fully understand and care for all the emotions you will experience in the quest to have a baby.

Let go of the idea that he will always say the right thing. Abandon the hope that he will always know exactly how to comfort you.

As much as my husband wanted children, he did not always understand my raw anguish or single-minded drive. Looking back, I shouldn't have expected him to understand all my emotions. It was a waste of time and energy I needed to put into my healing.

What I didn't understand was that, while my husband's desire to have children was strong, he manifested it differently than I did.

Sometimes I became enraged when I felt he was being a bit too clinical about the whole experience.

Don't try to get your husband to express his desire for a baby in the exact same way you do. It is pointless. Your husband cannot be the focus of your frustration right now.

Doing things to make your body healthier is where your energy needs to be, not in fighting with your husband over his perceived insensitivities.

Some husbands are just not able to fully grasp the intense passion, fervor and sometimes obsession a woman can feel over having a baby.

If your husband does understand, you are very fortunate.

If not, that's okay too.

Just remember--this journey isn't about him--it is about bringing the baby of your dreams to life. Wasting time arguing with him or expecting him to totally relate to your feelings is, well, a waste of time.

As much as you need his support right now, you need to empower yourself and find your strength within. If you can, build a network of support outside of your marriage, so that he won't be your exclusive source of comfort.

Don't expect him to rescue you from the pain and work involved in infertility treatments. Don't expect him to mother you, nurse you, or completely get what this means to you.

Do expect he may say exactly what you don't want him to say at exactly the wrong time.

Many husbands end up becoming true heroes to their wives during infertility treatments, but even those who rise to the challenge can sometimes disappoint--not because they are insensitive or uncaring, but simply because they might be tired, cranky, or feeling intense emotions of their own.

Infertility is tiring and sometimes people run out of steam.

For the times when perhaps he is insensitive, forgive him and let it go. Don't waste time moping and groaning about how he doesn't get it.

Remember: your husband cannot save you from the pain of this ordeal, or erase the frustration and rage you sometimes are going to feel.

Don't make trying to get him to understand your feelings your mission--you will be wasting precious time and emotional resources. Don't expect him to be driven in exactly the same way you are, although some men are.

Most likely all this infertility stuff is going to stress out your relationship, and you can't take too seriously anything you feel about each other at this time. The goal is to give birth to your baby, not make your husband feel the same maternal longing you feel.

Infertility treatments are extremely grueling work, and your husband may get impatient with the whole ordeal. Or you may be one of the fortunate ones, and have a husband as dedicated and motivated as you are.

My husband and I fought a lot during our infertility treatments, especially the first time. The stress was sometimes too much for us to handle. We often turned on each another. I'm not sure what would have prevented this. I needed him to be more tender and he needed me to be more understanding. We both needed to be a lot kinder to each other.

At my lowest points, I desperately wanted him to say some magic words that would make me feel better, and frankly, I was enraged when he didn't seem to have those magic words.

Looking back, most of our fights were wasted energy--just a place and a distraction to put all our anger and sadness over the situation.

I wish I had used that time more wisely. The second time around, I focused more on my battle to get healthy, instead of looking to my husband to rescue me. Issues with my husband faded into the background once I had my priorities straight, although in my darkest times, my darling, sweet, strong husband was my greatest ally, and ultimately, he worked just as hard as I did through the process. For his perseverance, I am forever grateful.

Once, after an IVF cycle didn't work out, my husband said he needed to go for a drive alone to deal with the pain. Somehow, knowing he hurt as much as I did helped me not feel so alone.

While my husband and I did turn on each other at times, especially when we were sad, ultimately he was my hero.

After a laparoscopy procedure when I woke up in excruciating pain, it was my husband who kneeled by my bed, rubbed my feet and did everything in his power to ease my pain. So as hard as infertility can be on a marriage, it can also bring you closer than you were before.

Your husband may support you in ways you never even imagined. Just don't be disappointed when he can't.

There are things, however, you can do to help him through this journey.

First, keep the happy chemicals in his brain going, and at the same time, enhance his sperm quality, with zinc, Vitamin C, Vitamin E, folic acid, magnesium, omega-3, lots of greens, vegetables, pumpkin seeds, oysters, selenium and L-Carnitine. Take relaxing walks together. Remember to say thank you and show appreciation for those times when he does help you in exactly the way you need.

As hard as it is, try to do some fun things together during this time. Maybe try golf or fishing or some other relaxing, non-demanding sport, like sand castle building or bird watching. Take a break, sometimes, and do something completely romantic. Always remember to kiss and make-up when times get tough.

The goal is not to turn on each other during this stressful time, and not to let unrealistic expectations about what your husband is suppose to do or feel cause problems in your marriage.

Hopefully, you will receive the support you need from your husband. When you don't, let it go and focus on your goal.

Chapter 8: Choosing The Right Doctor

Don't underestimate the importance of having a good doctor, and don't ever be naive about the damage the wrong doctor can do. Frankly, the wrong doctor can steal your chance of having a baby and the family you dream of.

Start by researching infertility clinics in your area. You want to choose a clinic with high success rates and an esteemed reputation. You want a doctor who is a fertility specialist and affiliated with a highly reputable fertility clinic with a high success rate. I would strongly suggest against using your gynecologist as your infertility specialist.

A gynecologist may not have as much experience as a specialist who focuses exclusively on infertility. They may also lack the resources and access to the latest reproductive technologies.

Research the success rates of various clinics within 30 minutes to an hour from your home. When choosing a clinic, weigh carefully the travel time and route to the clinic. You will be going to the clinic a lot, sometimes every day for weeks. If travel is no consideration, go to the best clinic within an hour from you.

When choosing a clinic, make sure they have a wide range of fertility treatments available and are familiar with the latest technologies. If you have choices, try to select a clinic that makes you feel comfortable, doesn't stress you out, and who can offer you the best and most choices. If you know others dealing with infertility, ask for their opinions and experiences at different clinics with different doctors. I found the doctor who helped me become pregnant with my son through a neighbor he also helped conceive and give birth to her son.

It is important that you select a doctor you feel comfortable with and who answers your questions. If a doctor refuses to answer your questions or seems to dismiss your questions, this may not be the doctor to select.

If they almost come off as disrespectful and arrogant, than perhaps then you need to ask yourself: will they listen if I request a certain test or change in medications? Or will they ignore my requests?

Ideally, you want a doctor who listens to your recommendations and orders whatever tests and medications you request.

A doctor who doesn't put the time into finding solutions for you may not be the right doctor.

While physicians in the infertility industry are very busy and it is not realistic to expect excessive emotional support, you should be able to expect one who listens and pays attention to your requests, is determined to help you, and is willing to try new procedures and medications. Some fertility doctors may seem cold because they have large caseloads.

Occasionally, doctors with high success rates can sometimes have a hidden agenda in trying to get you to quit the attempt for a biological child. Before following the recommendations of a doctor, always consider where their motive for your course of treatment might be coming from. If you are of an advanced age, every time you do an IUI or an IVF and it fails, their success rates for live births are lowered, and thus it is in their best interests to persuade you to try an alternative method that precludes the attempt at a biological child so their statistics remain high. Could your continuing to pursue the goal of having biological children lower their live birth rate statistics? Is this a doctor more concerned with their stats than with helping you achieve your goal? For those who can maintain high live birth statistics, it means higher rankings and more customers.

Also stay alert to how long you are kept on a medication, especially if it is not working. Is your doctor keeping track of your progress and alert to when a change in medication is needed? If you have suffered miscarriages, did your doctor prescribe or suggest progesterone for future pregnancies? Are they making an attempt to give you what you need so you don't miscarry again?

Do not stay with a doctor who is not producing results for you, or at least trying to find what is going to work for you. If your doctor stays with the same protacol repeatedly, despite no success, it might be time to get another doctor. Or at least see if your doctor is willing to sit down and reevaluate your treatment plan.

It is important that you don't get stuck trusting just one medical professional to the point that you waste years with someone who isn't getting results for you, or is just on the wrong track altogether. Be open to finding a new doctor, even one within the clinic you go to, when if time has passed and there is no progress or results.

You need a doctor willing to switch gears, and try different tactics to get you pregnant. You want a doctor who is willing to acknowledge when it is time to try something new in your treatment.

You don't need a doctor so tied up in ego, so stuck on one way of doing things, that they don't venture out and try every available medicine and procedure out there. You want a doctor who will investigate why things are not working out for you.

If you strongly feel you need certain tests and your doctor refuses to do them, by all means find a new doctor. If you ask for a change in medication and that request is ignored, it is time to find another doctor.

After an IVF that failed, I went to my doctor with a list of questions and a request for a new medication I had read about and researched that seemed like it would help me. This doctor refused to answer even one of my questions, told me my eggs were bottom of the barrel and I should quit trying, wanted to give me an ovarian reserve test to determine whether my fertility was over, and would not even consider trying the new medication.

I went home, called the clinic, and changed doctors immediately, thanks to some very wise advice from my mother.

I then chose a doctor within the clinic that my neighbor had. He had helped her become pregnant with her beautiful son. What a change!

My new doctor answered every one of my questions and immediately agreed that this new medication was one that he would definitely try and was considering before I even suggested it.

Two months later, I was pregnant with my son, who I gave birth to nine months later.

That other doctor was completely wrong. If I had listened to her, I probably would have given up. If I had taken that ovarian reserve test, and somehow it showed my ovarian reserve to be low, my insurance company may have then denied my right to fertility treatments. Why did she want to put me in such a position that my treatments would no longer be covered and I could not afford to pay them out of pocket. Perhaps she had too many patients and didn't have time for a patient like me. Maybe she got the ranking of 'best in' my area because she pushed patients towards using egg donors rather than their own eggs because with younger eggs comes a higher chance of live births, thus falsely elevating her success rate.

When patients of advanced age use their own eggs, the risk of failure is higher, and she did not want the failed IVFs that would lower her success rate.

Do you see how dangerous listening to the wrong doctor can be?

The first doctor didn't really care about me or the outcome of my treatments. She simply didn't want to be bothered with me anymore. She didn't think my desire for a biological child was worth one more try.

The next doctor was accommodating, hard working and willing to try a new treatment plan.

As I said before, the wrong doctor can steal your chance to have a baby, while the right doctor can play a significant role in making your dream happen.

Make sure the doctor you choose is organized. Does your doctor seem scattered, like they are more concerned with publishing in medical journals than actually practicing medicine?

Do they seem hassled, like they have taken on too many patients and cannot handle the workload? If so, they may make poor decisions when it comes to your care.

The doctor I mentioned above was named one of the best in New England, but she mistakenly diagnosed me as having fibroids. I underwent a procedure to remove them, but it turned out I did not have fibroids at all. She never apologized for the unnecessary pain and time wasted on this operation that she caused me. Because of this operation, my fertility treatments were delayed for months.

If you have friends who also are being treated for infertility, or were treated successfully, ask for their recommendations and feedback. But take note: while you can listen to suggestions, you need to follow your own gut feelings. A doctor might be right for one person, but not another. At the same time, if you have a friend you share a lot in common with, and they found success with a certain doctor, you might want to schedule a 'getting to know you' meeting with their doctor and see for yourself. Note how your body feels when you are with this doctor—do you leave feeling agitated or calm? Confident or unsure of yourself? Never overlook or deny nagging feelings of doubt.

How do you know you chose the wrong doctor?

You know you have the wrong doctor when the doctor does not explore every possible reason for your infertility, refuses to listen to your ideas, does not answer your questions, and does not try new medications and treatments to help you get pregnant.

The wrong doctor never admits when they are wrong, and they stubbornly stay tethered to a plan that doesn't work. The wrong doctor is not knowledgeable on all the reasons you may be infertile and is not aware of all the new medications available.

The wrong doctor is more concerned with their statistics than in trying to help you. The wrong doctor will try to push you in a direction you may not want to go. The wrong doctor will take away your hope.

Never take the word of one doctor as if they were God.

Even if you really like your doctor and have a wonderful relationship, be sure to question, analyze and investigate the course of treatment they give you.

You may be taking the word or accepting the decisions of one doctor who may be on the wrong track, or who might not have your best interests in mind, or might be a bit lazy, or have too many patients, or who may simply be too arrogant to realize a change in your treatment is needed. Or simply—your doctor might be great, but is still failing to get you on the right medication or treatment plan.

If you are not getting pregnant, and it has been a long time, try a new doctor, get a second opinion, don't stay tethered to any one doctor or clinic if you don't see results or they are not listening to your concerns. Even if you find a doctor you like, if they do not produce results for you after a certain amount of time, go and get another opinion. This is not the time for you to be stuck on one doctor to the point that you don't aggressively pursue every test, medication and treatment that will get you pregnant. Initially, I liked that doctor who led me down the wrong path. She was comforting during certain procedures and had a likeable personality. But ultimately, she was a danger to my fertility. That's why when it comes to choosing and staying with a doctor, keep your eyes open and keep close track of your progress.

Chapter 9: Common Mistakes You Need To Know About

Here are some common mistakes those suffering with infertility often encounter:

Waiting too long to get help: Stop listening to those people who tell you to simply relax and it will happen. Relaxing does help, but it is not the only solution. If you've been trying to get pregnant for awhile and it is not happening, see an infertility specialist immediately.

Not trying enough times and/or giving up too soon: When undergoing infertility treatments, never forget the old saying, "if at first you don't succeed, try, try again." Even if you have done several cycles, if you feel you can cope and want to continue, let yourself try again. Don't listen to those who say, 'you've tried X number of times and if it hasn't work yet it isn't going to.' The next try could be the one that works.

Not seeing the correlation between poor eating habits, and infertility: Don't get tricked into believing that you can eat any way you want and it won't impact your fertility. Everything you consume impacts your fertility—and it your responsibility to start getting this part of your life right.

Not strengthening every part of your body, from your liver, to your kidney to your adrenal glands: You know various ways to detoxify and strengthen your organs—so go ahead and do it.

Not participating in your own healing process and thinking it is someone else's responsibility: Your doctor and the infertility clinic can provide you with a treatment plan and medications to help you get pregnant, but the rest of the healing is up to you.

Not Trying To Discover The Root Cause of Your Infertility: Even if your doctor diagnoses you with 'unexplained infertility' the bottom line is there is a reason you are not getting pregnant—one that perhaps is so subtle that the clinics have no precise test that can diagnose it.

That is where it is in your best interests to seek out holistic and alternative medicine to address the subtle reasons your body is not conceiving naturally.

Chapter 10: Bye Bye Stress!

You've heard it a million times before. Now you will hear it again: stress is a huge enemy of your fertility. Stress weakens your body, impacts your hormones, and could be what is standing between you and your future children.

Stress makes your body a less welcoming and hospitable place. Some doctors believe that stress plays a role in 20 to 30 percent of all infertility cases.

The reason stress is so dangerous to your fertility is it elevates hormones like cortisol and epinephrine, which inhibit the body's main sex hormone gonadotropin releasing hormone (GnRH).

Stress inhibits the release of reproductive hormones. GnRH is responsible for the pituitary gland's release of luteinizing hormones and follicle-stimulating hormones.

Stress disrupts hormone communication between your brain, pituitary and ovaries, thus interfering with the maturation of the egg and ovulation process.

Stress can also kick the body into a fight or flight response that makes it difficult for the body to feel safe enough to get pregnant.

However, it should be noted that all around the world, lots of women are very stressed and get pregnant anyways. Stress is part of life, and yes, you will feel stressed sometimes during this process. I am not in any way saying: 'relax you will get pregnant' because there are many underlying, hard to detect physical reasons pregnancy is not occurring. It is disrespectful to suggest that a person going through infertility treatments would somehow not feel stressed.

Of course you are going to be stressed! How could you not? So, don't feel guilty if sometimes you feel stressed.

However, you deserve to stack the odds in your favor, and do whatever you can to reduce the stress hormones in your body.

Here are some suggestions:

• Take Some Time to Analyze Exactly What in Your Life Stresses You

For a few days, write down every time you feel stressed. What caused you to feel stressed? Where were you? Who were you with? What was happening that made you feel this way? Then, ask yourself: are these stressors something I can change?

Write down ways you can change the stress triggers in your life. If these stressors are not factors you can change, ask yourself: can I change my attitude or how I talk to myself about these stressors so I do not get as upset next time?

The goal is to identify your stressors and find ways to change your circumstances so these triggers are no longer in your life. Or, if you cannot change the stressful situations in your life, can you change the way you react, think, talk to yourself about, and cope with these stressors?

An example: you realize that your daily commute to work is very stressful. Is there an alternative route you could take? A co-worker you could drive in with? A form of public transportation that would be more relaxing? A favorite CD or book you could play while you drive to help change your mood and what you think about as you drive? Would your employer be open to a change in work schedule that might lessen the traffic you encounter?

Are there any opportunities for jobs closer to home or work-from-home days? What could you say to yourself during your commute that you can change? Start thinking of ways to address the situations that bring up feelings of stress in your life.

• Repeat Positive Sayings and Positive Words

 If you find you get stressed around a certain person or at a certain time of day, choose a saying or mantra that you can repeat over and over to yourself that will help calm you down.

Sayings that might help include:

Let go and let God
With God all things are possible
Everything will be all right
Been there, done that, all will turn out well
Breathe, breathe, breathe
Time for my bath
This too shall pass
Keep calm and carry on
Keep calm and love
I don't worry, I be happy
I s-m-i-l-e
I don't have to be perfect
I choose happy
I choose good
The sun is shining on me
Right now, a batch of warm chocolate chips cookies are coming out of the oven
I breathe peace
I breathe love
Stay calm—it will be all right
Inch by inch, life's a cinch
One bite at a time
Relax, God is in charge
God loves me and will take care of me
Love is here right now
It will be okay
I did good
Peace is mine
I will conquer

I smile with joy
My happy heart is light
Love is here, love is mine, love is everywhere
Courage is mine
My heart is smiling
Hope arrived!
I stand by you
Life is beautiful
Once upon a time there was a princess named <u>your name here</u>
I am happy
I feel wonderful
I am love

Choose a mantra that elicits positive feelings within you. For example, if you relax when you hear the word 'chocolate' or 'joy' create a saying you can repeat each day around those words, such as 'I have chocolate covered joy."

• Put Yourself In Situations Or Around People That Make You Feel Safe

Feelings of danger often bring up stress in the body. Do whatever you can to increase your feelings of safety at this time. If you feel safe wrapped in a certain blanket drinking tea, make that part of your daily routine. If hearing your mother's voice or cuddling with your cat make you feel safe, do those things more often. Feeling safe helps us relax. If you can, avoid situations where you feel you are in danger.

• Spend Ten Minutes Every Morning and Every Night Doing Deep Breathing Exercises

Inhale for a count of four, exhale for a count of four. Or, put one hand on your chest, one on your belly, and deep breath through your nose. Try alternate nostril breathing, where you hold the right thumb over your right nostril and inhale deeply. At the peak of inhalation, close off the left nostril and exhale through the right nostril. You can also try a long, slow inhale, and then a quick, powerful exhale from the lower belly.

• Start Swimming

Swim indoors, outdoors, at a health club, a gym, in the ocean, a lake, or a river. Swimming was a big stress reliever for me. I always come out of the water feeling better than when I go in. If you have a yard, consider an inexpensive above-ground pool and start swimming daily.

Swimming relaxes the body because it requires alternating stretch and relaxation of sketal muscles, while simultaneously deep-breathing in a rhythmic pattern. A note here: swimming might be best before you do an IVF or IUI cycle in order to relax the body. After an IVF treatment, it might be best to stop all exercises that are too extreme or harsh on the body, and this could include swimming.

• Write Poetry

Write a poem, read uplifting poetry or choose an author and read all their poetry, either to yourself, aloud or start a poetry reading group. Some great poets include Walt Whitman, Maya Angelou, Robert Frost, Langston Hughes, Elizabeth Barrett Browning, William Shakespeare, Robert Browning, Henry Wadsworth Longfellow.

• Get Your Hands Dirty

That's right—research has shown that touching dirt relieves stress. Plant some flowers, grow a potted herb garden, dig up some weeds, plant vegetables, flowers, grass. Just put your hands in the dirt and enjoy.

• Spend More Time in Nature

Many studies have been done on the healing effects of green space on reducing stress and tension. The natural world offers some of the best relaxers available. Levels of serotonin, a neurotransmitter that regulates our moods, rise when we are outside in nature. Make it a goal to be outside at least 15 to 30 minutes a day, even if it just means sitting on the front steps of your apartment or in your driveway.

Smell nature, stare at nature, sit in nature, and be in the moment with nature.

Go barefoot. When you are unable to get outdoors, take some pictures of natural scenes and display them in your home or workplace, so you can enjoy the peaceful serene feeling being in nature can bring.

Take daily walks in a park. Sit under a tree. Put your hands in the dirt and garden. Sit on your front lawn and take in the sunshine. Bring a sketchpad to a park and draw. Feed the birds, the deers, the seagulls, the turkeys. Hike a local trail every morning. Choose a spot and stare at a tree. Sit on the beach. Lay down in the grass. Have a picnic at a local lake. Swing on some swings. Read a book outside. Grow some grass in a pot and sniff it. Touch a tree. Pick up some pine needles, or sticks.

- **Bring Flowers Into Your Life**

Buy yourself flowers weekly. Various studies have shown that we feel less negative and more energized when we are around flowers. At some local supermarkets, bouquets of flowers can often be enjoyed for $5 or less.

Put flowers in a visible place where you can see and enjoy them, such as by your bed, on the kitchen table, or on your desk at work.

- **Hum Your Way to a Baby**

Music can be a powerful tool in lifting our moods and relaxing our bodies. Music has been used as a healing tool for thousands of years, and it can be a healing therapy for you too. Research has shown that music sets off a neurological chain in the body that alleviates stress and induces relaxation.

As you undergo infertility treatments, begin using music as a way to relieve stress and elicit feelings of joy and hope. Commit to bringing more music into your life. Buy and play music from happy times in your life. Play music that lifts you up or relaxes you.

Avoid sad, depressing music that makes you melancholy or reminds you of sad events in your life. Play Broadway show tunes, inspirational music, music that you love to dance to. Play whatever type of music calms you and helps you feel happy. Try some classical music. Play Italian love songs at dinner.

Keep a stereo in your living room or kitchen, and listen to music while cooking dinner.

Replace half an hour of TV watching each day with a half an hour of listening to music. Write a song or lyrics to a song. Play music when you feel worried or anxious, start listening to music as a way to distract you. If you play an instrument, sit down and play along to a favorite artist or song. Create a favorite play list you can listen to while driving to the infertility clinic. Keep sheet music nearby that you can play or sing along to. Get a karaoke machine.

If you've had formal music lessons, take out your instrument and play for your own enjoyment. Or purchase a set of drums, a piano, an organ, a flute, keyboard, or a guitar and just bang away. Let yourself enjoy creating sound for nothing more than the joy of creating sound.

Take some time to find the music that makes you feel like nothing can stop you. Play music that makes you feel like you are on a winning momentum. Research various forms of classical music to see what best suits you. If there is a certain instrument that you love, make sure to get music highlighting that instrument's sound.

Join a drumming group, take piano or clarinet lessons, sign up for a music course at a local college. Get a CD with the sounds of the ocean, wind or other forms of nature. Listen to musical theatre if it puts you in a great mood or study the works of a favorite band, singer of composer.

- **Watch What You Watch**

If the evening news brings you down, stop watching it for now. Horrible images, frightening scenes, upsetting events, are not going to help your body heal and become strong. If you get news updates on your phone, stop them if they shake you up and leave you depressed.

There is some evidence that when you are sad, your adrenals become weakened, which impacts the entire hormone system in your body.

From now on, watch movies and TV shows that make you laugh and generally leave you with an optimistic, positive, upbeat feeling.

When you feel happy, you have a better chance of keeping your adrenals strong. Organs, such as the thyroid can also be weakened by a sad mood. If not keeping up with the news makes you feel guilty, realize that you are just doing it during this time in your life. It is important to give your body a chance to feel safe and watching unsettling events that attack your feelings of safety is not what your body needs right now.

- **Begin a Mild Exercise Routine**

Find an gentle exercise that gets your body movingl. Nothing too demanding or harsh. Walk three or four times a week for a half hour. Note here: once you do an IVF cycle, I would suggest stopping all extreme swimming, running and aerobic work-outs. This is not the time to push your body too hard with aerobic, running, or cardio-work-outs. Extreme exercise at this time will not aid your body in conceiving, but could negatively impact the outcome of your infertility treatments.

- **Reduce the Time You Spend Looking at Screens**

Too much time on your phone, computer, television, video games affects melatonin production and throws off the circadian rhythms that lead to deep, restorative sleep. As much as you can, reduce the time you spend with the technology in your life. Don't text as much, watch as many movies or TV, or play as many video games. Try to cut your screen time down in half.

- **Move the Stress out of your Body**

Take walks, dance in your living room, get a massage from a trauma release specialist.

• Thank God Every Day for Everything Good in Your Life

Say thank you for all the beauty around you. Say many 'thank you' prayers each day. Say thank you for things you never noticed before.

• Start Keeping A Gratitude Journal

Keeping a gratitude journal will help get in the habit of focusing on the positives in your life.

Studies have shown that those who keep gratitude journals and practice gratitude experience lower blood pressure, strengthened immune systems and higher levels of positive emotions in their life.

Write at least three things you are grateful for at the end of each day. Keep an eye for the subtle things that you might overlook. Don't worry about what you write—there is no right or wrong way to do this, and no one is grading you on the quality of your entries.

• Appreciate the Special Moments in Your Life

Get a poster board and write: Moments In My Life I Appreciate. Tape it to the refrigerator. Then every day, write what you experienced that day you appreciate. It could be something as simple as 'I had a nice day at work' or 'I really enjoyed going out for pizza with my friend' or 'loved talking with Mom on the phone today.' Start keeping track of all the positive things that happened in your day—even small things you previously overlooked.

• Get an Aquarium

Some studies have shown that looking at an aquarium reduces stress and lowers blood pressure. Major retailers often have affordable tanks that come with all the basic items you need to set up. Place the aquarium in a spot where you can spend time watching it. Add a few plants in your fish tank to create a pleasing environment.

• Sing More!

Start singing as much as you can everyday. Research has shown that singing can put you in positive state of mind and reduces depression and anxiety. The use of song as a calming influence in everyday life has taken place in cultures around the world since ancient times.

Hormones such as oxytocin and endorphins are released when we sing, and those who sing have lower levels of the stress hormone cortisol in their body. Singing also lowers blood pressure and heart rate, because when we sing oxygen enters our body.

Singing has been known to increase energy levels and boost the immune system. Some believe that blocked energy in the body is released through the tonal vibrations that come from singing. When we sing, we breath differently than when we are talking.

Join a local choir or start your own singing group. Set up a karaoke machine or a microphone in an easy-to-access place in your home. Get a Wii sing-along game. Join a local chorus, show choir, or vocal group. Take singing lessons. Start a singing club with your family or friends. Choose a morning song to start your day, sing on the way to work, sing on the way to your fertility treatments—don't judge yourself or your voice, just sing!

• Keep A Journal

Give yourself ten minutes a day to write out whatever is bothering you. For just ten minutes, let whatever is within pour out on to the paper—and then leave it there, out of your body.

• Get A Pet

Get a dog or a cat. More and more research is showing the stress-relieving benefits of having a pet. Petting your cat, walking your dog, listening to your cat purr, caring for another living being, provides social support, stress relief, a strengthened immune system, and many other health benefits. Pets ease pain and lower blood pressure.

Note: if you have a cat, once you are pregnant, you want to be sure someone else is cleaning the litter box so that you do not contract toxoplasmosis, a parasitic infection carried by cats, that can cause problems to the growing fetus. Make sure the litter box is changed daily and whoever is cleaning the litter box should wear disposable gloves.

• Read Uplifting Books

Read books that inspire, books that relax, and books that make you smile. Read classics you enjoyed in high school. Read personal growth books that encourage positive thinking and emotional healing. Read stories that give you courage, strength and hope.

• Pray

For me, nothing helped release my stress like prayer. Being able to pray to God is and was a grand privilege that helped me like nothing else. Being able to communicate with God was what helped me most during my journey through infertility. I prayed on the way to the clinic. I prayed while I was at the clinic. I prayed on my drive home from the clinic. I prayed while my husband gave me shots, and I prayed when I waited for news from the clinic. I prayed day and night. I prayed when I felt despair, I prayed when I felt hopeless, and prayer is what gave me the strength to continue on during the hardest, most dismal times. I thank God that He gave us the privilege of prayer.

• Do Something You Always Wanted To Do

Sometimes stress builds up when we are forced to do things we don't enjoy or really want to do. Start doing something you really want to do – something that gets you excited and thrilled.

• Get Creative

Set up an art expression center in your home. Keep all your art supplies in an accessible bin, container or basket. Creating art is a positive way to express your emotions and release deeply buried unconscious feelings.

Paint, draw, sketch, color, sculpt, glue, sew, design. Do art projects that relieve your stress and put you into a state of flow. Don't critique your work, but use these mediums as a way to release and express. If you get the urge to put your fingers in paint, smoosh away. Draw the tree outside your window. Cartoon, knit a blanket, make a collage.

Buy some coloring books and color. Make I-Love-You posters for your friends and family. Buy a journal and draw pictures. Make a colorful mosaic. Stencil, quilt, use stickers. Make greeting cards, draw animals, do collages, take your photographs and create collages of pictures and words.

So, put on some music and create! You'll feel a positive change in your body's physiology and attitude.

• Take a Vacation

Consider taking a vacation, a mini-vacation, or a one or two night getaway to a nearby area. If you are doing an IVF or IUI, it might help to spend a week before or after at a local beach, lake, or beautiful inn. Only consider a vacation if it will relax, not stress you. For some people, a change of scenery and escaping everyday life can help them relax. Escaping to somewhere with natural beauty, such as an ocean, mountain or river, can be very soothing.

• Do Something Nice for Someone

Helping another person is a great way to relieve stress. When we do altruistic deeds, we experience a 'helper's high' which lowers our stress levels and improves our health. Doing kind deeds triggers our brain's reward circuitry—and 'feel-good' chemicals like dopamine and endorphin are released. Buy a friend flowers, make cookies for an elderly neighbor, treat your mother to lunch, knit a blanket for a local homeless shelter, write a loving letter or card. Set a goal that you will do one kind deed a week – or everyday if possible.

Kind deeds can include writing a poem for someone special, putting together a healthy fruit basket, putting a coin in an expired meter, paying the toll for the person behind you, dropping a favorite coffee off for a friend, creating a recipe book for someone who wants to learn to cook, writing a thank you note to a teacher or professor who changed your life, weeding someone's garden, cleaning someone's house, making a bagged lunch for someone.

Doing something nice for someone can cost nothing to very little, but can make someone in your life feel happier, loved and thought of.

- **Feed the Birds**

Hang a bird feeder and welcome some birds into your life.

- **Smile as Much As You Can**

Then smile some more.

- **Join A Group**

Join a book club, knitting club, garden club or some other activity that gives you a chance to be with people.

- **Spend Time With Others**

We are happier when we spend time with others. Even if you are super busy, try to make some time every day to enjoy tconversation and companionship of others. If you find yourself alone a lot, try to invite someone over at least once a week. Make a lunch date, meet in a park for a picnic, go walking or shopping together.

- **Distract Yourself**

Distraction can be a way to alleviate stress. Instead of sinking into feelings of stress, start distracting yourself with fun, interesting activities. Learn cake decorating and donate cakes to brides. Start a bird sanctuary in your yard. Volunteer to beautify your town.

Learn to knit, crochet, or do needlepoint, and with each stitch, say positive words like "love" "miracle" "safety." Get a greenhouse and become an expert gardener. When I was going through infertility treatments, I kept a seed catalog by my bed that I looked at every night. Somehow, looking at all the varieties of vegetables and flowers calmed me tremendously. Try difficult puzzles. Learn an instrument. Take singing lessons. Write a book. Create a new cartoon. Photograph every tree in your town. Learn to make jewelry. Make scrapbooks for friends. Learn a new language. Go to local plays or musicals. Offer to make costumes or set designs for a local theatre company. Volunteer at a local animal shelter. Join a local singing group.

Learn a new language or about every animal native to your area. You get the idea: distract, distract, distract. Put your brain into something that will give you a break from thinking about what stresses you.

• Write One Love Note a Day

A love note can be written to anyone in your life you care about, your sweetie, a best friend, a former co-worker you lost touch with, or a teacher you had as a child. The goal is to spread love, appreciation, and good will.

• Massage Can Help Release Stress

Massage can help release stored memories impacting the body. So get a massage or give a massage! Either way, you'll find yourself a lot more relaxed.

• Cuddle More

Cuddle with your spouse, your pets, your Mom and Dad, your best friend. Hug, hug, hug. Hold hands. Let yourself touch and be touched. Experience the power of a good long cuddle.

- **Don't Forget To Kiss**

Yup, kissing relieves stress too!

- **Spend $3 A Week On Someone Else**

Spend $3 a week on someone else. Buy a friend a pair of earrings, a bag of jelly beans for a neighbor, a book of stickers or crayons for your niece. Doing small acts of kindness relieve stress.

- **Do Things That Made You Happy As A Child**

Your original self holds many keys to what makes you authentically happy. This part of you knows what genuinely feeds her soul, without all the adult voices and restrictions telling her what she is suppose to do or suppose to like. Ask yourself: what did I love to do most as a child? What activities, places, games, hobbies made me totally relax and lose track of time? Try to bring some of your childhood passions into your life now.

Chapter 11: Freeing Your Body from the Traumas and Painful Memories That Might Be Destroying Your Fertility

Our body is a walking history of our life. There is always a very strong and direct relationship between your emotional life and your physical health. You may not realize it, but trauma and painful experiences in your life can impact your fertility in a very significant way.

Your body contains and records all the traumatic and painful experiences you have endured. It then stores these traumas and sad memories in your cells and tissues.

Traumas, from rape or incest, to being bullied, criticized or rejected, can form negative pockets of energy in our cells and organs. Our bodies remember and trap feelings of fear, sadness, rejection, loneliness, betrayal, abuse, or disrespect in our cells. Our vitality and overall health is severely weakened once these negative pockets of energy inhabit our body.

Even if a trauma occurred long ago, its negative energy can remain stuck in our cells for decades.

Our brain produces neuropeptides in response to our emotions, and these peptides interact with the cells in our body, firmly connecting our mind, emotions and body. The feelings and thoughts then trigger physiological responses in our body that affect the chemical and neurological balance of the hormones involved in reproduction.

Never underestimate the brutal and destructive power that traumatic and upsetting life experiences can have on your fertility.

Since everything we have experienced since birth accumulates within us, to regain our health and fertility, we need to release and let go of these trauma pockets in our body that weaken us.

By releasing trauma pockets in the body, we are giving our body a chance to be restored to its true fertility potential.

When you release trauma, you are giving your body a chance to let go of the negative energy pockets stuck in the body.

Once these negative energy pockets are released, our bodies are free and unburdened from energy-draining emotions like hurt, anger, grief or shock.

Letting go, moving forward, forgiving ourselves and others, are all part of the release that is needed so that the traumas stuck in our body can no longer impact our infertility in a negative way.

Do not ignore this aspect of healing. You might have gone through a trauma or an extreme emotion that is altering the state of your body and ultimately stealing your fertility.

Here are some ways to rid your body of the traumas, painful memories and destructive emotions that could be interfering with your body reaching its maximum health potential and your right to have a baby:

- One of the best and most powerful ways to release and unblock emotional traumas that have physically lodged themselves within your cells and tissues is through body work. Various forms of holistic treatments are available that can unblock emotional traumas. These include: chiropractic adjustments, myofascial release, cranio sacral therapy, Somato Emotional Release, deep tissue massage, trauma release massage, neuromuscular therapy, Neuro Emotional Technique, Thought Field Therapy. Zero Balancing, therapeutic touch, reflexology, kinesiology, fascia release, trauma touch therapy, Somatic Experiencing, EFT, therapeutic body work, emotional release bodywork, or light therapy. You can do an online search using these terms, adding your city or town, to see what is available in your area.

- Consider applied kinesiology, a very powerful form of trauma release. It can be done by a kinesiologist, chiropractor or other holistic practitioner skilled in kinesiology, also known as applied kinesiology.

First, write a list of the traumatic and painful events you have experienced in your life, including names of the people who have hurt you. Give this list to a kinesiologist and ask that they muscle test each item on your list. If the kinesiologist finds that you are storing trauma associated with a certain person or experience, they can then apply an activator instrument that looks like a small, hand-held gun type mechanism, to release the emotion or trauma at its location in your body. This is a non-invasive treatment that can help you let go of long-held traumas and painful memories. If you have gone through a lot in your life, you may want to consider doing at least three or four treatments, or going on a weekly basis.

• Homeopathy and flower essences can be used also as a way to release traumas within the body.

• Write the experiences and events in your life that caused you a great deal of grief, trauma and fear, put them in an envelope, seal them and say goodbye to them. Mail them to an unknown address or to yourself. In these letters, say what you need to say and stand up for your right to voice out loud whatever you feel needs to be said.

Your memories do not have to stay locked up inside of you. You have a right to write letters stating the truth of your pain. Even if you blame yourself or think whatever happened is your fault, trust me, whatever happened is not your fault—and feelings of shame need to be sent on their way—because you have a right to your emotions, a right to your anger, and shame no right to keep you prisoner any longer.

• Write down all your painful memories, burn them in a fire and bury the ashes. You can do this outdoors in a fire pit, a bonfire, or in an indoor fireplace. You can do this alone, or with family and friends. Whatever you choose, it is a chance for you to physically see the end of the painful memories in your life. As they burn, consider these memories as disappearing so now you can allow health, happiness and vibrant fertility in your life.Throw the ashes of these memories into the ocean, a lake, or bury them. The hold these traumas have over you is now gone.

- Write a letter to yourself that gives you permission to say goodbye to your painful memories. When writing this letter, show love, compassion, forgiveness, and kindness to yourself. Let yourself know it is safe and okay to let go of the traumas of the past—that you are not safe by holding on and reliving these traumas over and over again. Let yourself know that you are not to blame for these events, nor should you keep holding yourself hostage to their power because of misguided shame you might be carrying.

- Pray about these old memories and ask God that their hold on you be released so that your body can heal and move forward.

- When you swim, walk or work-out, imagine that you are releasing and sweating away toxic, negative patterns in your body. For example, if you are taking a walk, with each step repeat: I am walking away from my pain, I am walking away from my pain, I am walking away from my pain. If you swim, with each lap affirm: My traumas are floating away. My traumas are floating away. My traumas are floating away.
Or you could say: My hurt is being washed away, my hurt is being washed away, my hurt is being washed away. Exercise can be a way to physically release emotional pain.

- Write letters to the people in your past who hurt you or let you down. You never have to mail them, but in writing to them, you will energetically be releasing some of your pent-up feelings. Pour out your emotions, especially if there are people or incidents you think of often. Don't do this exercise if you have already moved past painful incidents in your life, because regurgitating old memories sometimes resurrects the pain and makes it worse. But if you find anger, sadness or other emotions pertaining to these incidents coming up often, then it is time for some cleansing and releasing. Don't be embarrassed that you are still hurt by an incident that occurred decades ago, or one that may not seem significant to others. If it hurt you and you still think or dream about it, then it deserves to be acknowledged and released.

We humans feel deeply, and we should not be ashamed of our sensitivity, our emotions or the impact that negative, toxic people and events can have on our lives.

• Volunteer to help others who have suffered or been violated in the same way you were. Helping others is a very powerful way to heal yourself. For example, if you are a victim of some form of childhood abuse, find a way to help other victims of abuse. Or if you need to heal from bullying, volunteer to help stop bullying in your area. Empowering and helping others is a form of taking back your own power. By using your energy and insight to heal others, you will also begin to heal yourself.

• Write a play starring yourself as a main character and tell the story of how this character releases her sad memories and goes on to give birth to a beautiful baby. You may want to act out this play before very trusted family and friends, or it might be a play for you alone to enjoy. Either way is fine. Just remember: don't be afraid to write a happy ending to this story.

• Buy a bouquet of balloons, write your painful memories, tape them to the balloons, and then let them go one-by-one, saying goodbye to the negative impact these events had on your life.

• Plant a garden and name each flower a positive emotion growing within your body, such as joy, self-love, self-acceptance, an ability to see beauty, or an ability to experience joy. As your flowers grow, see them as a physical manifestation of the positive emotions growing within you.

• Write a song about the memories that weigh you down, but be sure to end the song with your letting go and moving past these memories, and on to the life you desire, surrounded by your children.

• Get a pet and talk with your pet daily about the memories that hold you prisoner. Keep an image that your pet is listening, silently healing you and unconditionally accepting you.

• Pray, pray, pray. Then pray some more.

- Have a conversation with yourself, making sure you know that whatever trauma you went through is not your fault. I repeat: NOT YOUR FAULT. Write a letter to yourself making sure that every part of you knows IT IS NOT YOUR FAULT.

- Write to characters in literature or history and tell them your life story. Select characters that you feel may have experienced some of the same difficult experiences you have. Ask for their advice and support in moving on to the next stage of your life. Then, write back to yourself as these characters, giving you support and advice

- Take a dance class and utilize the motion of dance to release toxic emotions.

- Paint a picture of the emotional pain that lives inside your body. Name the pain. As you paint, let your inner knowing come forward to paint where your cells have stored these traumas. Use colors that express your pain. Paint pictures of the energy trapped in your cells being healed. Paint positive images of peace and joy entering your cells and tissues, allowing your fertility to blossom within you.

- Aim to forgive. Aim to forget. Aim to accept all the imperfections in this world and still see the beauty around you. Aim to forgive even those who don't deserve your forgiveness. You might start a forgiveness journal, and each day write: I forgive _____, I forgive _____. Allow yourself to feel the relief and joy that forgiving another—even someone totally undeserving—can bring. It is understandably hard, but you deserve a future free of the pain and anger that not forgiving will bear upon you.

- Buy or make yourself a blanket of safety. Make a blanket that symbolizes being safe—using colors, pictures, images, quotes and fabrics that give you a feeling of safety. You could make a blanket with pictures of people and places that soothe you and make you feel loved. Use material that you find pleasing and welcoming to touch. Or buy a blanket that appeals to you—it can be a kid's blanket, a lovely floral blanket, a big cozy blanket—and call it your 'safety' blanket. Sew some words on the blanket, such as 'It Is Safe For Me To Have A Baby' or 'I am Safe.'

During times of stress or sadness, wrap yourself in this blanket and let yourself feel safe. Envision this blanket providing you safety from the pains of the past.

- It is time to give yourself the empathy you deserve, whether you ever received it from others or not. If you find yourself thinking: I am insignificant, I am a failure, I am unlovable, I can't trust anyone, I am broken, I don't deserve to be happy, you need to replace these statements with: I am significant. I am a success. I am lovable. I can trust good people. I am strong and whole. I deserve to be happy.

- Spend some time looking for what positives may have come from the traumas in your life. Are you a kinder person because of the cruelties you experienced? Are you more sensitive to the feelings of others because your feelings were disgarded? Are you a good listener because you know what it is like not to be listened to? Do you try not to hurt the feelings of others because of the betrayals and rejections you experienced? Do you look for the good in others because the constant criticism you received was so painful? Did your negative life experiences make you more determined? Hard-working? Self-sufficient? Intuitive? Wise? Forgiving? Empathetic? Generous? Write down all the ways you are a nicer, kinder, stronger, person because of difficulties you endured. Let yourself see the positives that these traumas brought you—not because you deserved to have these traumas happen, but because your body deserves to start feeling some peace.

- Write 'forgiveness cards' to those who have hurt you, and when writing them, try to see the hurt and pain those who have hurt you may have felt that led them to such injurious actions. In seeing their pain and wishing for a healing for them, you will begin to heal yourself. Through forgiveness and understanding the pain of others, compassion can begin to replace anger. You don't have to mail the cards, but you can release them in some way, sending forgiveness into the universe.

- Next time a traumatic memory comes into your mind, give yourself support by repeating words like: 'I am safe' or 'life is beautiful.' Other supportive statements you can repeat include: Love Is Here. Love Is Now. Love Is With Me.

- Your story deserves to be told. Write it, videotape it, share it with others, blog it, say it. Tell it in the form of a book, a play, a journal, an essay, a musical or in song. Let yourself be heard. Share it with friends, family or strangers.

As you tell your story, make sure that you note the gifts, values and strengths you maintained despite the hurt you endured.

- Write a Declaration of Independence from your pain...stating your inalienable right to happiness, peace, feelings of security, safety and fertility! Then sign the document and make it official: you are free. You might even want to have a signing ceremony, with a fancy document and pen, making your freedom from emotional pain official!

- Get in touch with the beliefs that sprung up within you due to the pain you experienced that might be in some way holding you back. Begin seeing those beliefs as counterfeit balloons that need to be popped! Actually, go out and get some balloons, write these limiting and constricting beliefs on the balloon and then pop them!

- Begin to live a lifestyle where your vitality and adaptive energy can be restored, so that you have the energy to release the traumas in your body. Make sure to eat and juice a lot of greens to better alkalize your body, which can help give you the energy you will most need to heal from life's injustices and traumas.

- Ground your energy by getting in close contact with the earth. Walk barefoot outside. Put your hands in water. Start gardening. Your body needs the healing the earth itself can provide.

- Flood your life with positive experiences, positive words, positive images, and positive events. It has been said that the mind can only hold one thought at once. That being said, try pouring more joy into your life than you ever have before. Plan a party for someone you love, or a child at a group home, or a loved one nearing a big milestone. Learn a new skill that puts you into a state of flow. Plan a wonderful trip to a location you have always wanted to visit. Repeat the words: Life is beautiful. Life is beautiful. Life is beautiful...about 100 times a day.

Buy a bouquet of flowers for someone every week. Plant 1,000 tulips in your backyard. Start a band. Write a musical. Bake a different flavor cupcake every week and give them to strangers.

You get the idea. Fill your life with so many positive, generous acts and experiences that you tip the scales towards joy more than you ever have before.

• Let yourself feel and then take action. Acknowledge your feelings. Then commit to an action that will make a difference in your life and in the lives of others who may be suffering too. No act is too small if you can relieve the pain of another who is suffering.

• Write a congratulations card to yourself. Congratulate yourself on how you endured so much and how you are not allowing traumas from the past to hold you down anymore.

Chapter 12: Letting Go Of the Secret Thoughts and Hidden Beliefs That Might be Holding You Back from Getting Pregnant

You may find this hard to believe, but hidden within your subconscious could be some negative perceptions of pregnancy, childbirth and motherhood that are holding you back from having a baby, without you even knowing it.

You may have some hidden fears or beliefs about becoming a mother that conflict with your desire to have a baby.

Sometimes, the body can hold two very different desires at once. One part of us wants one thing, another part of us wants another. Consciously, you may want to become a mother more than anything in the world. Subconsciously, you may have fears that are making it hard for your conscious wishes to come true. These two very different parts of you could be playing a tug of war: who will win? Who will get their way? Whose needs will be met? This conflict can make it hard for us to really commit and do the work needed to get what we want. This tug of war steals energy away from what your body really needs to be doing—and that is healing and getting pregnant.

Ultimately, the goal should be that all the different parts of you are working harmoniously together and have the same goal: to conceive a baby.

Deep fears and childhood issues sometimes need to be acknowledged, listened to and healed so you can move forward in having a child. It is important that you discover and acknowledge all your feelings and beliefs about becoming a mother—even the ones that are not all warm and fuzzy. Our conscious self might want something, but if our subconscious does not want it, it could be off doing a dance of its own. If your subconscious doesn't want something, your body could follow suit.

Subconscious fears about pregnancy, child birth or raising a child could even at times influence your hormones and the physical processes required for conception.

Does having doubt, fear, or hesitance about having children mean you won't be a great mother? Not at all. Millions of great Moms once had doubts or fears about becoming a mother. Millions more worried about pregnancy, childbirth and how their life would change. Embarking on a new life path naturally brings up feelings of doubt and fear.

To find out what your subconscious really thinks about getting having a child, start by asking yourself what you think about becoming a mother, and then write down whatever response comes from you without editing yourself. Allow your subconscious to voice its feelings on the subject without judgment or criticism.

Negative feelings or beliefs left unexpressed or unresolved hold considerable energy which can block conception. If you ignore your subconscious, it might stage a rebellion within your body—not allowing you to get pregnant because it wasn't given the respect and attention it deserved.

Begin by writing: "I will become pregnant soon" or "My womb is ready to receive" and then after you write that, start writing whatever comes up from deep within. Let whatever comes up from within you come up, come out and be heard. Write without editing or judging what you are writing. Do not consciously think about what is coming up, or try to force something you don't really feel or think. Just write.

This exercise can help you uncover what you are feeling about your infertility on many levels. It can also reveal if there is a part of you that wants to sabotage your efforts to become pregnant, or feels that you are not worthy of a baby. By knowing your innermost feelings, you can then work on bringing together the different emotions within you, so that you can achieve your goal. Later on, reread what you wrote and thank your subconscious for opening up.

Try not to judge your subconscious, even if what comes up is not exactly what you want to hear.

You could also write down the words: 'I deserve to have a baby' and then type or handwrite whatever comes up. Remember: No judging. No editing. No thinking this out. Write without restraint and let your deep internal self say what it needs to say.

Other writing prompts include:

- My body is ready to conceive and give birth to a baby
- It is safe to have a baby
- I deserve to have a baby
- I am good enough to be a mother and give birth to a baby
- My body is capable of giving birth
- A woman like me deserves to be a mother
- I am ready to be a mother and have children
- It is safe for me to become a mother
- Being a mother is a good thing for me

Honestly listening to every part of yourself shows your courage, because you are not going into denial.

Every part of you needs deserves to be listened to so they can all work together. If you ignore the needs of your subconscious, it could sabotage all the hard work you are doing to get pregnant.

Here are some questions to ask yourself, write responses to, and spend some time thinking about.

- **Are you afraid of repeating the same mistakes your parents made?:** Do you fear repeating some of the negative and dysfunctional family patterns you grew up with? Do you sometimes find yourself thinking, 'when I become a parent, I never want to do to my child what my parents did to me' or 'I never want to put my kids through what my parents put me through.'

- **Are you scared of becoming a mother?:** Do you have fears about becoming a mother, such as or 'I'm afraid of who I will become when I have a child' or 'I'm afraid I don't have what it takes to be a good Mom' or 'I'm afraid I won't be able to care for my child properly.'

- **Are you worried about losing some of your me-time once you have a baby?:** Are there aspects of your life that you really like that you are worried you will lose once you have a baby?

- **Do you fear that once you become a mother, you will turn into your own mother?:** Did your Mom behave or act in a way that you don't want to repeat and hurt you a lot as a child? Or did your Mom do things that you promised yourself you would never do? Did you long ago make a silent pact with yourself that you would never become your mother?

- **Do you sometimes feel infertility is a deserved punishment, either from yourself or from God, for something you've done or didn't do, in the past?:** Could infertility be something you think you deserve to suffer? Did you do something, or not do something, you believe merits you being infertile?

- **Do you feel God is mad at you?:** Do you feel God is judging you harshly for something you did in your past that you still feel guilty about?

- **Were you a victim of physical, sexual abuse or emotional abuse? Did you have an abusive parent?:** Do you ever fear that you will become an abusive parent like they were? If so, you might fear repeating negative family patterns.

- **Did you ever experience a trauma that has left you feeling unsafe and weary of new experiences?:** Are you open to new experiences or does doing something for the first time unnerve you? Do you often feel scared and worried about your safety?

- **Are you a bit of a control freak?:** Do you need to control everything in your life? Or are you able to let life flow naturally towards you? Does the idea of having a baby make you feel too out of control? Are you the type of person who needs to control everything in your life, and letting life happen is not something you are comfortable with?

- **Do you feel you really deserve a baby?:** Or do you feel unworthy of this joy? Is there something about who you are, or what you have done or experienced in life, that makes you think someone like you doesn't deserve a baby? Do you feel worthy of getting what you want?

- **Does yearning for something feel more natural and comfortable than actually getting what you want?:** Have you spent a lot of your life yearning? Are you the type of person who feels more comfortable when you are yearning, wanting or suffering over something you can't have?

- **Are you more comfortable when you are the one giving, rather than the one receiving?:** Do things like getting a gift or a compliment make you feel uncomfortable? Are you in the habit of being able to be on the receiving end of things?

- **Do you feel confident in your body's ability to give birth, or did you ever suffer an illness or injury that has shaken your belief in what your body can do?:** Do you see your body as weak and incapable? Have you ever suffered from a trauma or an illness that has left you doubting your body's strength and capability? Does physical pain of any sort bring up bad memories for you?

- **When you think of being pregnant, does the word 'fat' come to your mind?:** Do you consider pregnant women beautiful or unattractive? Do you fear losing your shape or physical beauty once you have a baby? Do you fear that pregnancy will ruin your body? Do you see pregnancy as an empowering event for your body or something that will steal the hot body you are proud of.

- **Does the work of caring for a baby seem overwhelming? Are you afraid of the demands that a child will make on your life?:** Do you ever see mothers with their children and think 'I could never do all that work.'

- **When you hear the word 'mother' do positive or negative images come to your mind?:** Do you associate the title 'mother' with positive, loving images or negative, frightening images?

Do you think of the positive words associated with mothers, such as loving, protective, warm, or do you think of the negative connotations surrounding motherhood sometimes promoted in the media, such as being controlling or demanding?

- **Do you fear going through childbirth or did your mother go through a very hard delivery with you?:** Do images of a woman screaming in pain come to your mind when you think of childbirth? Did you grow up hearing horror stories about your own birth? Did your mother talk a lot about the difficulty she had giving birth to you or a sibling? Do you have any negative thoughts about childbirth, due to media images or experiences of family or friends?

- **Did your own mother enjoy having children or did she complain about how hard it was to be a mother?:** Did you grow up with a mother, or a father, who found being a parent very difficult? As a child, could you sometimes sense how frustrated or overwhelmed your parents were with raising children? Did their experience taint your view of parenthood?

- **Do you fear that your body can't survive childbirth? Does being pregnant or giving birth seem dangerous to you in any way?:** On some level, do you fear you might die during childbirth? Do you think being pregnant hurts? Do you have concerns about the physical dangers of child birth? Do you see woman as being in danger when they are pregnant or give birth?

- **Do you feel ashamed because you want a baby?:** Does your intense desire to be a mother make you feel ashamed? In general, do you often feel the emotion of shame, especially when it comes to your own desires and needs?

- **Do you feel capable of caring for a child and being a good mother? Did someone ever say or suggest you would be a terrible mother? Or that you are not capable of being a mother?:** Sometimes people can see us in one way only, and because we've never done something, they cannot imagine us doing it.

- **Were you ever at the mercy of a female who was cruel to you?:** Have you somehow equated the cruelty of a mother, stepmother or female caretaker with a role you are about to step into?

- **Have you spend a lot of your life trying not to get pregnant?:** Have you told your body that it is now okay to get pregnant? Have you given your body permission to get pregnant?

- **Do you respect your feminine self and genuinely like being a woman?:** Or do you see things defined as feminine as dumb, stupid or unworthy of respect? Do you respect the feminine body that has the ability to carry and give birth to a child, or is there a part of you that disrespects the feminine body?

- **Do you trust yourself enough to become a mother?:** Or because of your family history or childhood experiences, do you distrust yourself?

- **Do you fear that becoming a mother will change you in a way that you don't want to change?:** Do you fear having a child will change something about who you are, or a part of your personality, you value and like about yourself?

- **Do you worry a lot about having a child with birth defects?:** Do you think a lot about the 'what ifs'?

- **Do you fear that you don't have what it takes to be a good mother?:** Is there some aspect of your personality or character that makes you think that women like you are not cut out to be good mothers? Have friends or family ever joked that you would be a terrible mother?

- **Is your husband/partner truly the person you want to have a baby with?:** Or do you have doubts about raising a child with him? Do you think your partner will be a good father or not?

- **Do you worry about certain choices you might be forced to make when you have a child, such as what religion you will raise them in, or how you will pay for college?:** Do you find yourself worrying about the choices that will face you when you have a child?

- **Do you link being a mother to having to endure some type of suffering?:** Did you ever, somewhere along the way, get the idea that being a mother equals some type of physical or emotional suffering?

- **Do you think having children ruined your mother's life or trapped her in some way? Do you fear becoming a Mom will trap you also?:** Did you ever see your own mother as being trapped because she had children? Do you think your mother was trapped in a bad marriage because she had you? Or did she suffer economic hardship because she was raising children? Did she give up a promising career because she was a mother? Did you ever see your mother struggling and think, 'I never want to trapped like my Mom."

- **Do you fear you are too old to have a baby?:** What are your views on aging? Do you sometimes think that only young women can have healthy babies?

- **Do you fear that this is an unsafe world to bring a child into?:** Do you worry about bringing a child into a world with problems? Do you watch the evening news and think 'how could anyone bring a child into this world'?

- **Do you feel guilty bringing a child into this world?:** Do you ever feel selfish for wanting to have a baby?

- **Do you ever feel like you can't afford a child?:** Do you think a lot about how you will afford to raise children? Are you worried about the financial responsibility of raising a child?

- **Do you fear that having a child could destroy your marriage?:** Do you worry that your relationship with your husband will change once you have a baby?

- **Do you worry that your sex life will end once you become a mother?:** Do you think that Moms are sexy? Or do you think the sensual part of a woman disappears once she becomes a mother?

- **Do you fear that having a child will destroy your career?:** Do you love working and worry a lot about how you will continue your career once you have children to take care of? Do you fear that having a child will put an end to all the other goals that are important to you?

- **Do you fear that having children will threaten some of the important relationships in your life?:** Are there relationships in your life that you fear will be threatened once you have kids? Do your friends have children or are they childless?

- **Are you a perfectionist who thinks you need to be perfect and everything in your life should be perfect before you become a mother?:** Do you feel you should be perfect before becoming a mother? Do you want to be a good mother so badly that a part of you believes only being perfect is good enough?

- **Do you welcome change into your life?:** Or are you the type of person who fights change and finds any type of change very difficult?

- **Did your own mother abandon you, either due to divorce, death or neglect?:** If you were abandoned in any way by your mother, having a child and becoming a mother yourself may bring up a lot of fear. Secretly, you may fear that you are going to be like your mother and abandon your children also. You might fear repeating your mother's negative pattern of abandonment.

You might still feel so angry at the feminine role model in your life, i.e. your mother, that having anything in common with her, a.k.a. both being mothers, might be something you want desperately to avoid.

Within you, might be a little girl still longing for her mother—so much so, that becoming a mother might be something your 'little girl within' resists. Or, you might blame yourself for your mother leaving, and subconsciously you equate children with pain because on some level, you believe your mother's leaving you was justified on her part. So why would you feel comfortable having a child—when a part of you believes children deserve to be left?

- **Was one of your parents an alcoholic or drug addict?:** If so, you may fear that having a child will kick off this cycle again. Maybe you blamed yourself for your parent's addiction—and now you wonder if having a child will spark an addiction within you.

- **Do you tend to shy away from responsibility?:** Does the responsibility of becoming a parent scare you? Are you often scared of taking on new responsibilities in general? Do you have confidence in your ability to take on new life assignments, or do you doubt yourself?

- **Do You Say No A lot Easier And Quicker Than You Say Yes:** Do you more often say no than yes?

Here are some thoughts that might help you heal some the fears and beliefs that could be blocking your infertility:

- **You don't have to be perfect to be a good mother.** Let go of the idea that for you to be a mother, it is perfect or bust. There are millions of kind, loving mothers who are not perfect in any way and make lots and lots of mistakes—and yes, their kids turned out fine. You will make mistakes and that is okay. Let go of the notion of perfect. It doesn't exist. You are not perfect right now, nor will you be once you have a child…and that is perfectly okay. Millions of children grow up to be happy, functioning adults and none of them had perfect parents. Remind yourself that being a good mother is one who tries hard, admits their mistakes and learns from them.

- **If you feel your parents made a lot of mistakes in raising you, remind yourself that learning from the mistakes of others is something we humans can do very well.** If your parents behaviors or choices hurt you deeply and resulted in your having a difficult childhood, set out to make a conscious decision to make different choices than they made.

Remember: you are not your mother and father. You can learn from their good choices and from their bad ones. You are not a prisoner of your family history or family patterns. You can do it differently. You have choices about how you will live your life. You are not pre-destined to do what your parents did.

You can educate yourself through the thousands of books on healthy parenting. You can find a person you consider a good parent to mentor you. You can do a form of therapy that heals you and helps you formulate a plan of how you will handle some of the challenges your parents didn't handle so well. You can pray to God everyday to be a decent, kind and loving parent.

You have the right to write your own life script, one very different from your parents.

You've got the key—now let yourself out.

There are resources within you and in the world around you that can help you be the parent you want to be, regardless of the family you come from. You can acknowledge the weaknesses that existed within your family—and then you can work hard to avoid the behaviors and choices that fueled the negative behaviors.

Simply making the decision that you will try to be a loving, kind and hard-working parent is a great start. If you feel you face a special challenge due to your family background, such as a history of alcoholism or sexual abuse, don't be ashamed to look for help in breaking destructive family patterns.

- **Remember that being a mother does not mean you have give up all the other parts of yourself that you value.** There are millions of mothers who live a life that is true to who they are. Many mothers continue being artists, writers, poets, doctors, lawyers, teachers and whatever else they choose to be, while raising their children.

You have a right to hold on to the parts of you that you hold sacred and dear, and in being true to yourself, you will be setting a great example for your child. While being a mother does require hard work and sacrifice, it should not mandate giving up all the parts of yourself that you cherish.

- **You are allowed to have more than one dream.** It is okay to dream of being a mother—and okay to have other dreams too. More than one life dream is allowed.

- **If you worry about losing me-time once you have a baby, create a plan that will give you some of the alone time you need.** Are there grandparents or relatives nearby who are willing to babysit? What childcare options are available to you?

Remember: you are not a bad Mom if sometimes you need time for yourself. But, you might actually enjoy spending time with your little one much more than you now realize.

- **Did your mother behave or live her life in a way that hurt you?** If you fear that having a child will turn you into your mother, remember once you consciously acknowledge something and bring it into the light, its hold on you is significantly lessened. If you believe you have qualities or personality traits like your Mom that you don't want to repeat, seek help and learn how to break negative behaviors and patterns.

Be aware that no two people are exactly alike even if they are alike. Your situation and life experience doesn't have to be the same as your mothers. In fact, you can learn from your mother in what not to do. You can spend some time analyzing what your mother might have needed that would have made things easier for her. Did your mother need some type of medication to address a mental health issue? Did she need exercise, a creative outlet outside the house, a different diet that would have better suited her needs?

You also have to realize that times have changed since you were a child, and challenges your mother faced might not even exist today.

You are not sentenced to recreate the dysfunction of your Mom if you choose not to.

- **If something within you makes you feel unworthy or undeserving of being a mother, remember that as a human being, you are worthy and this is your natural birthright.** Remind yourself daily that you deserve to have the baby of your dreams, and you don't need to be perfect to enjoy this role. Let go of the idea that you deserve punishment in any way. Love yourself, forgive yourself, and repeat: I deserve a baby, I deserve a baby, I am worthy of having a baby.

- **Many women, before becoming mothers, wonder if they are capable of caring for a baby.** It is a natural concern, and yet step-by-step, day- by-day, millions of women learn how to care for their babies with great and profound knowledge, insight, strength and love. You have within you the capacity to learn and grow.

You don't need to know everything all at once. You have to trust the learning process your life as a mother will provide you with. There are hundreds of books on childcare that you can read, and you can talk and get tips from other mothers on how to care for children.

- **If doing something new feels unsafe or frightening, start saying to yourself: 'new experiences are safe for me' or 'it is safe for me to have a baby' several times a day.** Often, the most frightening aspect of doing anything new is the time before you actually do it, when you are thinking about and imagining yourself doing it. Did you ever worry about something you were going to do that you never did before, but once you dived in and started doing it, a lot of the fear disappeared, becasue you realized it was not as hard as you thought it would be.

Many of your fears will disappear once you actually have a child. Fears of changing a diaper, feeding a baby, keeping a baby safe, will dissolve as you actually do it. Before I had children, I really believed I could not endure changing a diaper. Once I had a baby, I actually loved changing diapers and had no problem with it at all.

- **If you tend to be a control-freak or just someone who likes a measure of control in your life, set up things ahead of time that will give you a feeling of being in control.** Then, trust. Just trust. It will be okay. You may need to learn how to let life happen, rather than always trying to control.

- **If you've had health issues in the past, remind yourself that the human body is strong and resilient.** If there are aspects of childbirth that worry you, talk with your doctor about planning a birth experience that you will feel safe with. It is okay to do whatever is necessary to reduce the pain you will experience. No guilt please on that one.

While some women are okay with no pain medication, other women welcome relief from the pain involved with childbirth—and that is perfectly okay too. Even if your mother had a very difficult delivery with you, remind yourself that times have changed, medical procedures have advanced, and that you will probably have a different doctor and experience than she had.

• **If you worry constantly that you are not going to be a good mother, relax and take the pressure off yourself.** In the media, we are presented two very different versions of motherhood. One is the perfectly sweet, kind, loving mother and the other is the evil, controlling, wicked selfish mother. The reality is most mothers are not all-goodness or all-evil. Take the pressure off yourself. Yes, you have a responsibility to treat your child with love and kindness, but nobody is perfect—even the most perfect of mothers are not perfect. A side note here: this does not give you permission to be abusive, cruel, neglectful, or dismissive to your child, but it does give you permission to be human.

• **If sometimes you fear that having a child will be too much work for you and that you are not capable, repeat and think about these affirmations: I am capable of being a Mom.** I am capable of learning. I am capable of working hard when I need to. I am capable of trying again when I make a mistake. I am capable of improving on skills I already have and acquiring skills I don't have.

• **If you have worked hard to be in shape and fear that pregnancy and childbirth will ruin your body, remind yourself that there are many, many hot Moms out there.** Women who work out and eat well usually look great, whether they have no kids or five kids. The habits that put you in good shape will still be available to you, whether you are a Mom or not. Think of it this way: when you are 80 years old, do you want to have a human being beside you or a picture of how great you looked way back when.

Start to see pregnancy and childbirth as an empowering event for your body, where you get to tap into your body's full potential.

- **Start thinking about all the fun you will have with your child, rather than the pain and loss you imagine you will experience.** Spend time thinking about what you will gain when you have a child, rather than what you will lose. Start thinking about all the positive changes that come with having a baby, rather than dwelling on what you think will be negative changes in your life. Positive changes can include: having someone to love, having another person to become stronger for, having someone to teach, nurture and do lots of fun things with.

Spend some time thinking about all the fun, life-enhancing things you will do with your child. Focus on the pleasure, not the pain, of having babies. Think about cuddling and holding your baby, baking with your little girl, playing baseball with your son, building with blocks, reading stories, spending a day at the beach, going to a park.

Think about the traditions, hobbies, and family heritage you can share with your child. Think about the beauty of creating a family, and having as your legacy your role as a mother.

When the fears start to invade your head, turn it around by thinking about the positives. Maybe even create a scrapbook entitled: The Fun I Will Have With My Child and cut out pictures of all the fun, wonderful things you plan to do together. Look at this book often, so anticipation and joy replaces the fear.

- **If your mother didn't enjoy being a mother, it doesn't mean you will feel the same way.** Think about it: is your life right now exactly like your mothers? Are you exactly like your mother? Are your circumstances identical to your mothers? When you have children, will your life be just like hers? Probably not. Repeat: I am not my mother. I will live the life I want to live, not the life my mother lived. You can also spend time analyzing what aspects of motherhood your might have found hard, and do what you can in advance to prepare yourself for such challenges.

- **If you find yourself excessively worrying about things like will my child have a birth defect, stop, read up on all the things you can do to maximize your chances for a healthy baby.** Find out what foods you can eat and supplements you can take before you get pregnant, such as folic acid. Schedule 'worry time' once a week, rather than allowing worry to crowd your thoughts on a daily basis.

- **If you have concerns about your husband being a good father, take steps to address the issue.** Talk with your husband about your concerns, attend parenting classes together, read parenting books and seek male role models that can mentor your husband in his new role as a father.

- **If you worry a lot about everything, just stop.** That's it. Stop projecting into the future. You can plan. You can take positive steps to address certain concerns, but worrying about every little thing won't serve you or your child. Stop projecting into the future. Stop playing out negative scenarios. Stop focusing on all the bad stuff. Just stop.

- **When you feel overwhelmed by negative thoughts or fears, do affirmations, such as: it is safe for me to have a baby. It is safe and okay to be pregnant.** Childbirth is easy for me. Childbirth is safe for me. I am looking forward to a beautiful birth experience. My baby and I will enjoy a beautiful birth experience.

- **Begin to link the idea of pleasure to being pregnant and having a baby.** We as humans run towards pleasure and run away from pain. To help your subconscious get over its fears, you need to begin to convince it that having a baby will mean more pleasure in your life than pain. Do a collage with positive words and images about childbirth and motherhood. Talk to your subconscious often about all the joy, happiness and contentment you will experience as a mother. Make a list of all the activities you can look forward to doing as a mother and read this list often.

- **If you have a lot of concerns about how your life will change once you have a baby, begin a preparation plan that addresses your concerns.** Bring in the support you will need.
You'll feel better, more in control, and you'll see the possibilities for creating a life with your child that pays respect to your needs.

- **If you have gone through a trauma in the past that has left you feeling perpetually unsafe, begin to do body work to release the trauma so that your body can relax and let down its guard, and allow you to have a baby.**

- **If your mother abandoned or rejected you in any way, you have seen the dark side of motherhood.** For you to become what you may hold great anger and hatred towards, you need to try to forgive your mother, and at the same time, hold the confidence that you are going to tap into the positive side of motherhood, something perhaps your own mother never did. Rather than looking at the woman who left or rejected you as a mother, you need to see her actions as a result of who she was as a person, disconnecting the link to motherhood in any way. She did not leave you because she was a mother—she left you because she was a person with flaws, deficiencies and most likely great emotional and mental pain.

It was not motherhood or being a mother that made your mother hurt you, it was something within her that most likely manifested itself in various aspects of her life, including parts of her life that had nothing to do with being a mother.

- **Feeling afraid of a big life changer like having a baby is normal.**
Having some fears, wondering if you are really ready to be a mother, does not mean you are not ready—it means you are human and millions of women throughout history have gone through similar feelings of doubt, fear and hesitation, before becoming the amazing, wonderful mothers they turn out to be. Having some natural fears and apprehension is not a sign that you are not ready, capable and able to be a great mother.

Believe it or not, it is completely normal and okay to desperately want a child and, be afraid and hesitant at the same time.

Feeling two conflicting emotions at once doesn't mean you are not ready to welcome and care for your baby. It just means you are human, and sometimes we are afraid of new experiences and changes in our lives.

Chapter 13: 50 Creative Projects To Help You Tap Into Your Fertility

Creativity is a powerful anecdote to feelings of hopelessness and depression. Doing creative activities can help you unlock and release negative energy patterns and paths in the body. Tapping into your creativity can help you transcend emotional blockages that may exist within your body.

Exploring your creativity can relax you, de-stress you, and give your body a dose of happy, healthy chemicals that can assist in healing infertility.

Here are some creative exercises and activities to try while undergoing infertility treatments:

1. Make a collage representing birth, babies, and the body's ability to conceive and have a baby.

You'll need a poster board, construction paper, or whatever kind of paper feels right to you. Cut out pictures from magazines, books, newspapers, or download and print pictures from the Internet of babies, pregnant women, along with images and words that represent what getting pregnant and having a baby means to you. Then, glue them in whatever pattern you choose on the paper or poster board of your choice.

When I was trying to get pregnant with my second child, I made a huge collage that affirmed my body's ability to get pregnant. I cut out pictures of babies and words like "the princess has arrived" and "mother love." I used lots of positive words that meant a lot to me and I personally connected to having children. My collage had pictures that represented new life emerging and the upcoming and most definite arrival of my child. I hung it in my office so I could look at it and feed off its positive energy every day.

Making this collage was a very joyful experience for me, because I had been trying for over a year to get pregnant and was not successful. I was extremely depressed, but while making the collage, I entered a very optimistic and hopeful state of mind. Every time I looked at my collage, I felt renewed hope and a surge of power—something that I needed desperately to gain back at that time. A few months later, I did become pregnant and gave birth to my beautiful son.

So, collage away. I used a huge poster board which I felt made my collage something powerful to look at. Make sure to use whatever images, pictures, words strike a personal note for you.

2. **Make a collage celebrating babies.** Cut out photos of babies from magazines and write something at the top like: Welcoming All Babies—Including Mine! Or: Welcome To All The Babies and My Baby Too! Put a picture of yourself in the middle of this collage along with something that represents your baby's arrival. In doing this, you'll be setting out the welcome mat for your baby's arrival and reminding yourself that babies are born everyday and soon yours will be too!

3. **Make a collage on the topic of fertility.** Use words and pictures that represent your body enjoying a healthy state of fertility. If you see pictures that symbolizes fertility to you, add it to your collage. Make sure to put a picture of yourself in the middle of the collage, with words like: "My Body is Fertile" or "The World Around Me Is Fertile and I Am Fertile Too" or "I Am Part of A Fertile World." Surround your picture with powerful and meaningful images of fertility that you can personally relate to.

4. **Create a scrapbook titled "My Successful Journey To Motherhood"** and include in it whatever pictures, quotes, experiences or items reflect your story of having children.

5. **Go to a crafts store and purchase pink and blue buckets and make flower arrangements that you will have in your hospital room when you have a baby.** Get flowers and decorations that you want in your room when you have a baby.

6. Play inspiring music, like the theme to the movie 'Rocky', and march around your living room, picturing your ovaries turning out a healthy baby. Play music that puts you in a state of positive expectation and joy. Allow the music to help you transcend all doubt, if even for just a few minutes. Let the music carry you into a state of being where you allow yourself to feel your dream of being a mother coming true. Play a song that represents triumph and victory as you see yourself giving birth and becoming a mother. Then, as you play this song, move, march, dance in a celebratory way that says: my baby is on the way to me soon.

7. Make a collage of all the goals and dreams in your life that came true, as a hefty reminder that good things do happen to you and will happen to you again.

By reminding yourself that you can get what you want, you'll be triggering the thought of 'it happened once, it can happen again.' Along with words and images of goals and dreams that came true, include a picture of yourself next to a baby and write on the collage, "my dream of having a baby is my next dream about to come true." Hang it in a place where you can see it often.

8. Write a song about your victory over infertility. Songwriting is a way to express your feelings about having a baby in a hopeful and positive way. Write and sing a song about the triumphant way your body was able to conceive and give birth to a baby, as if it already happened. Write a song inviting your baby to find a home in your womb. Write a song to your future child about all the wonderful things you will do together. You don't have to be musically inclined to pen a song that speaks of hope and the happiness that awaits you.

9. Cut out words that describe the strength of your body and glue them onto a large piece of poster paper. Put a picture of yourself in the center of these words, which can include words like: Fertile. Reproducing. Wise. Strong. Healthy. Ripe. Hang it somewhere where you can look at it often.

10. **Imagine you are a coach and let your inner fertility coach give you tips on how to get pregnant.** See getting pregnant as a game and listen to what your inner coach has to say about what you need to do to win this game. You can ask your inner coach to create a playbook, with what 'plays' or actions need to be taken for you to win at this fertility game. Draw a picture of your inner fertility coach and write down your inner coach's five best pieces of advice, and hang it somewhere you can see it often.

You know more than you think and this is one way to tap into that inner knowing.

11. **Make or buy a kite and write your wish to have a baby, attach it to the kite, and send the kite out into the universe.** Or attach to the kite a message inviting your future child to come to you and let it go into the world. Create as many kites as you wish and send them off with whatever message about having a baby you want to send out into the world.

12. **Write a story about the day your child is born.** Imagine the sights, the smells, the sounds, of this beautiful experience that awaits you. Write about the faces you will see, the emotions you will experience, the feeling of touching your child for the first time. As you write, let your body feel the story as if it were a reality, that already happened.
Go into detail: what hospital will you give birth in? What words will your partner, mother, and doctor say to you on the day your child is born? What will you wear to the hospital? How will you pack your suitcase? Write as if it already happened.

13. **Paint a picture of how you feel about having a baby, using colors, symbols, words and images...whatever comes up from within you about your child.**

14. **Draw a picture of yourself holding a baby or holding hands walking with your child.** Look at the picture often as if it has already come to pass.

15. **Pick a song that will be you and your child's theme song someday and play it often.** Dance to it and imagine you are dancing together at your child's wedding. Imagine you are at your child's high school graduation party and you're explaining to all the guests how this was a song you played when you were wishing and hoping for the arrival of your child. Imagine dedicating this song to your child at their kindergarten or middle school graduation party. Keep a CD in your car or download on your phone and play this song often—always imagining you and your child dancing and celebrating your love for one another.

16. **Write a story about your journey to have a child--and give it a happy ending.** Write about how you finally got pregnant, carried full term, and delivered your baby.

17. **Make a collage using images and words representing living things that reproduce, such as animals, plants, trees.** Put a picture of yourself right smack in the middle of this collage, reminding yourself that you too are part of this life cycle--a living being born with the ability and right to reproduce. Write something like: All Living Creatures Reproduce And I Can Reproduce Too!

18. **Write a story as told by your body about your problems getting pregnant.** Have your body explain what healed it and enabled it to conceive and give birth. Don't think this out--just write whatever comes. Even if it makes no sense, let whatever your body say what it wants to say. Let your body tell the story of how you healed from infertility, whether it makes sense or not.

19. **Make a collage that says 'Thank You' for all the babies that will be born on this earth in the next few years, including yours.** Say thank you for the millions of births that occur every day throughout the world, including the upcoming birth of your own baby. Include pictures, images, colors and words of gratitude that express a thankful heart for the births happening everywhere at this time—and the birth that will occur in your own life soon.

20. **Choreograph a dance that symbolizes your fertility.** Choose a song that represents your body giving birth. Create movements that mirror this amazing journey of birth that you will soon experience.

Use music, costumes and props that show your body in the state of receiving a child into your womb and then giving birth.

You could also take a dance class and ask your teacher to help you create a dance that symbolizes your journey to becoming a mother. You might want to consider taking a ballet, hip hop, jazz, belly dancing or some other type of dance class and incorporate what you learn into the dance you will create.

Once you have created your dance and chosen the music, do this dance often as an invitation for your body to follow suit. If you like, perform it for family and friends, as a way to express your fertility.

21. **Make a collage showing all the ways you are a mother right now to your family, friends, and the world around you.** Place a picture of yourself in the center of the collage and surround yourself with pictures and images of the way you now manifest your mothering ability. As you do this collage, let yourself see how you are ready and capable you are of being a mother, because in many ways, you have begun the mothering process.

22. **Draw a rainbow with the colors you associate with birth.** Put your picture in the center of the rainbow.

23. **Buy a drum and beat out the news of your child's upcoming arrival.** Play this drum in whatever way your body intuitively wants to play it, announcing to the world the soon-to-be arrival of your baby.

24. **Take walks in natural settings as much as possible, and take pictures every time you notice the birth cycle in your environment.** Say aloud, "thank you that I am part of this natural process of conceiving life and giving birth." Then, write a two-page essay on your observations regarding the birth cycle in the world around you and include your photographs in it.

25. **Get a box and each day put items inside it that symbolize the gifts you are going to share with your future children.** These gifts can include words that you will impart to your children, pictures of places you plan to visit together, lists of things you will do together, books you will read, hobbies you will pursue. It can also be items that symbolize spiritual and emotional gifts you plan to share with your children.

26. **Make a storybook of the kind of mother you want to be.** Let your inner maternal voice shine as you write, draw and paste pictures of the type of mother you plan on being to your children.

27. **Write a letter welcoming your child to the world.** Your letter can include your hopes and dreams for your child, favorite memories you want to share, and information about yourself. Put the letter or letters in a box with the words: Letters to My Child.

28. **Buy a beautiful chest and make it your baby hope chest.** Paint and decorate this chest in ways that inspire you. Then each day, put something in the chest that symbolizes your hope and confidence that your child will be born. You can put items, such as a picture of a flower that you will grow in a garden together, recipes you want to make with your child, pictures of the places you will go together, books you will to read to your children, and favorite pieces of music you want to share. Consider this box a place to put many of the dreams you have for your child and the childhood you will create for them.

29. **Go somewhere in nature, such as your backyard, and put your hands in dirt and feel the pulsating life that lives right beneath you each day.** Or buy a big pot and fill it with soil. Sit outside and let your hands dig in the soil and feel the rich fertility of the soil, reminding yourself that you are as fertile as this soil. As you feel the soil, say: I am as fertile as this soil.' Do this often.

30. **Invite family and friends who have supported you in your journey to have a baby to participate in a parade, where you all will march through a forest or your backyard, singing songs affirming that your body is healing and able to have a baby.** Invite everyone to make posters welcoming your future child. Let your friends and family nurture, love and support you, as you state aloud your firm conviction that your body can and will conceive and give birth--and that, yes, you will find a way to fulfill your desire to parent.

31. **Write a message to your future baby, put it in a bottle, and release it into the ocean.** Ask whoever finds the bottle to send you positive thoughts in your quest to have a baby.

32. **Plant a garden dedicated to your future child.** Give your garden a name and a theme. Put figurines of children in the garden, symbolizing that you are welcoming living beings into your life. Keep a journal about your experiences with this garden. Then, take a picture of your garden and put it aside as a gift to give to your future child.

33. **Get a bunch of washable paints and allow your body to completely relax as you release your feelings about giving birth through color and finger movement.** The painting doesn't have to look like anything, but simply is a way to express.

34. **Create a birthing rainbow with colors that heal you.** At the end of the rainbow, draw a picture of your baby or cut out a picture of a baby and place it there. Look at these healing colors daily--and then look at that baby at the end of the rainbow. Visualize these colors healing your body and helping you produce your 'baby at the end of the rainbow.'

35. **What do you look forward to doing with your future children?** Make a scrapbook with all the fun activities you are excited to do with your kids. This can include games you want to play, brochures of places you want to visit, and arts and craft projects you want to do together.

36. **Every morning, step outside your door, raise your arms to the sky and say, "I am ready for my baby!"** "I welcome my baby' 'Thank you for my baby.'

37. **Decorate a t-shirt with the words, "I Am Fertile."** Use colors and pictures that express your innate fertility. Wear it proudly!

38. **For one day, act as if you are pregnant.** Eat, drink, walk, sleep and move like you are pregnant. Talk as if you are already pregnant. Say right out loud, "I am pregnant." Let your body think it is pregnant.
At the end of the day, write about how you felt being pregnant. Write it as if it was a reality. Call this essay: Today I Am Pregnant.

39. **Buy a dollhouse and work on furnishing and decorating it for your future child.** Make the house something either a boy or girl would enjoy, perhaps making some rooms 'superhero' themes and other rooms more of a girl-oriented theme.

40. **Design the backyard of your dreams for your future child.** Make a collage with pictures of swing sets, pools, doll houses and more.

41. **Sing! Sing! Sing your way to pregnancy!** Select songs that imbue you with the feelings of joy and hope. Have the words of the songs in front of you, and each day, sing them aloud. As you sing, envision yourself pregnant and giving birth to your baby. Choose songs that reflect your positive vision of becoming a mother.

42. **Create a special dance for you and your husband.** Choose a song that makes you both feel very hopeful about having a baby. Choreograph this dance as a moving, living symbol of how you two will make a baby together.

43. **Paint some dishes for your future child and imagine that someday your child will eat delicious meals you prepared on them.**

44. **Create positive, hopeful greeting cards for other women experiencing infertility.** Make sure these cards offer words of hope and healing, and donate them to an infertility clinic, or give as a gift to a friend also experiencing infertility.

Or leave them in the waiting room of the clinic you go to, as a way to share and impart hope to others.

45. **Get your camera and go out and take pictures that are Proof That Miracles Happen.** Then, make a photo collage with the title: Proof That Miracles Happen. Make sure one of the pictures is of you wearing a t-shirt that says: I am pregnant!

46. **Write a one-woman play about your experiences with infertility.** But….end the play with you talking about how you became pregnant and had a baby! Speak this aloud with conviction and positive belief.

47. **Begin a daily diary that you will give to your child someday.** Start your entries by writing: To My Child or Dear Baby and share with your future child whatever you like to share about your day or your life.

48. **Set up a place in your home where you can paint your body healing from infertility.** Paint whatever colors, forms, images come to you. Let your inner artist paint whatever it wants to express about the physical and emotional healing your body needs to experience to become pregnant.

If it helps, paint the pain, emotional wounds and physical parts of your body that are calling out for healing in your infertility journey.

49. **Knit, crotchet or sew blankets, hats and clothes for your baby.** Allow yourself to picture your baby wearing them as you create them. Or, begin to sew maternity clothes for yourself, including what you want to wear the day you give birth. Sew clothes that include patches with sayings like: 'can't wait to meet you!' 'Mommy loves you!' 'So excited to see you!' on them.

50. **Make a quilt representing your journey through infertility with your desired destination of becoming a mother as part of your journey.** Create a quilt that is positive and hopeful, and conveys the idea and energy that yes—you will become pregnant and have a baby soon! Don't worry if your quilt is not perfect. Be sure to choose images that align with a positive vision of your baby's arrival.

You could also make a wreath, with items such as rattles, bath toys, pacifiers, teething rings, representing your baby's arrival. (p.s.: when your baby arrives, hang this beautiful wreath on your hospital door!)

51. **Create artwork for your future children's bedroom.** Draw or paint pictures. Put together a book of pictures with quotes you want to share with your child.

Chapter 14: Making Your Home Into A Fertility Nesting Center

Transporting yourself to an island paradise tomorrow may not be possible, but creating a world at home that is a nurturing incubator for you and your baby is possible.

Your home can be a helper in your fertility. It can be a nest where you feel safe enough to conceive, receive, give birth and care for your babies.

Sometimes, just a simple change can turn a home into a loving nest: painting a room a color you love, putting a sweet teddy bear or cozy quilt on your bed, hanging a photograph that calms or inspires you.

Envision yourself as a mother bird preparing a nest for her eggs she must keep safe and warm.

Feeling safe and in a nest will help you at this time, since the body finds it easier to procreate when it does not feel threatened or in a state of fight or flight.

Look around your house and ask yourself: Do I like it here? Do I feel safe here? Do I feel like I can safely keep and 'hatch my eggs here'?

Try to find ways to make your living space one in which you feel safe and comfortable. This could include: displaying a tea cup or doll collection, hanging photographs of people, places and memories that leave you feeling happy and warm inside.

Create a room that reminds you of things you loved as a child. How about a shelf in your kitchen with Raggedy Ann and Andy dolls? Or a 'Disney Dreams Come True' room with memorabilia from the various Disney princesses if that is something you love.

Walk around your home and try to find ways to increase the feelings of safety, joy and comfort.

Even if you don't live in an ideal setting or particularly like where you live, there are small things you can do to make your home feel more like a warm incubator for yourself and your baby.

Start by looking around home, and ask yourself: where do my eyes spend most of their time?

Notice where your eyes go each day—during breakfast, dinner, where you watch TV, and try to make your where your eyes spend their time more conducive to positive feelings.

Whatever areas of your home get your 'eye' time offer key opportunities for healing.

For example, if you often find yourself sitting in a certain room, looking at a certain wall, could you hang a positive saying or beautiful picture that inspires you or just make you feel happy? Example: When I was trying to get pregnant, I hung a picture of a little girl playing with a bunny in my bedroom. The picture made me feel soft and hopeful, even during very painful moments.

Ask yourself: what could I bring into my home that would bring pleasure to
my eyes, ears and body each day? Think about items you could put in your home that would bring you a renewed sense of joy every time you look at them.

In whatever ways you can, make your home a place of healing, a nest where you can rest and rejuvenate as you prepare to conceive, an environment where you can access the positive emotions within you.

Here are some ways to turn your home into a comforting nest for you and your baby:

• Color

What colors make you sparkle? What colors give you a feeling of peace?

Don't worry about what colors are popular or 'in' right now—think about how different colors make you feel and put colors in your home that give you the type of feelings you are looking for.

When I was trying to get pregnant for the second time, I realized that the yellow paint color in my living room annoyed me. I never felt quite right in the room. So we went to the big hardware store and picked out a beautiful tahiti green paint color—wow what a difference that made! My spirits lifted every time I walked in that room. Granted, it was an unconventional color and not one that an interior decorator might have recommended, but at that time, it suited my soul perfectly. In fact, most people who came to my home liked the yellow color better, but it was draining me. I needed Tahiti Green's vibrance!

Two months later, I got pregnant. The color of my living room, of course, was not the 'cure' for my infertility—but I do credit it with lifting my spirits and helping me on some level, which is exactly the point: every little thing you can do to raise your spirits and reduce your stress matters.

If certain colors lift your spirits, bring those colors into your life. Look around: could you paint your bathroom a brilliant orange, the kitchen a soft pink, your living room a relaxing lavender. Think out of the box. Are you in the mood for bright, vibrant colors, like green or orange that bring about a friendly, happy feeling? Some color experts believe the color orange can help balance the adrenal glands, red provides energy and vitality to the ovaries, and violet is nurturing to the pituitary glands. Pay close attention to what colors you are drawn to and then bathe your home in these beautiful colors.

• Photographs

Photographs are a powerful way to relive positive, happy memories.

Instead of keeping your pictures locked away in boxes, or on your phone, print them out, buy a few frames and hang them throughout the house. Take photographs of places in nature that soothe you and people that you love. Display photographs that are reminders of life's beautiful and joyful moments.

• Make Sure Your Home Is Healthy

 While paying attention to the aesthetics of your home, take some time to investigate whether or not your home is healthy. An unhealthy home can contribute to your infertility. Is there mold or mildew in your home? Have an air quality test done in your home. Do you need to invest in a air purifier or HEPA filter system if you live in a high pollution area? Some studies hve suggested that the air inside most house is 5 to 10 times worse than the air outdoors. Does your heating system need to be professionally cleaned? Do you have professional lawn care services that might be bringing lots of pesticides and chemicals into your life? Do you live in an older home that could still harbor lead paint, asbestos or arsenic? Do you have cabinets, paneling, plywood, particle board, carpets or furniture made with volatile organic compounds (VOCS)? Are the carpets in your home full of chemicals that emit VOCS? Do you have moth balls in your home that contain the chemical paradichlorobenzene? Is there lead in your plumbing fixtures?
Do you use air fresheners that contain ethylene-based glycol ethers and terpenes? Could you have radon in your home or a carbon monoxide leak coming from a furnace, generator, or appliances? Be aware of the chemicals that you bring into your home and start using natural cleaners that are non-toxic or even make your own homemade cleaning products. Filter your tap water, use a vacuum cleaner with a HEPA filter to get as much dust as possible, and change your furnace filter often.

• Bring Nature Indoors

 Did you know that just touching a houseplant prompts a relaxing response in the brain? Create an indoor herb garden. Put plants all around your house. Buy yourself flowers every week.

Note: if you have pets, do not bring in plants that are toxic and could hurt or kill them. If you have pets, you may want to consider a small greenhouse that your animals do not have access to.

- **Healthy Scents**

No, this is not the time to buy air fresheners or any other type of scent that is not natural and could bring toxins into your environment, but you might want to consider bringing natural healthy scents into your home. Simmer orange peels, cloves, dried lavender, apple peels and cinnamon over the stove. Consider natural essential oils and grow fragrant herbs on your windowsill, such as rosemary.

- **Bring In The Pillows**

Create comfort whenever you can.

- **Make Music Available**

Get an iPod or even an old-fashioned stereo and set it up in the living room. When you are doing chores or cooking or put on some CDs. Make your home a place where music is readily available and accessible.

- **Tap Into The Power of Words**

Think about what words, sayings or quotes you can use to decorate your home and lift your spirits each day.

When I was trying to get pregnant, I put a poster in my kitchen entitled: "Relax..God is in Charge." It was filled with quotes that reaffirmed my faith and lifted my spirits whenever I was in the kitchen. The poster cost me less than $10, but it was a daily form of therapy for me. I grew to love that poster, because whenever I felt down, I would walk into my kitchen, see it and feel more peaceful than I felt before. If you have a lot of favorite quotes on your phone or in your social media space, print them out, glue them on a poster board, and create an inspiring display of words that empower.

Or stencil your favorite quotes on a wall or on furniture. How about creating a wall of great quotes in a hallway or bathroom?

• Welcome Some Water

Set up a plug-in tabletop fountain, buy a fish tank and fill it with beautiful fish and aquatic plants, hang photographs of the ocean or a beautiful lake. The sound of water can lower heart rates and stress levels. Studies have shown that just looking at a picture of water can induce feelings of relaxation.

• Make Sure Your Bedroom Is As Dark As Possible

Getting a good night's sleep is key right now, so make sure your room is as dark as possible and no light is creeping into your bedroom at night. Get shade darkeners, heavy curtains, and unplug all electronics.

• Make Your Home A Place Where You Are Free To Be Yourself

Do you feel authentic in your home? Or is it set up to impress others? Is it decorated in a way that is true to who you are? Or does your home look like someone other than you should live there? Make your home a place that is authentically you.

• Display It

A favorite doll, a momento from a great trip, your collection of seashells from a walk on the beach. If you have items that make you happy, and bring up feelings of peace from times gone by, put them out where you can see them. On my kitchen counter, I have items from my beach vacations that mean so much to me.

• Make Your Workspace Pleasurable Too

While you may not be able to say goodbye to your annoying boss, you may be able to put a saying or a quote on your desk at work that gives you a measure of joy and peace.

- **Display Reminders of the Beautiful Relationships In Your Life**

A gift from someone you love, a blanket your Mom made you, a loving card from a friend. Frame and display cards and letters from friends and family. How much happier our environments would be if we hung our cards instead of putting them away in drawers. How about making a collage of all your favorite cards from different times in your life?

Diary Excerpt: The First Ultrasound

When I started infertility treatments, there was one moment where I almost gave up before I even started and detonated my chances of having a baby.

Recalling that moment is very painful, because I was seconds away from running away and giving up before I even gave infertility treatments a chance.

I never liked pap smears or invasive procedures. I've done then before, reluctantly, but I can't say I ever felt entirely comfortable with them.

The first time I had to do an ultrasound at the clinic, I was hit with a wave of fear. I never had a vaginal ultrasound before, and suddenly, surrounded by medical personnel, I felt overwhelmed

"I can't do this. I need to leave," I told Christine, one of the ultrasound technicians.

My fight-or-flight response had kicked into high gear: I wanted to run, escape, get out of there.

My mind was on one track and that was: I want out of here. All the appointments, the driving, it was too much.

All I kept thinking as I lay on that table was: 'I can't do this. I just can't do this. Maybe it was a mistake coming here. I'll find another way to get pregnant.'

Everything in me wanted to jump up from that table and run, and if it wasn't for the patience of Christine, the ultrasound technician, I probably would have left the clinic that day, and maybe blown my opportunity to get help getting pregnant.

"I need to leave," I told repeated. "I can't do this."

"Yes, you can," she said gently, never making me feel pressured or forced in any way to continue with the procedure. "You can do this."

She tenderly talked me into feeling more comfortable, and with her patient loving support, I didn't runaway. I started to calm down and despite feeling scared, I was able to get through the ultrasound. Christine looked and spoke to me with such compassion and gentleness, that the hammering fear inside my brain stopped, and I regained a measure of safety.

There were many, many more ultrasounds after that. Many IUIs and other procedures that were invasive and painful, but with the help of Christine and other technicians, I successfully did each one and became more and more comfortable, to the point that eventually doing a vaginal ultrasound or any other test almost felt like nothing at all.

I shudder to think of what might had happened had Christine not chosen to be so kind and patient with me that day. Would I have continued at the clinic if Christine had lost her patience, or been more concerned with rushing to the next patient, and not taken the time and care to help me stay put and get that much needed ultrasound?

What if I had run out due to my overwhelming fear, would I have ever gone back to that clinic--or any clinic for that matter? Would I have given up on having children, thinking I wasn't strong enough or brave enough to go through infertility treatments?

I shudder at the possibility that maybe that day, my fear could have resulted in a life changing decision. Had I run out, because some fight-or-flight trigger had gone off inside me, maybe that would have been my last attempt to go through infertility treatments. Maybe I would have resigned myself to defeat, never knowing I had it in me to endure the many painful tests infertility treatment requires. I did not realize that proving I could go through this first test would pave the way for my successfully going through dozens and dozens of painful tests later on.

That day, Christine wasn't just an ultrasound technician, she also became my infertility hero. She didn't have to give so much or try so hard to help me.

She could have said to herself: this woman is way too scared and too paranoid to endure the trauma of all the tests she will have to endure. Why should I give myself so much extra work in trying to keep her here? Let her go. Let her deal with her problems somewhere else. She seems like a paranoid person and I have a long list of patients waiting for their ultrasounds who won't take so much time and won't be so slow. Instead, she cared enough to slow down and gently coach me. She didn't make me feel like a freak or flawed in any way. She didn't shame or embarrass me for my fear, or insinuate I was weak, ill, or crazy. She was respectful and kind, and gave me exactly what I needed to endure this first test.

That would not be the last time Christine helped me and it would begin a very special friendship that continued for the next four years.

I beg infertility clinics across the country to look closely at their support staff, assistants and technicians. Is their staff truly understanding and are they trained to deal with the anxieties that patients may experience during treatments? Does the support staff take the extra time when needed to help a fearful patient?

Are they taught that it is important to treat clients with patience because certain tests and procedures can ignite complex emotions in infertility patients? Does the staff actually care about the person enduring these tests--or are they just consumed with their own work load and agenda? Do they slow things down, if it means getting a woman over the first rough initial stages of infertility testing? When hiring, do they not only look at the technical qualifications of their support staff, but also the emotional qualifications? Is the staff truly kind? Compassionate? Empathetic to what infertility can cause a woman to feel?

To work in this field, you not only have to be medically and technically astute, you need tolerance, patience and understanding of the emotional hurdles patients like me must conquer to walk down this path.

Throughout the years I dealt with Christine, she was always kind and never once did she make me feel like a fool for being so afraid. With her, I never felt judged or put down. She didn't dismiss me, pity me, or treat me like I was odd or overly flawed.

She never showed anger at me for creating more work for her. She was caring enough to take the extra time to go very slowly with me.

Do you know how much I respect and completely admire this woman? She is one of the bright and shining stars of the medical profession. She talked me through that first day, which allowed me to continue my infertility process. That first day, it could have all ended. I never again after that felt a desire to runaway and escape the clinic.

 That day, I might have allowed my fear to halt the whole process, but thanks to Christine, I kept going and didn't give up.

If it had not been for Christine's extraordinary patience, understanding, and kindness, I don't know where I'd be today.

Thank God Christine was doing my ultrasound that day. Thank God the clinic I went to had the insight to hire someone like Christine.

Thank you Christine.

I Have Polyps

All the tests have yielded one explanation thus far for my not getting pregnant: I have a polyp on my left ovary.

This is good news—finally some type of answer.

Last night, I went to the clinic to have some type of thing put in my vagina to prepare me for the operation...but when they found out I had a bad flu, the whole procedure was cancelled and rescheduled. I feel a bit relieved.

A Month Later...

A month has passed, and I'm back to have this thing put in my vagina to prepare for tomorrow's polyp removal.

It is so uncomfortable. Actually it hurt really bad. Tonight, I laid in bed and Chris rubbed my back until I went to sleep. This is so uncomfortable and awlful.

The most upsetting part of this procedure is the idea of going under anesthesia. I almost didn't want the operation because the whole anesthesia thing is frightening to me. I probably drove everyone crazy today asking about a million questions about anesthesia and the dangers of it. I talked to the anesthesiologist and he explained that now they insert a tube in your throat so they always know whether you are breathing or not, when in times past, they didn't have that precaution. That eased my fears a lot, because I remember all the horror stories about people going under anesthesia and never coming out.

The procedure turned out not to be bad at all. When I woke up, I barely felt sore.

Actually, I felt pretty good after the operation, except it was extremely boring to lay in the ugly recovery room waiting to be sent home. The room was gray, with metal pipes on the ceiling, and it looked like something left over from World War II. When we got home, Leah was waiting to greet me.

I am excited because maybe that polyp was my trouble all along--the hidden reason I was not getting pregnant. Maybe I will get pregnant next month! Good thing I came to this clinic or I would have never known about this polyp. Next month I can start on a new cycle. Maybe pregnancy is close behind.

Chapter 15: Journal Your Way To Pregnancy

Journal writing is powerful way to release trauma and heal from infertility. It is a way to express and let go of painful emotions, and give yourself the gift of hope when you need it most. In this chapter, we'll discuss different forms of journal writing that will help you express, release, get in touch with, and heal from your innermost feelings.

Journal Writing Through Your Subconscious

Doing journal writing exercises that allow your subconscious to speak can be a powerful and life-changing experience, because a subconscious that is shut down and forbidden to speak can wreak havoc on the body.

Becoming aware of all your emotions surrounding pregnancy and motherhood, especially the ones that might be hidden, can free up trapped energy that might be stifling your body's ability to relax and conceive.

If you have any ambivalence, fear or hesitation about having a baby, subconscious journal writing will bring to light these feelings. When you allow your subconscious to speak freely, you will begin releasing emotions that may be trapping negative energy in your body.

A side note here: having fears or conflicting feelings will not prevent you from getting pregnant. If healthy, a woman can become pregnant even amidst lots of hesitation and fear (think of women who are raped and end up pregnant, or women who get pregnant in the middle of a famine or war), but giving your subconscious a chance to be heard through writing will help you to understand and harmonize conflicting feelings within your body.

To begin, type or write a sentence such as: 'I am excited to be a mother' or 'I am deserving of a baby' and then type your responses to these statements without editing, analyzing, or thinking too long about what you want to say back. Just let whatever bubbles up come out.

Give your subconscious unedited, nonjudgmental, uncontrolled room to speak. By listening to what your subconscious has to say, you'll be helping your body release pent-up fears, frustrations, confusions or conflicts.

Let your subconscious speak openly about any reservations it may have about becoming a mother. Then comfort this part of you that needs some reassurance. Disguised conflict within could interfere with your goal to be a mother. Your body might even be physically weaker if fear and doubt about having a baby lurks in your unconscious mind.

I feel most comfortable typing. Others may prefer writing in long hand. Letting my subconscious speak was a very freeing experience for me. When I did it, I could feel parts of me loosen up and get soft, because I wasn't rigidly trying to silence a legitimate part of myself that deserved to be heard.

Whenever I did this type of journal writing, I was often very surprised at what my subconscious had to say. As hard as it was to hear what this part of me had to say, I needed to hear it. I did not want a saboteur to live within me that I didn't know about, especially one who might quietly work against the goal I was working so hard towards. The subconscious needs to be allowed to rage and scream sometimes. It can be dangerous if you have unacknowledged feelings and beliefs roaming around your body that you have no conscious clue about. If you silence your subconscious, you might be starting a potential war within yourself.

Listen to this part of yourself. Comfort this voice within. Once you are aware of deeply held beliefs and fears around pregnancy, childbirth, motherhood, you can then work to heal and release them.

For some of you, after doing this exercise, you may find that you have no conflict at all, and that every part of you is open, ready and willing to be a mother.

But if you do find conflicts within yourself, that is okay too. It is okay to be afraid. It is okay to have doubts.

Having these feelings will not stop you from getting pregnant and having a baby.

Millions of women are scared and not completely sure about becoming a mother. Yet, they get pregnant anyways and go on to be wonderful mothers who raise great children.

So if emotions like fear, doubt, and worry exist within you, they cannot stop you from having a baby--but knowing if they are there can help you create harmony within yourself.

Ask your body: 'why am I having trouble getting pregnant?' or 'why have I not conceived yet?' and let whatever answers within you come up and be heard. Do not judge yourself as you are writing. There is no right or wrong answers to these questions. Just allow whatever is within you to speak.

Some questions you may want to ask your body include:

What prevents me from getting pregnant?

Do you want me to be pregnant?

What can I give you so I can get pregnant?

What do you need to get pregnant?

How can I help you get pregnant?'

Why am I not pregnant yet?

Should I get pregnant?

Do you want me to have a child?

Are you afraid of having a baby?

How do you feel about getting pregnant?

Do you think I deserve a child?

Do you want to be a mother?

What scares you the most about becoming a mother?

Is becoming a mother something you feel ready for?

Why haven't I had a child yet?

Do you think mothers are good or bad people?

Are you afraid of being a mother?

Do you think you need to be perfect to be a mother?

Is there something dangerous about becoming a mother?

Am I good enough to be a mother?

Write some of the following statements and then let your subconscious respond in any way it wants:

I am having a baby.

I am pregnant and in nine months I am going to have a baby.

My body is ready to create babies.

I deserve a baby.

I deserve to be a Mom.

I am worthy of being a mother.

I am pregnant.

I am getting pregnant soon.

My body is healthy and ready to have a baby.

I am having a baby.

I am going to get pregnant soon and have a healthy baby.

I can carry a baby for nine months and give birth to a healthy baby.

It is safe to have a baby.

I like myself and I believe I can have more babies.

I have permission to have a baby.

Having a baby is good for me.

It will be fun to be a mother.

I am excited to raise my children.

I am looking forward to holding my child.

Now, I'm going to let you in on the conversations I had with my subconscious. Take a look at the self-hatred that was living within me.

Journal 1

Me: I am having a baby.

Subconscious: A baby--you? You big loser? You know what a loser you are. A baby? You couldn't have a pet cat if you tried. *(Note: today I have four pets cats so I guess my subconscious was very wrong!)* A baby--oh my God, everyone knows you are too old and too worn out. You can't handle anything. Do you realize what a screw up you are? Paula, the road to hell is paved with good intentions, and you are that road to hell. I can't believe you think this can work out. Get a grip.

Me: I am having a baby. I am having a healthy beautiful baby. I am pregnant right now.

Subconscious: Oh God, you are nothing. I can't believe you buy this optimism crap. I think you better give up my dear, because you are worthless.

Me: My vagina is strong and my baby is growing healthy inside me. I can carry a baby.

Subconscious: You can't carry a baby. Hasn't it been proven your eggs are too old and too messed up? You have some problem--maybe mercury, but give up weirdo. You are indeed a big weirdo. You are not like all the other women who had babies young. You are too old. You are very old.

Me: I am pregnant and in nine months I'm going to have a baby.

Subconscious: Wishful thinking. You are meant to struggle and get nothing. You are meant to be perpetually punished for your sins. No one ever believes in you.

Me: I like myself. I believe I can have more babies. I am strong. I make good eggs.

Subconscious: Stop the bravado. It isn't working on me. I feel like you can't have any more kids. Dr. M said you were too old--and I believe her. You look old. You feel old. You seem like the world has gone by you on this one. God hates you too. How could He like you? How in the world could you think God would help you?

Me: I can have babies. I am having more babies. My body is creating more babies. *(Note here how after repeating positive statements, my subconscious began to change and become more positive too.)*

Subconscious: Your friend had a baby with one ovary, barely made any eggs, and somehow got a baby out of the deal, a nice boy baby. You are not looking for gold--you want one more baby. You can do this. Look, it may be hard. It may be a long road. No one said this will be easy. You need help along the way. But ultimately, you can have a baby. You won't do stupid things. You'll rest a lot.

You'll go to Eileen and Dr. Deutsch a lot. You'll get help.

Journal 2: In this journal entry, I asked my body why it was having trouble getting pregnant.

Me: Why can't I have a baby?

Subconscious: Because you are bad. Because you are not worth anything. Because you get envious and anxious and something is wrong with you. Because you are not worth anything. Because you deserve nothing

Me: Why can't I have another baby?

Subconscious: Because you only get one shot at happiness. Because you can't escape your fate.

Me: I hate my life. I am stuck. I am in a hole. I am disappearing. I'm tired of people telling me to give up and accept. I am never giving up! That is not me. I am not giving up at all. I never give up when I want something.

I want a second baby. No! I want ten babies. Two is not enough. I want many, many, many, babies. Give me more babies! Give me more! *(Note how at first, my conscious self was starting to agree with my negative subconscious, but then began to argue and fight to my right to have more babies.)*

Subconscious: No! You are a bad girl. Other girls will get everything-- you get nothing. You are a loser. You can't escape your life. You are a weirdo. A loser.

Journal 3: I wrote this when I was pregnant with my son.

Me: I am going to have a second baby in nine months.

Subconscious: Bull! Nothing ever goes right for you. You are a big loser. You always have bad things happen to you. That is your lot in your life. You try and try and get nothing. Everyone sees you as a loser.

Everyone still sees you as that girl who can't get anything she wants. Why would this be different?

(Note how I now argue with this negative part of me, in the attempt to remove some of these counterproductive ideas.) Me: Shut up! You are wrong. I am having this baby. For your information,
people believe in me. I am not a messed up. I am a strong woman. A good mother. I am a determined person. I have worked hard to earn this baby. I have gone through test after test, shot after shot. I earned this baby and I'm going to see my reward.

Subsconsious: How? How are you going to see it?

Me: Because I am a strong person. Because my body is strong. Because this time, I am arming myself. Because God is on my side. Because my vagina is strong, my uterus is strong, and I love my baby. I love this little baby inside of me. I adore him. I love him. He is already my best friend.

This child will be my daughter's best friend. They will play house together and love each other. She will have a ready made support system. She will have what other people have: a built in network of people to love. I will be an example to others that what you put in you get back--that if you work hard enough, and try hard enough, you get what you want. When we go to weddings, my daughter will have a companion, she will not be at the mercy of bratty children who ignore her. *(Note how I am now clearly defending myself and my abilities.)*

Subconscious: Honey, I see you are sad. You are such a wonderful girl. You will have your own babies. *(Notice how when I argued and gave solid points to my subconscious, it began to advocate for me and be on my side.)*

Journal 4: Here, I ask my body what it needs.

Me: Okay vagina and uterus, talk. Tell me what you are feeling.

Subconscious: I am feeling helpless. I am not feeling loved. I want to hear 'Rocky.' Do you understand what I've gone through? It is hard on me. *(Note: it is a good idea to ask your subconscious what it needs. There might be something this part of you needs that it is not getting, or a deep need that is being ignored)*

Me: What do you need?

Subconscious: Bring me an afghan. Bring me peace. Bring me time in the Artic with penguins. Bring me good books. Bring me love. Bring me Rona Jaffe. *(Note that my subconscious gives specifics as to what she needs and in knowing this, I can help calm her down and comfort her.)*

Journal 5: Note some of the self-hatred that I had to work through in order to feel worthy of receiving my goal.

Me: I want a second baby.

Subconscious: No you don't. Only young women deserve babies. You are too old. You can't have it all-your fun and then all the children. You can't get everything in this world. You need to choose either one or the other.

Me: I want a baby.

Subconscious: So what? Lots of people want things they can't get. What makes you any different? Aren't you the same as everybody else?
Me: I deserve to have a baby.

Subconscious: Nope, sorry. Only good girls get babies. You ruined your liver kidney channel. You deserve nothing.

Me: I am going to have a baby.

Subconscious: Nope. Sorry. the answer is no. You don't want a baby deep down. To start all over again--oh Lord no. I can't go through that again. I can't go through the scare of the nine months, the delivery, the horrible recovery, the bleeding, the stitches, the whole thing is too much for me.

Let my body alone--we are tired and we try too hard. *(Note that my subconscious is expressing its fatigue and fear of going through another pregnancy. Because I knew that, I knew I had to give myself the rest and security I deserved throughout this pregnancy.)*

Me: I am going to have a baby.

Subconscious: Nope, your eggs are old. You used them up. That is what you get.

Me: I am going to have a baby. *(Note: I repeated my wish over and over, as a way to bring up from the subconscious conflicts and to bring my subsconscious over to my conscious side.)*

Subconscious: No, sorry. You deserve nothing. The baby thing is over and done with. Forget it. Don't drive yourself crazy. Enjoy your daughter and forget about it. No one listens to you. No one believes in you. I don't want to go through invitro again. I don't want to have to put under, and have my legs opened up, and to have to hold my urine for seven minutes--they are going to kill me with that. My bladder can't take it. It is too hard. I am too tired for this.

Me: I am going to have a baby. *(Notice that I ended with a positive statement as a way to counter subconscious fears)*

Journal 6

Me: I am going to have a baby.

Subconscious: No goofhead--you are going to have heartache. You are going to cry. You are a big nobody who nobody loves. You are a loser. Your husband is going to leave you. I wish you would just give up. I am tired of doing stuff, tired of trying. Does it really matter?
You are never going to be happy anyways. You are a loser. Everyone knows that. You are a big loser. You are never going to change. You are a joke. I think you are a weasel. Everyone sees through you. Nobody actually likes you.

Me: I am going to be pregnant soon and have a baby.

Subconscious: A baby? No way! You are alone now and will always be alone. You are a weirdo and you've never been able to hold on to any relationship.

Me: I am going to get pregnant and have a baby. I am strong and my body can do this. I have good eggs inside of me.

Subconscious: No way! You heard Dr. M--you are bottom of the barrel. It is a joke. Why do you keep doing this? Putting yourself through this? You are a glutton for punishment. Paula Paula--the girl who works hard for nothing.

The girl who keeps going even when she should give up. Why do you make everything so hard for me? Why do you keep me working and working for nothing? You are always out there, chipping away, doing too much. I feel sorry for you. (*Note that this part of me doesn't really want to put forth the work and effort needed to heal and get pregnant— and if left to her own devices, might have stopped me from doing everything in my power to get pregnant.*)

Me: I am going to get pregnant soon. Then I'm going to have a beautiful pregnancy and have a baby soon.

Subconscious: You--a beautiful pregnancy! Honey, nothing ever goes that smoothly for you. You are not the type to enjoy that much smoothness. For you, life is one big down hill rollercoaster ride. Other people get good stuff--you just try and have a good heart, but can't really pull it together. You keep trying, old good hearted one, your efforts are nice, but you can't get results. *(this part of me refuses to see that positive efforts reap positive results, a key to getting healthy for anyone.)*

Me: I am going to get pregnant soon. I am going to have a healthy, beautiful pregnancy and then give birth to a healthy baby. I am going to enjoy this whole process.

Subconscious: Maybe. Remember: you are a big loser.

Me: I am going to get pregnant soon. I am going to have a healthy, beautiful, safe pregnancy, then I'm going to give birth to a healthy baby.

Subconscious: You are going to have a sick, damaged baby. You are going to have a weird deformed baby. You are a weirdo dear.

Me: I am going to get pregnant soon. I am going to have a healthy baby, and a beautiful, safe pregnancy.

Subconscious: Only young girls can have healthy babies. You were different and weird to begin with, and you'll always be different and weird.

Me: I am going to get pregnant soon. I am going to have a healthy, safe, beautiful pregnancy. I am going to have a healthy baby.

Subconscious: How in the world are you going to do that? You are almost 37 years old---3 years from 40. You are no spring chicken. How would this happen? Do you think your old body can really do this? You are a stressed out, unhappy, overworked and underpaid girl.

Me: I feel so tired. I can't possibly keep going. I am so so discouraged inside of myself. I am so so so tired. I am beyond tired. I want to stop, get on my knees, got to the water and swim. I can't keep going. Will I ever get peace in my life? When will peace come to me? *(Note that now my conscious is starting to reveal its own fears and doubts.)* I have no idea when peace will come? I dream of having a life I want. I am willing to work for it, but I'm so tired. I am so emotionally tired. I am tired of dealing with jerks and prickheads. I am tired of dealing with stupid people. I am tired of the subtle rejections and hurt feelings all around me.

Journal 7

Me: I am pregnant.

Subconscious: No ! You? You who mess up everything. I can't be pregnant. I'm afraid to be pregnant. So much can go wrong. I'm going to scream. What if I miscarry? My husband will kill me. I can't take this. I can't take the nine long months. I want the baby here now. I want the baby here right now. I can't wait. I need to see the baby, touch the baby, feel the baby. I need to grow a baby. Oh God, I am not up to this. I am a delicate little flower who wilts in the sun and wind. I am not strong enough to have a baby. I am not tough enough. I am just a woman. A small woman. A frail woman. I'm a woman who tries hard and who messes up and doesn't seem to be the right kind of woman. I am a messed up woman. I am so messed up. I hate myself. I hate everything.

Me: I am going to have a baby. Maybe two or three babies.

Subconscious: Everyone will hurt you. You are the mercy of everyone. You will end up being hurt. You always start out on the right foot and end up goofing up. It is amazing you even have one child. Why should you have more than one beautiful baby when some people get nothing?

You deserve nothing. *(Note a deeply held belief I needed to heal from and overcome.)*

Me: I am going to have a baby. My babies are growing strong.

Subconscious: The stress is too much for me. What if something goes wrong? I can't bare to disappoint anyone. I am just one person. I don't want to disappoint anyone. I want this to work out. I am going to scream. I need to see Eileen every single day. I need to see Dr. Deutsch every single day. I need to do too many things.

I need to scream and yell, and scream and yell some more.

Me: I am going to have a baby. Maybe two or three babies. I am a strong mother. I am a very strong woman. No one perseveres like me. *(Note that I continue to speak positively as a way to counteract the negative emotions of my subconscious.)*

Subconscious: Oh God, I'm so afraid. Please God, let this pregnancy be normal, safe, happy, noneventful. Let the time pass quickly. Let it fly by. Let my baby be okay. Please God, Help me, without your help, nothing can work out. What if God hates me? God must hate me. Why would He love me? Why in the world would God love me? What have I ever done to have God love me? If anything, God must hate me. I must be hated. I deserve to be hated. I am a hateful person. I am an evil person. I deserve only bad things to happen to me. I am a bad woman.

Me: I am going to have a baby. My body is strong. I eat good, I exercise, I take my vitamins. I walk, I sing, I dance, I think positive thoughts. I need to keep going. I need to pray constantly. How will I live? How will I keep going? How will I not think about the baby inside me? I am so stressed out being pregnant. So much pain around being pregnant. I can't take all the pain. I can't take all the possibilities in my life right now. What if they all end up being nothing? What if they end up being one big mess up? What if I lose all my chances? I'm right at the door of everything I want. Will I go in that door?

Me: Yes! Yes! Yes! I will walk in that door. No one and nothing will stop me from walking through that door of joy. *(Note how I progress from a lot of fear around being pregnant, to a state of confidence and joy.)* I've been here before, and I never realized that I deserve--yes really deserve--to walk in this door. I'm doing good things. I'm giving my daughter siblings. When she is old, she can go food shopping with her siblings.

Me: (continued) When she goes to the meeting or an assembly, she will not be alone, but with her sibling. When she comes home from school, she'll have a pal to talk with, laugh with, play with, and be there if friends hurt her. No way! My daughter will have someone to love. She will have someone to play with. She will have someone who invites her over on special days off, someone who will love her and hopefully watch out for her like I do. I deserve this! I'm a good person.

I deserve this! I deserve joy. I've wasted so much time in sadness, and it got me nowhere. I want the joy. I want the happiness. I want the good stuff. (Note that once I express my negative self-doubts, I am then able to move on to feelings of worth.)

I want all the good stuff I can get. I am ready to get. I'm
tired of always waiting for good stuff to happen. I deserve good things. I am a good person. I deserve good things. I worked very hard for this. I sacrificed, I kept going, I spend money, I didn't stop. A big screw you to anyone who wants to take this from me.

Subconscious: I am anxious. I want it all now. I want my baby now. The journey, thus far, was easier when I wasn't so near everything. Now I'm near to getting everything and I'm incredibly scared and incredibly nervous. It is scary to come so close to having everything you want. Oh God, what am I going to do? How am I going to do this? What if I kill myself in the process?

Me: I am going to have a baby. My baby inside of me are growing strong and healthy.

Subconscious: You Paula couldn't grow a cucumber big and strong. You are a big loser. You are not an earthy Mama. You are not a fertility queen. You are not a baby producer. You are a dried up little nerd. You are different than other woman. You are not allowed to be like other women. You are bad to want a baby. You are bad to want babies. You don't need or deserve two or three babies. You deserve nothing. You are nothing.

Me: I am going to have babies. There are babies--beautiful babies--growing inside of me--strong and healthy. Yay! I deserve this! I'm a servant of God. God loves me. God answers my prayers. God knows my heart. God is helping me.

Subconscious: God doesn't want you to have babies. How could you do this? Are you sure God wants more babies in this world? You are a selfish person. What a selfish prick you are. You are ordinary. You are a selfish lady Paula. Who are you going to help now? How are you going to help save mankind? You deserve nothing. You deserve to suffer. I hate you so much--that is what you deserve. You think things are so easy. I say that you are a weirdo and you deserve nothing in this world.

I would like to see you suffer some more. I would like to see you miscarry just to prove what a bad person you are. I hate you. I want to see only bad for you. You deserve nothing in this world.

You were and are a bad person. God only blesses good people and you are not one of those good people. Do you understand? I hate you. I hate you so much.

(Note how my subconscious sees only negatives for me, but as she speaks, she begins to express her need for help.) I am stressed! Help me! God, help me! Get me through this time! I am going to scream! I am trying to escape, wishing I was somewhere else. The journey is so long, and I beg for help. I cannot be sent back there. I need to stop thinking.

Me: I am going to have two or three babies. My babies are growing strong. They are nice babies. They are kind babies. They are good babies. They will make the earth a better place. My daughter's life is going to be better. I am a strong mother. I am a wise mother. I am a woman who is ripe for baby-making. Wow--I am a baby making machine.

(Note: the internal fight between me and my subconscious.)

Subconscious: You can't do this.

Me: Yes I can.

Subconscious: No you can't.

Me: Yes, I can!

Journal 8

Me: I am having a baby.

Subconscious: No! You don't deserve a baby. You are no good. Remember how nothing you were? Remember how completely horrible you were? Remember? You don't deserve everything. You have to suffer for the rest of your life for your sins. Do you think you can just have so much fun? Good people deserve to have working vaginas and working ovaries. You are all dried up now, a curse from God above for your sins. You are an ugly, nondeserving, stupid person. You are nothing. I won't let you have a baby because I don't think you deserve it.

I think you need to suffer more. You need to suffer and suffer and suffer. I hate the life you created for me. This isn't what I wanted.

I want respect. I want love. I want quiet peace. Nothing went right for me. Everything that could have gone wrong went wrong. I'm so tired of trying. I'm so tired of trying for things. A baby? Why--so one day I can wake up and be bleeding. Does anyone understand how much I have lost?

Me: I am having a baby.

Subconscious: Why? Why do you want a baby. I don't want a baby. I want to go to Channel 2. I don't want to go through all the hell I've gone through. I am ugly. I can't take nothing happening anymore. I can't take any more disappointment. I need this to work. I need it all to work. *(Note that my subconscious enjoys work and doesn't want to miss work due to a pregnancy—acknowledging this is a step towards resolving inner conflict and setting up situations that work for all parts of me.)*

Me: I am having a baby.

Subconscious: You? You loser of the year. You having a baby? No one thinks you can have a baby. Everyone knows you are a nice goodhearted person who simply will never get anything. Everyone knows that. Special people who deserve everything are the ones who get the babies, not you. You are the weird girl. You are a loser, a weirdo.

Me: I am having a baby.

Subconscious: Yah--and do you think your vagina is strong enough to hold a baby? Do you think your measly stupid little vagina could actually hold a baby?

Me: I am having a baby. My baby is growing inside of me. My baby is growing strong.

Subconscious: That affirmation stuff never works.

Me: I am having a baby.

Subconscious: Yah--and you think about chocolate, don't you?

Your Daily Happiness Journal

To get on a road of hope and healing, it is absolutely necessary to feed your mind positive thoughts each day. Your Daily Happiness Journal will help you do that. Filling out this Daily Happiness Journal will help you recognize the good things happening in your life right now, as you walk, run, and sometimes crawl, towards your goal of having a baby.

Thoughts of hope are what you most need at this time--it is those thoughts that will lift your body to a higher level of health and give you the extra energy you need to keep trying when all looks dim. Don't underestimate your body's ability to listen and respond to every uplifting message that it is sent.

This Daily Happiness Journal will subtly change the way you experience your day, and the way your body interprets the stress it experiences.

By digging deep within to complete these sentences, you'll change the track your thoughts are on from negative to positive.

Think of this journal as adding a positive-feeling antenna to your brain. It will help you be ever-alert to everything good within you and around you.

Even on days when you might feel discouraged, and it is difficult to feel even a smidet of hope, take the time to fill out this journal and force your mind's eye on to hope and possibility.

Read what you wrote out loud at the end of the day, once, twice or even three times, to imprint these thoughts in your mind. Or photocopy the following and put it on your fridge, as an reminder to fill it in each day.

Your Daily Happiness Journal

I am happy today because_____

I am thankful today because_____

I am hopeful today because_____

I am peaceful today because_____

I am contented today because _____

I am enthused and joyful today because _____

I am healthy and fertile today because_____

I am excited today because_____

I feel good today because_____

I feel strong today because _____

I want to thank my body today because_____

A beautiful moment I experienced today was_____

Today my body is able to conceive
because_____

Today I want to tell my body that I love it
because_____

_____

Today I can feel my body becoming more fertile
because_____

Today I have evidence that life is wonderful
because_____

Today, I know my body is strong and capable of giving birth
because_____

Today my ovaries, my vagina, my hormones, and my entire reproductive system feels great because_____

I am very fortunate today because_____

My world is beautiful and becoming more beautiful each day
because_____

Good things are happening to me today and everyday
because_____

Life Affirmation Journal

In your Life Affirmation Journal, you will start taking note of all the ways birth and life take place in your environment.

Start by observing and taking note of the reproductive cycle that occurs in the world around you each day. Record all the forms of birth that you see in your daily life, including those you might never have noticed before. Note especially when nature finds a way to give birth, even in bleak circumstances. Notice the birth and rebirth of trees, flowers, weeds, insects, birds and animals in your surroundings and record them in your journal.

As you spend time outdoors observing the birth process in the natural world around you, make sure to remind yourself that YOU ARE PART OF THIS NATURAL BIRTH CYCLE.

When you record these instances of birth, write: "Just like BLANK reproduced this week, I will reproduce soon" or "Just as BLANK is involved in the birth process, I too am part of the birth process around me."

Observe a new leaf growing, a flower blooming, a branch blossoming, baby birds, bunnies and squirrels. Start a garden or simply buy a plant, and write down what you observe about how living things grow, multiply, develop, sustain themselves and thrive, even after a long period of time being barren.

Plant something and record how the tiny seed you planted grew. Watch as that tiny seed turns into a stem, a leaf, a flower, a plant. Get a greenhouse and become an expert at observing the natural birth flow that occurs in nature.

Look for all the ways in nature that reproduction occurs-- even when it looks like reproduction of any kind is no longer possible.

Understand that your body is part of the miraculous birth process that occurs around you many times a day.

Your body contains the same potential and is similarly programmed to give birth, just like the weeds in your yard that won't stop growing or the ants in the driveway that seem to come out of nowhere.

Your body, like the natural world around you, contains the ability to rejuvenate itself and give birth, even after a long barren. Note that barren tree in the winter: the leaves are gone, it is bare, but a few months later, as the season changes, the tree sprouts with new buds. You, my dear, are no different from that tree. While at times things may look sparse and hopeless, with the right conditions, your buds can bloom again.

Remember: it takes the spring conditions of warm sunshine to bring the barren trees to life—a change in the conditions the tree is in enables it to reproduce again.

When you notice birth and life around you, remember that it is not something separate from you, but something you are intrinsically connected to and have the power to experience.

Carry this journal with you, and be on the look-out for the blossoming of new life. Remember: whenever you record birth, add the words: I am part of this birth cycle too."

Life Affirmation Journal

Today I saw _____giving birth in the world around me. I _____ am part of this birth cycle.

Today in my environment, I saw the birth cycle at work in the _____. I _____ am part of the birth cycle in the world around me.

Today the birth cycle presented itself to me in _____. I _____am part of the birth cycle in the world around me.

My Child & I Journal

In this journal, you will voice your most optimistic and confident dreams for the future. It is where you will write your happiest dreams of a future with your children by your side.

Journal about the wonderful adventures you plan to have with your children. Cut out pictures of projects you plan to do together, and paste them in your journal.

Write a list of the '100 Things I Am Going To Do With My Child.' As you write this list, feel yourself experiencing these activities with your children.

Write about all the places you want to take your children.

Write about the traditions you will pass on to your children.

Create a list of all the recipes you want to make with your child. Are their family recipes you want to share? Recipes you want to teach them? Childhood favorites you want them to experience? Favorites from celebrations and traditions you want to pass down?

Write letters to your future children, with advice and ideas that you want to share. Tell them how excited you are to meet them! Let them know you believe you will be together soon. Tell them about all the fun things you plan to do together. As you write, envision the day when your child will read this letter.

Chapter 16: Keeping Track of Your Emotions

It is important as you go through infertility that you understand what triggers your positive emotions, as well as what brings up your most negative emotions. One way to do that is called emotional tracking.

Here's how emotional tracking works: each day, you will begin to keep a record of when you feel positive and when you feel negative. By doing this, you will gain insight into the people, places and events, that evoke negative emotions, and what brings up your most joyful, positive, emotions.

Emotional tracking goes something like this:

Experience A Place, Person, Event=Feel The Emotion That Accompanies or Follows: Is this an emotion to release and say goodbye to or one to hold onto, pursue, repeat and chase down again?

When you begin to see that a certain place, person or experience empowers you to feel positively, pursue that place, person or experience.

By understanding what triggers your emotions each day, you will be better
equipped to understand what ignites positive emotions and what brings up negative emotions.

Once the root cause of a negative emotion is discovered, it is less able to take you off guard and derail you.

Simply put: if something evokes a positive feeling, pursue it, chase after it, try to repeat it.

If something evokes a negative feeling, learn how to experience it differently, change it, let it go, release it, heal it, avoid it, replace it, forget about it, or distract yourself from it.

Use the sheet below to do Emotional Tracking:

Emotions Tracking

Emotion:
Time It Happened:
What I Was Doing When I Felt It:
Did An Event, Experience, Person or Place Trigger It:
What Were You Thinking About When It Occurred:
What were you eating or drinking?

What Can You Do To (choose the ones that fit what you want to happen)
Change It:
Avoid It:
Alter How You Think About It:
Distract Yourself from It:
Repeat It:
What Situations, Events, Experiences May Have Triggered It:
What I Can Do To Experience It Again

More Emotional Tracking Exercises:

Morning:
Waking up I feel:
Breakfast I feel:
Preparing for the day I feel:
Ways to change, alter or slightly shift the morning routine to encourage more positive emotions:

Noon:
I feel:
What I am doing:
Do I want to continue feeling this way, or do I want to change it, repeat it, alter it:

Mid-Day:
I feel:
What I am doing:
Do I want to continue feeling this way, or do I want to change it, repeat it, alter it:

Early evening:
I feel:
What I am doing:
Do I want to continue feeling this way, or do I want to change it, repeat it, alter it:

Late evening:
I feel:
What I am doing:
Do I want to continue feeling this way, or do I want to change it, repeat it, alter it:

Bedtime:
I feel:
What I am doing and thinking:
Do I want to continue feeling this way, or do I want to change it, repeat it, alter it:

Some questions to help with emotional tracking:

- If you could change five things about your life, what would they be?

- What type of activities do you wish you had more time for?

- When was the last time you truly felt joy?

- What is one thing in your environment that bugs you each day? What can you do to change that?

- What time of day are you the most unhappy? What are you doing at that time? What could you do during the time that would put you in a different mood? Is there anything you can do to change the pattern of unhappiness you experience during this time?

- Draw a circle with a timeline of your day, labeling morning, afternoon and evening. Now, write down the activities, responsibilities, and patterns that make up your day. At what time of the day are you the happiest? What time of day do you grapple with feelings of depression? What are you doing or not doing at those times?

- What routines and responsibilities bring up negative feelings within you?

- What is one thing you can do each day to start your day on a happier note?

My Diary: Hard Time of Year

It is the week of Christmas and reminders that I have no children in my life are everywhere I turn.

I have no one to buy toys for, no one to bundle up and take sledding, no one to make hot chocolate for. Everywhere I look, there are commercials with beautiful little girls in pink and white dresses marveling at some wonderful new doll their mother has bought them.

Seeing it dangled before me constantly, I feel far removed from this normal and beautiful part of life.

I go in the Disney store at the mall and I run out almost immediately. When do I get a child to buy toys for? A child to tell whimsical fairy tales to? When does the magic I am seeing and hearing about all the time get to be mine to enjoy?

This feeling culminated when we visited my parents a few days ago for dinner.

I went there feeling depressed. It is December, and I am not pregnant yet. I am surrounded and constantly assaulted by visions of big families with lots of children gathering together. I see these images and ask: will I ever have this or will I always be so alone in this world?

When we got to my parent's house, I was feeling sorry for myself. I couldn't help feeling that this dinner shouldn't be so small.

The feeling was so overwhelming that I made a decision that day: this will be the last December I ever experience without a child in my life. If I don't get pregnant soon, I am going to adopt.

I was feeling pretty down, so I escaped to the upstairs bedroom. My husband followed me and asked what was wrong. I started to cry. He held me, and I told him it hurts so much to not have a baby yet... to month after month not be pregnant.

Just then, my father knocks on the door and wants to know what is wrong. I tell him about how hard it is for me to have yet another December come and go without a child in my life. He looks at me, obviously a bit confused, and says, "Can't we just have a nice day? We don't want the day ruined."

That was it for me. I was feeling very depressed to begin with, but this was too much. I storm downstairs, shouting a few choice words about his insensitivity, and lock myself in the downstairs bathroom.

I was not coming out until dinner was over and it was time to go home!

At that moment, I was already struggling to fight off my extreme disappointment and I had no stomach for my father's inability to understand the validity of my pain. I felt safer in the bathroom than being with someone who didn't fully get how beaten down a woman can feel when she is ready to welcome new members into her family, and those new members are not arriving as expected.

My mother and husband tried to get me to come out and enjoy dinner, but I just couldn't. I felt ashamed…a total loser…angry..So, so angry. I just wanted to stay hidden.

Maybe this wasn't the most mature response or the most considerate action to take, since my mother worked hard to prepare a lovely meal, but lately my emotions have been building towards a boiling point and once heated, I am unable turn them back.

I have little tolerance for all the people who take my feelings about being childless so lightly.

It seems everywhere I go, no one understands how painful infertility is-- a raw, blistering, heated pain that never lets up.

I need at least my family to understand how bad this feels.

Today I desperately needed them to understand just how hard it is for another family dinner to arrive and still it is just my tiny little family with no children.

Why couldn't my Dad see how hurt I am? How alone I feel? How horrible it is to experience life without a baby to love, when it seems every other family is overflowing with new babies, new children, a never ending supply of new life?

Where are the children who are suppose to be running around our family dinner table? When does new life get to come into our family?

On TV, I am barraged with images of big loving families with lots of adorable little children sitting at long beautifully set tables. I need that in my life.

I live in a dead zone with everything so stagnant and unchanging.

I need new babies at our family dinner table. I don't want another family dinner with the same cast of characters.

Give me new life, give me babies.

I want my Dad and everyone else to know that I feel like the loneliest freak in the world because I am without children. I feel like life is passing by me. Somehow, along the way, I got on the wrong track and something I was suppose to have has been stolen away.

I hurt so much. It was impossible for me to come out of the bathroom and pretend everything is fine. Nothing is fine.

It felt a lot less painful to lock myself in the bathroom than experience another family dinner with no children.

Chris eats quickly, thanks my mother, and we leave.

A Few Days Later

Now that a few days have passed, I understand a bit more clearly where my father was coming from when he said 'can't we just have a nice day.' He was excited to have us over for a visit and he wanted enjoy a good time. No dramatics. Just a quiet enjoyable dinner with his family.

He probably doesn't understand what the big deal is about having kids, especially since he only had me and what I have been to him is mostly trouble and upset. It must be very difficult for a logical man like my father to have a daughter like me--dramatic, sensitive, super emotional, always ready to launch into an emotional tirade about this or that.

Normally, my father is an incredibly loving man, but perhaps this time, he just didn't feel like dealing with my issues (trust me, over the years I have had a lot of them.) Maybe for once he wanted things to be easy, pleasant, simple. I can't say I blame him. Easy, pleasant and simple are words that do not in any way describe me.

I know he meant no harm. Still..I'll get over it. He's my Dad. He calls and apologies. A very nice apology. I accept and we make up.

But I meant it when I said this will be the last December I ever experience without a child in my life.

A Visit to the Nutritionist

I decide to get an appointment with an iridologist/nutritionist in Maine. I want to compliment my infertility treatments with holistic medicine so I can get to the root of my problem.

The nutritionist/iridologist is named Sarah M. and she comes highly recommended. She spends almost three hours with me. She starts by analyzing my body through iridology, which is taking an x-ray of my eye and looking at what it tells about my body. She asks me lots of questions. I tell her that I have no energy. Sometimes, by 1 o'clock in the afternoon, even if I've done nothing all morning, I am exhausted and just want to watch TV in bed.

She recommends a large number of vitamins and herbs. Since I can only afford to buy about five bottles, I ask her what are the top five supplements I need. She said not to worry: my father had called ahead and offered to pay for everything. That's my Dad for you—always so generous and obviously very sorry that he hurt my feelings a few weeks ago. I was so surprised and relieved—now I could get all the vitamins and herbs I needed! It seems my liver, blood and colon all need cleansing. I went home with about 15 bottles. I didn't even want to look at the bill since I felt so guilty that my Dad was paying. I know he spent a lot.

Shivering At Night

It is now the third day on Sarah's program and every night, I shiver in bed for hours before falling asleep. I know all the herbs and vitamins are cleaning me out in some way, removing toxins from my body, but it still feels horrible.

Rocky and Me

My treatment is not progressing the way I would like. It is has been a year since I started infertility treatments, with still no results.

So... I am marching... marching around and around my living room, to the theme song "Rocky."

I am doing this to psyche myself up to ask my doctor, Dr. P to start doing IUI's each cycle.

Time is passing and I feel panicky that I need them to do something more to increase my chances of getting pregnant.

A few months ago, I was a lot more relaxed about this—but now I am wondering: why am I not pregnant yet even though I have been taking Clomid for almost four months and my polyp was removed? Why am I still not pregnant?

I am so worried that Dr. P is going to refuse my request.

I've heard of people being kept on the same medications, doing the same procedures, for years without result, and I don't want to fall into that trap. I need an IUI.

Medication alone won't get me pregnant.

What if he says no? What if he feels it is too soon to move on to another level of treatment?

I play the theme song to 'Rocky' almost everyday on the CD player in my living room. I love this song. The beat, the tempo, bring me up to a victorious place, where even a loser like me can win.

I kind of feel like I am Rocky right now.

I put on the CD and I start marching around: trying hard now…trying hard now…I am trying hard now. Its so hard now…The drums beat…the trumphets announce a person is trying harder than they ever dreamed they could….

Give me a chance, Dr. P. Please give me a chance.

Getting strong now…Moving on now…Getting strong now…and the music starts to sound hopeful..like this man/me can climb this mountain, scale the wall, hit this victory…

I listen to the song over and over again. I march around my living room, picturing my ovaries turning, a baby sliding out, Dr. P saying yes to my request.

I listen and I march around the living room, my own homemade motivation clinic.

I have to be strong…strong enough to ask…to demand…to push…The medicine is not enough…I need more assistance…

Will my insurance cover an IUI?

What if Dr. P thinks I don't need to do this?

What if he says no?

Trying hard now...

Then what...what are my chances then?

Getting strong now...getting strong now...

I feel like such a loser right now, a faceless,
anonymous zero, and he is the almighty and powerful doctor who has the power to decide my future.

Come on try

I need an IUI...and he needs to okay it.

I march some more, around my couch, my coffee table, up and down the living room, around the table one more time.

It is raining out. I feel ridiculous, but something inside me is changing. I'm pumped! The music moves me. It gives me hope, makes me imagine that like Rocky, a big zero like me can somehow end up a winner.

Getting strong now

I imagine my baby. I see my ovaries turning and babies coming out.

I march.

I let the beat of victory pulsate through my tired sad, body.

My baby, my baby, my baby...I am a warrior setting out to battle and the music beats strong....

Come on try...

The music is my coach.

Will I take the right turn in the road? Will I say the right words, act the right way, have the right insurance, to make Dr. P do this?

I march for strength. I march because I need to be stronger than the doctor. I march for power because I have to make him listen to me.

Flying high now

I listen over and over again to this song, knowing that it is up to me to start directing the course of my treatments.

If he says no, I have to fight for my rights.

If he says no, I have to convince him. Stomp, demand, shout if I have to.

I've sat passively by for too long and it is getting me nowhere.

I need an IUI: I know it, can feel it. I need advanced help.

What I am doing now is leading me nowhere.

I need them to time my cycles, do everything to up my chances. I need help.

The music plays on and I am reminded that Rocky wins.

The music plays on and I don't know the outcome for me.

A baby, a baby, a baby....

This is my training ground. I am gearing up for a hefty battle. I am beat up, bloodied, and not a reigning champ by any means.

Around and around my living room I go, marching, walking, imagining myself victorious--ha!

I pump myself up, imagine Dr. P saying yes and me getting what I want.

I picture my ovaries churning around and around, like the wheels in an old mill, and babies coming out.

I march some more.

My baby....There is a point in the song where the music gains momentum.. where you can actually feel the hero rising to the occasion, stepping towards the exact moment where victory and defeat split in a fork in the road, and somehow the right road is taken leading to victory.

Will I take the right turn in the road?

I see my ovaries turning, churning, children jumping out of them. I see children..holding hands with one another...

Come on fly now...flying high now...Come on, fly...Fly...Fly....

A Meeting with Dr. P

Chris and I enter Dr. P's office prepared for battle. I have typed out all my reasons for wanting an IUI. I speak very slowly and seriously, anticipating denial and objection. It takes oh, about three minutes, for Dr. P. to say yes, of course, moving on to IUI's is fine. He shakes our hands, thanks us, instructs me to call on Day One of my next cycle, and in five minutes, we are done.

We both leave feeling relieved. We actually laugh a bit, feeling slightly silly that we expected such objection from him. Obviously, asking for an IUI is no big deal. He instructs me to continue to take Clomid and call on day one of my next cycle.

Chapter 17: Visualize Your Way To Your Baby

Here are some visualization exercises you can do to enhance your fertility.

• **See yourself standing in a field of colorful flowers.** The flowers are opening and blooming, just as your body is blooming. See flowers blooming from your vaginal area as flowers continue to open all around you. You are a flowering blossom, part of the earth's beautiful eco-system, and blooming is happening all around you.

• **See beams of loving light entering your uterus.** See this light healing all your organs. It is entering and healing your uterus. The light is entering your liver and clearing your liver of all anger. The light is now entering your adrenal glands and giving all your glands energy and love. The light is shining into your stomach and taking away any nervous tension or stress that once lived there. The light is going into your head, your neck and your chest. Feel how good it is. See the light working its way through your body. It enters your chest and you can breath. It enters your ovaries and they can do what they are meant to do. The light travels through your body healing and soothing every part of your body.

• **See yourself walking hand-in-hand with your child.** Look at your child's hands. Touch your hand, and imagine how it will feel when your child touches your hand.

• **Visualize walking into your baby's nursery and looking into a crib and picking up your beautiful baby.** What do the windows look like in your baby's room? What type of bedding did you choose for your baby's crib? Imagine lifting your baby from the crib and sitting in a rocking chair. Ah, it feels so good to sit and rock your baby. Let yourself feel the peace and contentment of holding and rocking your baby.

- **See your husband/parter's sperm traveling up your vagina, meeting your egg, connecting, and then exploding with new life.** See the embryo implant itself firmly into your uterus. See it growing into your baby.

- **Picture your ovaries turning and children jumping out from your ovaries.**

- **It is the day of your child's wedding. Can you see yourself there?** What are you wearing? See your child walking down the aisle. Your eyes are bright with happiness and you cannot stop smiling. Envision dancing with your child at the reception. Close your eyes and listen to a song you would like played at your child's wedding.

- **It is the day your baby is born. The nurse has just handed you your baby.** Feel it. For one moment, let yourself experience the emotions you are going to feel. Picture it as if it already happened.

- **Look down at your stomach. You are pregnant.** Say it out loud: I am pregnant. I am pregnant.' Pat your stomach. Doesn't it feel great to be pregnant? Tell your stomach you love it. Tell your baby you love him or her. Sit down and feel what it is like to be pregnant.

- Imagine the sun shining directly on your vagina and healing everything within you.

Diary Excerpt: First IUI

If I thought a lot of blood tests and ultrasounds were needed when I was on Clomid, an IUI demands more than I imagined. Although as time passes, I am slowly getting more and more okay with the new demands. I am feeling able to cope with whatever the clinic asks of me. I have finally got the reality in my head that if I want a baby, I have to do whatever it takes to heal and get pregnant.

We get to the clinic and Chris goes into a room alone to give his sperm sample while I read magazines in the waiting room. I thinking how separate my husband and I are at this time, when normally we would be together.

About a half hour later, I am escorted into a room for the IUI. I know that normally husbands are present during this procedure, but I asked that Chris not to be there during this time.
Sometimes during this process, I get angry at Chris for no reason at all, because it is easy to want to blame someone and put my anger on a target, and most often, my husband is my favorite target.

Sometimes, I find I all too easily to pin my stress, fear and anger on him—it is your fault, his fault, not my fault, and so during this procedure, I want to be clear of these negative emotions. With strangers, I will not get so emotional, won't give in to the anger so easily, will force myself to stay a bit more positive.

I am so nervous. A technician named Carol is there with a nurse named Melissa. They insert a speculum and screw it in tight. I am not accustomed to this. It hurts and makes me feel trapped. Carol sees my fear and asks if I want to hold her hand. I do and it does help. Carol talks to me. She asks me questions to distract me and somehow I get through it.

The nurse removes the speculum, and tries a smaller speculum so it won't hurt me so badly. I so appreciate her gentle and extra effort.

Knowing that now my cycles will be timed by the clinic and I will be doing IUI's exactly when my body is ready and fertile is a huge relief. Pregnancy shouldn't be too far behind.

I return tomorrow for one more IUI. It won't be long now...

Trying Clomid

They have had me on Clomid for four cycles now, which because of the delays due to the polyp operation, and my needing to take a month off here and there inbetween cycles, seven months have passed. Seven long months...

The other day, Christine, the ultrasound technician, cued me into something I should have known: she told me that Clomid usually works in the first three cycles, and if it doesn't work by then, usually another medication is needed.

Thank you Christine.

And hello doctor: why didn't you bother to mention that to me?

This made me realize how little I know about these medications, and how if you leave your treatment in the hands of busy doctors, you might never know when precious time is being wasted.

It also made me realize how helpful it is to know a person like Christine who lets you in on the little 'secrets' of the infertility quest.

I'm pissed of right now. Why didn't they tell me this? Why are they wasting my time? I need to write my doctor a letter and request that we move on to the next level of medication. I also need to educate myself about the medications I am on. Sitting back and trusting the medical professionals isn't a great idea when everyone is so overworked and busy.

A Request

I know that something is wrong with me that the clinic is not catching. Month after month, it is the same thing. I do an IUI cycle and the answer turns out to be no. No, no, no. No pregnancy. No, no, no. Why is nothing working? I decided today I'm going to write a letter to Dr. P requesting they do a lapascropy to check for endometriosis.
Maybe I have that, and they are not catching it. I'll type the letter, let them know I have some of the symptoms of endometriosis, and force them to look. They are wasting time and I don't have time to waste. I'm taking this into my own hands. I also want a different medication. If Clomid should have worked by now, I need to move on to something stronger.

Very, Very Sad

It is June. One year and three months since I began infertility treatments. Such a long time and still no baby. I am sad. No, I am beyond sad--I am enraged, frustrated, full of yearning.

I am tired of yearning.

I long to hold hands with a baby...a baby that is mine.
I look at mothers in supermarkets, mothers who look angry, tired and annoyed at their rambunctious little brats and I think: God, why can't that be me? Why can't I be pushing around a cart full of loud, overtired, rambunctious children?

These mothers look so overworked, and yet they have no idea that I would do anything to have what they have.

These women look deceivingly ordinary in so many ways, and I think: why can't I have their ordinary life--the one that includes a grocery cart full of babies?

There is a woman I see occasionally who has four young children. She is beautiful and her children are lovely too.

When I saw her holding hands with one of her young sons the other day, I was struck with that image--the image of a woman holding hands with her son.

Hands to hold. I want little hands to hold.

When I see the little hands of a baby, I think: what in the world must it feel like to hold the little hands of a baby that you gave birth to? What I would give to hold such little hands, to know those hands were mine to hold, to know that those were the hands of my daughter or my son?

I am going to write Dr. P a letter to ask that he do a lapascropy to see if I have a problem with endometriosis. I hope he listens and does what I want. I have to word the letter in a way that will get him to do as I ask.

I need little hands to hold. Hands that are all mine. To all the women I see shopping in supermarkets, who see themselves as ordinary mothers, I say--you have everything I want and there is nothing ordinary about your role as the mother to those little humans who are driving you crazy.

Please God, give me a little human to tire me out. Please let me be an ordinary mother in a supermarket one day.

I can't imagine anything in this world more special or more fun than pushing around my babies at the supermarket. My happy-ever-after is so plain and ordinary, boring even, and yet it feels so hopelessly impossible and faraway.

Meeting with Dr. P

I met with Dr. P today and found out a few disturbing things.

One is that yes, he knew I should be moving on to a stronger medicine, but because I tend to get scared and stressed during the procedures, he didn't think I could handle moving on to shots. I want to scream at him! Instead, I force myself to stay calm and I explain to him that the more time that passes, the less nervous I am during procedures.

He seems skeptical, but I continue talking calmly, stating that while I may seem nervous, that is just my style of coping—and that the moment I leave the clinic, I feel completely calm and back to normal (which is true. I expulse everything and then I'm over it. It could be called being Italian, but I don't say that because it may sound weird.) He agrees to do the lapascropy and will schedule it soon. After that is done, depending on the outcome of the surgery, we will move on to shots. I am now waiting for a surgery date.

Date of Surgery

The surgery is scheduled for July 6. Almost two months away. I wish it could have been sooner, but at least I feel like progress is being made. Maybe I do have endometriosis and they never caught it. Maybe it is the reason I am not pregnant yet. As I write that, some anger comes up…Do I have to direct their every step? It is aggravating to think that if I hadn't spoke up, Dr. P might have kept me on Clomid indefinitely, all the time knowing that if it hasn't worked by yet, it probably was never going to work.

I feel a bit ashamed too, that my behavior made them think I couldn't handle shots. I can handle shots…Hell, I can handle anything if it gets me a baby…why would they assume that just because I am verbal about my fear it means I can't handle it?

If I silently suffer, does that mean I am handling the stress better than someone who is verbal about their fear? That is the odd thing about the culture we live in---people that hide their pain are presumed to be a lot stronger than those who verbalize it, but in some cases, the person who holds it in might be a lot more stressed than someone like me who gets it out and then is over it. It is hard to explain that to someone who doesn't cope in the same way, however, so I won't even try.

The Donut Incentive

They have ordered some new tests. This morning I was scheduled for a test I am dreading. I am so afraid of this particular test.
I don't think I have it in me to do this test. The whole drive down to the clinic, anxiety rattled around my body. How in the world am I going to make myself go through this test?

Then I got an idea: on the way to the clinic, I went to a drive-through Dunkin Donuts and ordered two of my favorite chocolate frosted donuts.

I get to the clinic, sit in the waiting room holding my donut bag, and soon am called in for the test. The nurse leaves the room while I change. When she comes back in, I am lying on the table, dressed in a johnny, with the donut bag sitting on my stomach.

"What are the donuts for?" she asks, straining to act like no-big-deal-so-what-if-a-bag-of-donuts-is-sitting-on-a-patient, but since she's not a professional actress, her irritation comes shining through.

"They are my reward for going through this test," I said.

My logic here is this: if I can lay here, endure whatever I have to endure, all the while seeing and smelling these two donuts that I am going to eat the moment the test is done, the test won't feel so bad or be so hard to take.

Nothing is a better reward for me than chocolate donuts.

The doctor comes in, and very politely asks if I want to eat the donuts sitting on my stomach before they do the test.

Again, he is trying to be nice, but obviously is a bit confused by the presence of the donut bag on my stomach. The great efforts everyone went through to show respect to me, even though I obviously looked eccentric, was both hilarious and touching. What a nice group of people at this clinic.

"No," I giggled. "I'll eat them later," and it felt good to laugh and see the humor in this whole situation.

They did the test, and all the time I kept focusing on was: if I can get through this test, I can eat my donuts. I tried to think of nothing else, not the pain, not the nurses, not anything but the reward coming: the donuts.

How I love chocolate donuts.

The test ended. Everyone left the room. Before I even changed out of the johnny, I devoured the donuts in about ten seconds.

Ah, the power of chocolate donuts.

Even the most unpleasant test was bearable because I had two grand and delicious donuts to look forward to. Maybe I'll try this again.

Teaching Experience

I have one more IUI before my surgery in July. How great it would be if I got pregnant this time and never had to go through the surgery at all. Today I taught a magazine writing class at the community college I attended in the early 1980s. Since I am a reporter, teaching writing is something I do occasionally.

Typically, I love teaching. I teach one-day classes on Saturdays. Sometimes I teach journalism, sometimes writing your family history, sometimes magazine writing. Usually, teaching these classes leaves me with a buzz, a thrill, a high almost. When I teach,
I am seventeen and in love, I am six and allowed to go on the merry-go-round one more time, I am 11 years old and sitting in my treehouse, I am 14 and someone (anyone) thinks I am pretty.

When I teach, the insecure, negative, self-hating part of me disappears and I emerge strong, confident, and full of possibilities. The girl in college who wore a white cotton dress and truly believed that anything and everything was possible returns briefly for an encore.

When I teach, I realize that my true calling was not working as a newspaper reporter, but being in a classroom with students.

But today, my teaching experience was completely different than usual and left me feeling pretty hysterical. Here's why.

The class started out as usual.

First, I introduce myself, and then I call each student up to my desk to talk one-on-one about why they took the class and what they hope to learn from the class.

The students come to my desk one at a time and share their goals for the class.

Now it is the turn of the woman sitting in the front row who looks to be in her mid-30s. Immediately, I like her. She seems spunky.

Then she opened her mouth, "I'm here to write about my seven year hell with infertility."

Wham--I am in for quite a ride.

For the next seven hours, eight counting lunch, all I hear about is her horrible experience with infertility and how it DIDN'T work out.

Her voice and desire to share her story was louder and more fervent than any other person in class. She had enough anger and fury to dominate the entire class discussion.

"The clinic tricked me."

"I tried everything and it didn't work."

"I'm trying Reiki now, hoping maybe that will work."

"All my husband and I ever wanted was children."

Even during lunch, when I hoped for a break from hearing about her pain, which scarily mirrored my own, she sat with me outside on the picnic bench and continued her story.

I felt for this woman. At another time, the teacher part of me might have been glad she took my class in order to share her pain.

But the infertility patient part of me wanted to tell her to shut up.

I struggled all day to remain professional, calm and not interject with my own experiences with infertility....but inside I was screaming was IS THIS GOING TO BE IN SEVEN YEARS? Am I going to turn into her eventually? Will I try and try like she did and never get a baby?

Was her lot my lot?

No, no, no, I kept saying to myself. I won't make the same mistakes she made. I was going to a highly reputable clinic. I was already working on improving my overall health.

But still....I felt panicked and scared. Hearing her story just confirmed all my worst fears: that I could do infertility treatments year after year after year with no result.

All she ever wanted was a baby. All I ever wanted was a baby. Were we two peas in the same hopeless pod?

I hid my feelings all day, knowing it would open a can of worms if I told her I too was in the midst of fertility treatments.

But now back at home, I am burning with pain. Will this be me in seven years?

She reminded me yet again of the terrible statistic that not everyone who goes to a fertility clinic ends up with a baby. I can't stand to hear these statistics. They make me crazy.

I can't go seven more years without a child in my life. I won't be her, because if I don't get pregnant in one year, I will adopt.

I will always and forever keep trying for my own biological baby, but I will adopt before I let seven years pass without a child in my life. Hell, if I end up with both an adopted baby and a biological baby, what an incredible blessing that would be.

Everywhere I turn right now, I feel I am confronted with one hopeless infertility story after another.

Throughout the class, her pain was raw and rageful in a way I clearly understood, but surely didn't want to see, hear or understand. Why did she have to take my class? Was I suppose to hear something she said?

Was I suppose to know that sometimes this doesn't work out?

God help this woman, God help me. Let us both get the babies we so desperately want.

Chapter 18: Fertility Affirmations

Words have power. Words can help heal the body. Words can provide your heart with hope. Saying, writing, singing, and reading affirmations everyday can lift your mood and help you physically manifest what you most want.

Go ahead, begin affirming out loud that yes, you are going to have a baby! Yes, your dream of becoming a mother is going to come true!

Doing affirmations will give you a chance to take conscious control of your thoughts. No longer will negative thoughts have free rein to take over and demoralize you. You deserve to hear affirmations that positively announce the arrival of your baby. Affirmations will help you combat the negativity, frustration and fear that often accompany infertility. They will give you a powerful way to tap into joyful, hopeful emotions that you deserve to feel as you walk down this exciting life path.

Affirmations can slowly transform a subconscious who may have given up, into a subconscious that really and truly believes a baby will be arriving soon. Your body then can easily move into a state of hope and belief. A body that believes will act accordingly, because it knows that a wonderful guest is about to arrive.

As you say your affirmations, breath them, feel them, visualize them coming true. Let them sink so deep into your body that your very essence soaks them in as if watching a dream come true.

Repeat your affirmations as much as possible. Speak them, write them, sing them, turn them into poems, repeat and do it all again. Write and speak them, even if you do not believe them at first.

By affirming your baby's arrival, you are emitting positive energy into the world—an energy working towards your goal, not against it.

When you say out loud, "I can and will have a baby" you are using the energy of words to manifest what you most want.

Some ways to state your affirmations include:

• Write your affirmations and post them on a mirror or wall that you can look at each morning as you get ready for your day ahead.

• Get a notebook and spend five to ten minutes a day writing your affirmations. As you write, speak the words out loud.

• Record yourself saying your affirmations, either on your phone, iPod of CD, and listen to them when you take a walk or simply are doing chores around the house.

• Listen to a recording of your affirmations and visualize what you are saying coming true as you listen to them. You can add background music if that makes the affirmations more powerful to you.

• Choose one or two affirmations that are easy to say and say them when you wake up each morning. They could be something simple like: 'I am ready to have a baby' or 'My baby is arriving soon.'

• Create a piece of art or draw a picture that includes one or two affirmations that are important and meaningful to you.

• Hang a chalkboard and write your affirmations daily. If you can, put the chalkboard in a place where you see it often.

• Buy a calendar or an appointment book and write affirmations in each date.

Below are affirmations that you can do daily. Choose the ones that strike you most powerfully and that you most feel your body needs to hear often. Think about what negative beliefs you hold about your fertility that need to be replaced with positive, hopeful words.

• I trust my body can give me a baby.

- I give myself permission to have a baby.

- I grant myself the power to have a baby.

- My body is making a baby right now.

- I am ready to have a baby.

- I am ready to be pregnant.

- I am ready to be a mother.

- I am good enough to be a mother.

- I now welcome my baby.

- My body is creating lots of healthy eggs today.

- I will get pregnant today.

- My embryos are successfully implanted in my uterus and my baby is now on the way to me.

- I am an amazing mother about to have an amazing baby!

- I enjoy bringing new life into the world.

- My pregnancy is perfect.

- I agree to have a baby.

- Love surrounds me as I welcome my baby.

- I am ready, willing and able to get pregnant.

- I have the power in my body and heart to create a baby.

- Hip, hip hooray there is joy in my day!

- Its okay to get pregnant.

- My body is fertile and healthy

- I am pregnant with a beautiful, healthy baby

- My body knows how to get pregnant and care for my baby.

- I trust in my ability to give birth to a baby.

- I know how to meet the needs of my baby and myself

- Today, I will allow myself to get pregnant.

- I am allowing myself to become a mother.

- I feel relaxed and confident about my pregnancy.

- The birth experience will be wonderful for me and my baby.

- I am going to deliver a happy, healthy baby.

- I can see myself playing with my beautiful baby.

- My body is beautifully nourishing my baby.

- I conceive my baby with love, I carry my baby with love, I deliver my baby with love, and I welcome my baby with love.

- My body is a healthy perfect place for my baby to grow.

- I love getting pregnant.

- I love being ripe and fertile.

- I love being ready to welcome my baby.

- Every part of me is ready to have a baby.

- My body is fertile and full of healthy babies.
- My eggs are fertile, ripe and healthy.
- My womb is strong and fertile.
- I am completely deserving of a baby.
- My body knows how to get pregnant and carry my baby full-term
- Everything and everyone around me is helping me get pregnant
- My hormones are balanced and working just as they should
- My liver, ovaries and adrenal glands are strong and healthy
- I am ready to welcome my baby
- This is the perfect time and perfect age for me to have a baby
- I am strong enough to have a baby
- My uterus is safe and strong
- My ovaries are powerful, strong and ready
- I am worthy of having a child
- I accept the miracle of birth into my life
- I am part of the natural birth cycle
- I will successfully conceive and give birth to a baby
- I will have a baby, I will have a baby, I will have a baby
- My body says it is okay to have a baby
- My body has agreed to have a baby

- I am ready to have a baby
- I welcome my baby into my life
- It is safe for my baby to be born
- There is nothing blocking me from having a baby
- I am fertile
- I am full of hope and confidence that soon I will become a mother
- My baby is arriving soon
- I accept my right to be a mother
- Nothing from my past can hurt me anymore
- I am safe and I am loved.
- My mind, body and emotions are healed so I can now have a baby
- Having a baby is fun and relaxing
- My body says yes to having a baby!
- I deserve to be a mother
- I am going to be a great Mom
- My body has everything it needs to conceive a healthy baby
- I am healthy and ready to conceive
- I am able to receive and give birth to a baby
- Love and goodness follow me daily

- I am able to carry a pregnancy full-term

- I am able to conceive a child

- I am able to carry a pregnancy full-term and give birth to a healthy baby

- I am pregnant

- My body is ready, willing and able to be pregnant

- I can give birth whenever I choose

- Giving birth is easy for me

- Giving birth is safe for me

- I am capable of being a mother

- Nothing in my past prevents me from being a mother

- I give myself permission to be pregnant

- I am strong and able to conceive a baby

- My body is ready to lovingly produce a baby

- My ovaries are good and strong

- My ovaries are now making lots of healthy eggs!

- My baby is on the way to me

- I am a mother

- I am giving birth. I am holding life in my arms

- I can carry my baby for nine months

- Every part of my body is ripe for the birth and creation process.
- I am ripe and ready to conceive
- I am receiving my baby right now.
- I am holding my baby.
- I am ready to receive a baby.
- I am ready to give birth.
- I give myself permission to get pregnant.
- I grant myself the power to get pregnant.
- I have permission to be a mother.
- It is safe for me to have a baby
- It is safe for me to become a mother
- I have permission to have a baby
- My body has the power to conceive and give birth to a child
- My body is strong and deserving of a baby
- I deserve a baby
- My vagina, ovaries, kidney and liver are strong and healthy
- I welcome my baby
- My body is helping me get pregnant
- My body is ready to have a baby
- My womb is ready to receive a baby

- I am deserving of a child

Chapter 19: Your Personal Fertility Vision Statement

A personal vision statement is something you can read, record and listen to each day. When you listen, visualize what is being said so it can sink deep into your subconscious. Be sure to fill in your name.

Here is your personal vision statement:

It is a bright, warm, sunny morning and you are feeling really good. You walk outside, take a deep breath of fresh air, raise your arms to the sky and say thank you, thank you, thank you for my baby.

That's right, YOUR NAME_____, having a baby is easy for you. Your body and mind are ready, willing and VERY able to have a baby.

You smile, because being vibrantly healthy and super fertile feels good.

Really good actually.

You know on a very deep level that having a baby is good and right for you. You deserve this baby. You are completely and totally worthy of having a baby. You are capable of conceiving a baby, carrying a baby for nine months and giving birth, in the healthiest, safest, most wonderful way possible.

That's right, you are worthy of having children.

Because you ate so many healthy green vegetables, let go of the toxins in your body, and said goodbye to all the trauma, anger and sadness in your cells, you are now able to give birth to a baby whenever you choose.

That's right: you can have a baby whenever you want to. Today, next week, next month, whenever you choose. Your body has the power to conceive and give birth to a baby whenever you want it to.

You can see yourself smiling and holding your new baby. You see yourself kissing your baby and feeling so thankful that your baby has arrived.

You look in the mirror and smile, because being a mother feels right to you.

Your baby is here. You are fertile. You are super fertile today! You are actually over-the-top fertile right now! You are creating super healthy eggs this minute.

That's right: your dear sweet ovaries are right now producing ripe, rich, healthy eggs. Feel how strong and good your eggs are!

Your body now has everything it needs to get pregnant. All the organs in your body are working at maximum capacity to help you get pregnant. Your liver has let go of anger and is now balanced and calm. Your kidneys have let go of sadness and are happy now.

Nothing in your past can block you from conceiving and giving birth. You forgive those who hurt you. You released all anger and sadness. You have let go of all the bad memories, sad events, and traumas in your life. Only happiness lives in your cells now.

Love and happiness flow through your body now. Love flows into your heart.

That's right, there is immense power in your heart to have a baby.

You have permission to have a baby. You have permission to conceive. You have permission to enjoy a safe and successful pregnancy. You are ready to give birth.

Your hurt is gone. Your anger is gone. Your fear is gone. You are safe.

That's right, you feel safe all the time. Safer than you ever felt before. You know it is safe for you to get pregnant and safe for you to give birth and safe for you to be a mother. Life is safe. Motherhood is safe. Having children is safe. Everything is safe.

You feel safe all the time, because you know that having a baby is safe for you.

All fears and pain from your childhood are gone. All your anxiety is gone. All your frustration is gone.

You laugh and feel happy.

That's right, you laugh a lot lately, because feeling so healthy and fertile feels good.

Really good actually. Life is so good!

Your body is now full of pure and clean energy. Your bowels are clean and you eliminate easily. Your blood sugar levels are stable. Your hormones are balanced and communicate well with one another. Your pituitary gland, adrenal gland, thyroid and pancreas are healthy and balanced. Blood flows easily to your uterus. Oxygen flows easily to your ovaries. Your uterine lining is strong. Your vagina is open and ready to receive. Your ovaries are making lots of healthy eggs.

That's right, your ovaries are now making strong, viable healthy eggs that make it easy for you to conceive and give birth.

You now flow with life. You feel comfortable asserting your will. You let your authentic voice be heard. You welcome your real self. You respect yourself. You no longer feel shame or guilt. You honor and express all your feelings. You creativity express yourself, as having a baby is a creative expression you fully allow yourself.

You smile and feel relaxed.

You feel relaxed a lot lately. You slept so good last night. You sleep good every night.

That's right, you are relaxed and sleeping well because you know everything is going to be okay.

It is okay for you to get pregnant and have lots of babies.

You smile, because you always knew you would get pregnant.

That's right. You knew that infertility was just a temporary condition. You knew you would heal and be fertile. You always said, "I will get pregnant soon" and you were right.

You have already let yourself receive a baby. Your womb is a warm, welcoming place for your babies.

You are strong enough to receive and hold your baby.

Nothing in your past can hold you back having the children you desire. You deserve this! Go ahead. Let yourself have this. Let yourself have your babies!

You, my darling, are part of the world's unstoppable, undefeatable, always victorious birth cycle. See that flower blooming—you are part of that bloom. See that tree sprouting new leaves—you are part of that sprouting! You are part of life's beautiful birth cycle. You have everything you need within you to give birth to a baby, just like all the other living beings on the planet.

You got it kid! You do! Your dream of being a mother is now coming true. You are allowed to have a baby. It is good and right and okay for you to have a baby. It is safe for you to be a mother.

That's right—you are meant to have a baby. Things are working out for you, just as you hoped they would.

It feels right and good to receive your baby. Your body feels good doing this. Giving birth is fun. Being a mother is fun. Getting pregnant is fun.

Go ahead and have a baby! It is okay! You have given yourself permission! Every part of your body has agreed to help you conceive and give birth.

Getting pregnant is easy for you.

Go ahead, today is the day you can conceive your beautiful baby.

Then do it again whenever you want too, because getting pregnant and having children is easy, safe and fun for someone like you.

Chapter 20: Letters To Yourself

During your fertility journey, there are times you will need to be your own best friend. Here are some letters that you can mail to yourself, or leave around the house when you need a lift or just a reminder of how strong you are. Be sure to begin each letter by filling in your name and then signing it at the end.

_____

Dear_____

Congratulations! You are on your way to getting pregnant! Every day, you are one step closer to being pregnant! Every day, your body is getting stronger. I see you getting stronger! I can feel how ready your body is to conceive a baby. You are ready to have a baby! That's right-- your body can easily have a baby now! Congratulations!

Love,

_____

Dear _____

I know with all my heart that you will give birth to a baby soon. Your dear sweet ovaries, dear healthy healthy ovaries, can produce ripe, rich healthy eggs. Actually, right now they are making healthy fertile eggs! Your ovaries know how to produce good eggs. They are right now producing eggs that will lovingly grow into your baby. Thank you ovaries! Thank you for giving me healthy eggs!

Love,

_____

Dear_____:

You are ready to be a mother. I can see it—you are ready. Nothing in your past can hold you back from having a child. You deserve this! You are worthy of this! There is nothing to fear when it comes to becoming a mother. You can do this. Millions of women from various backgrounds, life experiences and families do this. So can you. You do not need to be perfect to be a good mother. Go ahead, let yourself have this. You deserve a baby.

Love,

_____

Dear _____

Your vagina, your dear beautiful healthy vagina, is ready to receive. Yes, sweet vagina, you are ready to receive. Thank you for welcoming my baby. Thank you for opening up and allowing my baby in. Thank you for being a safe place for my baby. I love you vagina. I love everything about you. Thank you for receiving my child and giving it a safe home to grow.

Love,

_____

Dear _____,

I think you know this, but I am to say it again: it is safe for you to have a baby. It is safe for you to get pregnant. It is safe for you to carry a child for nine months. It is safe for you to give birth. It is safe for you to be a mother.

Love,

_____

Dear _____,

Hello, I love you! I love you! I love you! I love you! You are going to have a baby soon! You are fertile and strong!
I love you! I love you! I love you!

Love,

_____

Dear_____,

You, my darling, are a part of the world's unstoppable, undefeatable, always victorious life cycle. You are a key part of the birth cycle that goes on around you each day. See that flower blooming: you are part of that bloom. You are an integral part of all the birth and life that goes on around you each day. You are part of life's most beautiful and welcoming cycle. You have everything you need within you to give birth to a baby, just like all the other living beings on this planet. You've got it kid! You do! You are part of the birth cycle of life that permeates the world. Congratulations!

Love,

Dear _____,

Your liver is healthy and clean. Your liver has released all the anger within you. It works hard to release the toxins within you. Amazing liver, I love everything you are doing to help me get pregnant. I love you liver! I love everything about you! Liver, you are calm and happy now. You have released all anger. Liver, you are doing a fine job of helping me get pregnant. Thank you for helping me make my baby.

Love,

_____

Dear_____,

Hello beautiful kidneys! I love you my kidneys! I thank you for releasing all the sadness that used to be in you. You, my sweet kidneys, are filled with happiness now. Thank you kidneys, for allowing yourself to be filled with joy, peace and hope. I love you kidneys. I love everything about you.

Love,

_____

Dear _____,

Congratulations! Your dream of being a mother is about to come true!

Love,

Dear _____

I give you permission to get pregnant.

You have permission to be pregnant.

It is right and good for you to have a baby.

You are allowed to have a baby.

Permission to have a baby is yours.

Love,

_____

Dear _____,

Your adrenal glands are full of energy. I thank you adrenals for being so full of energy. Adrenal glands, thank you for helping me have a baby. Thank you for your energy and your love. Thank you, adrenals, for giving me what I need to have my baby. Thank you for being powerful and full of good energy. I love you adrenals so much.

Love,

_____

Dear _____,

You are good enough right now in this moment to have a baby. You deserve a baby. You deserve to have a child. You deserve a baby right now—yes you do!!!

Love,

Dear _____,

Today, your life is filled with joy.

Life is good and good things are coming to you naturally.

You are happy. Your heart is happy. Your body is happy.

Your body is happy because it knows you are going to have a baby soon.

Wow, life is so good right now. Everything is so good right now. Joy fills your heart and all your organs—happy, happy, happy! Today that is you!!!

Love,

_____

Dear _____,

Stop being scared. It is safe for you to be a mother. It is good for you to be a mother. There is only good that will come from your experience of being a mother.

It is safe for you to be a mother.

It is safe for you to give birth to a baby.

It is safe to be pregnant.

It is safe to receive a baby.

Having a baby is safe for you.

Love,

Dear _____,

Soon, your baby will be growing inside of you! Congratulations!
Love,
_____

Dear _____,

You are going to enjoy a healthy pregnancy. I can see it for you. You are going to carry your baby full-term and deliver at nine months a healthy baby. Your body is going to stay balanced and give your growing baby everything is needs to be born healthy and strong. I am so happy for you.

Love,

Dear _____,

Your body is helping you have the baby you desire. I want to thank you, body, for healing. Thank you for being my friend and
helping me to have the baby of my dreams.

Love,

_____

Dear _____,

You deserve the best! You deserve to have a baby!

Love,

_____

Dear _____,

Things can work out for you.
Things will work out for you.
Things can go right for you.
Things will go right for you.

Love,

_____

Dear _____,

I love everything about you! I love your kidneys! I love your liver! I love your hormones! I love your adrenal glands! I love your thyroid! I love your ovaries! I love your vagina! I love your energy! I love your strength! I love you!

Love,

_____

Dear _____,

All trauma and sadness has left your body. Love is entering your organs and cells instead. Goodbye sadness! Goodbye sad memories from the past! Love is pouring in your body instead.

All difficulties from your childhood are leaving. Goodbye sad memories! Love is pouring in its place. Hello love!

Now, there is no trauma left in your body.

Now, there are no sad memories lodged in your cells.

Now, love flows through your body. Only love, love, love.

I can see love flowing through your body.

There is no more trauma, no more bad memories, to hold you down.

Your body has let go!

Now, love flows up through your vagina, into your stomach, up to your neck, down your legs. Love pours through your arms and into your hands. Love fills your breasts, your lungs, down to your feet. Love is flowing through your entire body!

The sadness is gone. The trauma is gone. The sad memories are gone.

Love is here and soon your baby will be here too!

Love,

_____

Dear _____,

All your hormones are in balance. Your hormones communicate well with one another. They are friends and they are helping you get pregnant.

Your kidneys are running perfectly. Your adrenals are filled with energy. Your ovaries are in perfect balance producing perfect eggs. Your uterine is open and welcoming.

Every part of your body is in sync.

Every part of your body is filled with love.

Every part of your body is running exactly and perfectly as it should be.

Love,

_____

Dear _____,

Everyone is here to help you.

We are all here to help you.

You are surrounded by help.

Love,

Dear _____,

Go ahead and have a baby! Its okay! You've got permission!

Love,

Dear _____,

I am here for you. You are not alone. I love you. I will help you. I will take care of you. I will help you every step of the way!

I love you. I am here for you. Don't be scared—together we can do this!

You are not alone.

Love,

Dear _____,

You are fertile! You are ripe and fertile! Your body told me so.

Love,

Dear _____,

We all love you. We all believe you can do this. Don't be scared. Together, we can do this.

Love,

_____

Dear _____,

Your desire to have a baby makes you powerful. Your desire to be a mother makes you strong. Your love for children makes you very, very fertile. Your desire to give birth makes you successful.

Love,

_____

Dear _____,

There is no reason why you can't have a baby. NO REASON! There is nothing that can stop you from having a baby. NOTHING! Don't be afraid. You can do this. Go ahead now—go have a baby!

Love,

_____

Dear _____,

I think you are ready to be a mother. I think you are good enough to be a mother. I think you are strong enough to give birth. I think you are ready to be pregnant. I think being a mother is right for you.

I think having a baby is going to happen soon for you.

Love,

_____

Dear _____,

Adrenal glands, you are strong and working well.
Liver, you are strong and working well.
Hormones, you are balanced and working well.
Kidneys, you are strong and working well.
Thyroid, you are strong and working well.
Ovaries, you are strong and working well.
Fallopian tubes, you are strong and working well.

All the parts of your body are strong and working well.

Love,

_____

Dear _____,

You are full of courage. All fear has left your body. You are able to move forward with your dreams. Being stuck is not part of you anymore.

You are peaceful. You are filled with love. You are happy. Your body is full of happiness. Sadness and grief has left your body. Goodbye grief! Goodbye sad memories from the past! Joy is pouring into you instead.

Frustration is leaving your body. All frustration has left your body. You are filled with power instead.

Love,

Dear _____,

All the parts of your body are ready to conceive a child.

All the parts of your body want you to know that they love you and are ready to help you give birth to a child.

Your liver, ovaries, adrenal glands, thyroid, vagina, are all in agreement that they can help you make a baby.

They love you. They want you to know they love you very much, and they will help you.   Love, Your Body

Dear _____,

You are not going to repeat the mistakes your parents made when you were growing up.

I repeat: you are not going to repeat the mistakes your parents made growing up.

You are aware and you know how to learn from the mistakes of others.

You don't have to be perfect to raise a child. You don't have to know everything. You can have flaws and imperfections.

You will raise your child in safety and love. You will not repeat the past.

Love,

_____

Diary Excerpt: A Door Opens...

Lately, I'm realizing that to get pregnant, I need to get as healthy as I can. When I first started infertility treatments, I thought that infertility medicine alone would do the trick. Then I thought doing an IUI would guarantee a baby.

Now, I am beginning to see that more is needed to make this all work.

Today at work, I started feeling so nervous and desperate that I prayed all day for answers. Every spare minute I could, I asked God to help me give my body whatever it needs to get pregnant. I prayed repeatedly that God would help me get as healthy as I can be.

I feel so afraid that even with everything I am doing, it won't work out.

After work, I went to pick up Chris at the salon where he works as a massage therapist on Saturday. I've driven that road dozens of times before, so it was odd that today, I noticed a sign I never noticed before: 'Chinese Herbalist'.

Something in me felt compelled to stop. I had recently read that Chinese herbs are sometimes used to help prepare the body for pregnancy. Maybe it wasn't an accident that my eyes landed straight on that sign, especially since I prayed so hard this morning.

I had to stop and see what this herbalist had to say about my condition, especially since I still had a few hours before my husband got off work.

Dr. Myung Kim would turn out to be an answer to my prayer. He turned out to also be an acupuncturist, and while he did not want to sell me any herbs, he recommended acupuncture. I tried acupuncture before and believe in it strongly.

He read my pulse, and told me that I had a weak gallbladder channel. I made my first appointment. He has even written a book on acupuncture.

It turns out that he has a second one about 15 minutes from my home, which I don't think is an accident considering how much I prayed this morning.

Although I have driven down this road about 100 times in the past year, I noticed his storefront today for the first time. Acupuncture needs to be part of my treatment, I am sure of it.

In A Waiting Mode

Getting pregnant has overtaken my thoughts like never before.

When I started infertility treatments last year, I felt an easy confidence: of course I will get pregnant soon, I thought, I'm going to a clinic, taking medication, this is going to work out.

Now that time has passed and I'm still not pregnant, a lot of fear has set in. I worry pretty much all the time.

What if I'm one of those women for whom infertility treatments don't work? What if I try and try and never get pregnant?

My desire for a baby has reached a point where what I think about and talk about most of the time is having a child: will I have a child? Why am I not pregnant?

Thank God that at work, we are allowed to talk during the day. I work in member outreach at a PBS station in Boston, MA, where we call members for donations. It is a part-time job that allows me to get insurance for me and my husband, the pay isn't bad, and it isn't so stressful that it takes up all the time and space in my life. It is the perfect job for this time in my life right now.

The best part of the job are the wonderful people I have met, Judy and Chelsea. We all are very comfortable with one another, natural friends and we share a lot with each other.

Judy has four children, and like myself, she cherishes children.

One day, out of the blue, Judy looked over at me and said, "I picture you with a daughter with corkscrew curly hair."

Hope! My dear friend was giving me hope! She was sharing with me a positive vision for my future! I can't thank Judy enough for gifting me with these words…words that I desperately need to hear. Hope is what I'm hanging on to by a thread right now…Hope…from a dear friend…much appreciated.

A Wedding

Today Chris and I attended the wedding of an old family friend. It was a beautiful wedding, and in the midst of it, one of my cousins heard a rumor that I was pregnant.

"Paula, are you pregnant?" she asked with a big, excited smile.

"Yes," I answered, knowing fully well I wasn't pregnant, but just wanting to feel for one moment how it feels to say 'yes, I am pregnant'. A second later, I told the truth: "No I'm not pregnant…but I could be."

"You are!" she said, as if she figured out a big secret and I realized I had gone too far.

"Well, I'm trying. I don't think I actually am right now," I said.

She smiled and walked away.

I felt like such a loser. All my cousins at this event have babies..had them pretty much without even thinking about it…What an idiot I am.

Visits to Dr. Kim

I have now started going to Dr. Kim for acupuncture every week. I realize that to get pregnant, I need to get my body healthy on a very deep level. I feel like I am stepping up like never before.

I would love to be pregnant this cycle—then I wouldn't have to go through the laparoscopy. I have an IUI next week, and maybe this time it will work.

How great would it be if it turned out I got pregnant on this time—then no surgery, no chance of endometriosis, no going under anesthesia.

That would be so easy…

June IUI

Today, my husband and I did the IUI. We were incredibly stressed. As we walked out of the clinic, down the long sidewalk to the parking lot, we started fighting. Literally we burst out into a fight the moment we left the clinic. Lately, we fight before, during and after most IUI's. The stress builds and builds and at a certain point, we end up attacking each other. I hate him on days like this. I need him to be safe, calm, sweet. Instead, he feels like the enemy. We walked down that sidewalk, bickering and bickering…and looking back, I'm not sure about what. I said something…he said something..I got annoyed at his tone..he got annoyed at my tone.

We are definitely not helpful to one another during these stressful times. This whole process has been tough on our relationship. Lately, I see him as the cause of my infertility. What if we are one of those couples who just don't mate very well naturally? What if my body doesn't like his sperm? Not the kindest thoughts, but having a child is such a priority to me, I can't help but analyze him this way. There is no softness between us during these times, when I know there should be softness, but there is only anger and more anger.

A Moment In Song

Something wildly odd and beautiful happened this afternoon in the parking lot at the supermarket. I was there to meet a friend for coffee, and arrived a little early. Stuck with about an hour to kill, I decided to just listen to the radio.

I started praying about having a baby, as I usually do whenever I have a spare moment.

While I was doing that, Will Smith's "Just The Two of Us" came on the radio. The song is a father singing to his son. The Dad gives his son advice about not swearing, remembering to say your prayers, and holding the door open for girls. I love this song, as you can feel the power of this father's love for his child.

As I listened to the song, a wave of joy came over me--like someday I would actually be able to sing this song to my child.

I imagined that on my child's wedding day, I would play this for him or her, and recount this moment in the parking lot where I was begging for his/her birth.

It wouldn't matter if my child was a boy or a girl--this song would still apply. "Just the Two of Us"--me and my child. I got so deeply into this vision, of me dancing and singing this song to my child at their wedding, that it began to feel completely real. Of course I will have a baby someday! No doubt..it will come to pass...

The song moved me to another time and place, and it felt so completely real, that it was as if it had already happened.

By the end of the song, I was on a wild high, visions of my child dancing in my head: their wedding, their birth, this song being our song. For a few minutes, I landed in such a place of hope.

A good place...

For those few minutes, all the desperation I usually feel was swept away by a tidal wave of faith and hope.

Do I dare think this song was maybe a kind of answer to my prayer?

For a few minutes even after the song ended, a feeling of certainty that I would have a child was mine, all mine.

My prayer, coupled with that song, brought me to a place of joy I haven't felt in a long time.

My child was real--our relationship was real--the future with my child in it all became real.

Could this be a signal?

I can't imagine the fullness I will someday feel if there was a little person on this earth I could actually sing and dedicate this song to.

Needing Validation

Everywhere I go, everything I do, in every conversation I have, I am looking for validation that yes, I am someday going to have a baby. I search conversations for clues, for hope, for someone to say "yes you Paula are going to have a baby."

People don't realize how their subtle words and expressions tell me volumes about what they really think about my quest to have a baby. A slight hesitation, a barely detected pause, the way they might casually say having kids is really no big deal, can send me plunging into a wordless, motionless depression. I am sensitive to the little nuisances in conversation that indicate the person doesn't really think a baby will ever come to me. I see it in that sort of shrugging expression people give when we get on the subject.

I need people to believe in me. I need friends to come right out and say: 'Yes You Can and Will Have a Baby!"

I want people around me to have no qualms about saying the most optimistic thing they can imagine saying to me.

I am hurt by all the people who see me as yet another statistic who won't get pregnant. The other day I was at the doctor's office getting a blood test when I came across an article on infertility and all the article did was rant on and on about the low success rate of infertility patients.

Why did they have this article available to all of us right their in the waiting room, while we are trying so hard despite the odds to get pregnant? Was it there to taunt and torment us?

I don't want to hear those statistics! I am tired of people imagining me a failure before I am ready to see myself that way.

One day at work, out of the blue, my dear friend Judy looked over at me and said, "I picture you with a curly-haired little girl." Imagine...out of the clear blue, she gifted me with a miraculous picture of hope! Judy sees me with a curly-haired daughter!

Does she know how much hope her words gave me that day? Does she know that her words released me from my sadness that day? Does anyone know how good it feels to know that someone else on this earth actually believes in my ability to give birth?

Why aren't more people like Judy? Why do so many people find it easier to believe I will never have a baby?

Lately, some people look at me like a lost cause. I am so tired of people who feel the need to share with me story after story of this person or that person who never could have children. Do people want to see me fail? Do they feel more secure in sharing bad news with me? Have they seen so much failure and disappointment in their own lives and in other people's lives, that they no longer believe a person can want something very badly and actually get it?

I don't know why their opinion means so much to me. I shouldn't need their validation so much. I know I shouldn't care what other people think, but I do.
I care because deep down, I agree with them: I don't believe in myself either.

A part of me feels this journey is going to be like lots of the other journeys in my life: me digging and digging for something, trying and trying, only to end up nowhere, and all my effort for nothing.

There is a part of me that has long believed my lot in life was to work and work for things, and end up with nothing. A part of me feels very comfortable on this path right now--doing lots of things without great hope or belief of ever reaping any reward for my efforts.

Many times in my life, almost reaching my goal has felt almost enough for me.

But this time, it has to be different. 'Almost' having a baby, 'almost' being pregnant doesn't count. When I was younger, sometimes I was content with 'almost'. I even found comfort in all the 'almost' in my life--I almost finished my book for young people when I was in my 20s, I almost had my children's book published, I 'almost' married a man I had adored for years.

Almost felt comfortable--like that was all I deserved. This time, 'almost' can't be good enough--because the reality is, when I am 80 years old, there will be no 'almost baby' sitting beside me. I can't 'almost' be a mother and 'almost' have a baby. This time, I have to go all the way.

God, I want a child so badly. I want to love a little person so much. Will I work and work for this and never see any results for all my efforts?

I need people to believe in me, because I don't believe in myself. I need people to help me silence all the voices in my head telling me this won't work out.

Sometimes, I don't think I am normal enough to have a baby, which is suppose to be the most normal thing in the world for a woman to do.

Getting pregnant and having a baby seem the natural right for other women--women who are better, stronger, more deserving than me.

I seem doomed not to have the ordinary things other women have. I'm not quite sure why, but I've long felt this. Things other women get easily and take for granted seem nearly impossible for me.

I wish I could say to everyone around me: please, tell me I am going to have a baby. Don't be afraid to be crazily-over-the-top-optimistic about my chances.

Don't feed me any more reality stories about friends who tried for years to get pregnant and failed. Don't--please, please don't--tell me that God might have other plans for me. I don't want other plans. I can't see why God wouldn't want me to have a baby. Please don't speak for God and please don't assume that He is always ready to deny me what I want. Believe in me. Hope with me. Kick the odds and the statistics out and see me giving birth. And please, don't tell me life can still be enjoyed without children.

For once, I wish people would err on the side of optimism. I want people to believe in me. Please everybody, tell me lies even. Even if you don't believe in my ability to have a child, lie to me and pretend you do. Tell me I am definitely going to get pregnant.

Waiting for An Answer

Of all the IUI's I've done since I started treatments, this is the one that I absolutely and completely wish would work. I have to face a surgery in a few weeks if this doesn't work out. I've been doing this a long time. I absolutely have to be pregnant. I've been going to acupuncture, taking lots of vitamins and I feel my body getting stronger. I am waiting for an answer: please, please, let this time be a yes.

Chapter 21: The Emotion of Deserving

Emotionally, it is important to root out every single thought that you may possibly hold about not deserving a baby.

If you are a person who s feels undeserving of good things, you might on some level not feel you are worthy of receiving a baby.

Many people say they want something, but on some level, they don't really think they deserve it.

Because of this deep subconscious belief, they prevent themselves from actually attaining what they want because a part of them simply doesn't think they deserve to get it. That subconscious feeling of not being worthy can lead a person to make the wrong choices, sabotage efforts, derail progress, to confirm the notion that they are not worthy of attaining their desire.

Not feeling deserving is a dangerous emotion—like harboring a spy who pretends to be on your side, but is actually working against you.

You need to convince every part of your body that yes, you deserve a baby.

All your thoughts and feelings of not being deserving must be eliminated.

If you think you are unworthy of having a baby, you may not put forth all the effort needed to achieve your aim. A person who feels undeserving may "prick their own balloon" sabotaging their efforts. If you think you don't deserve something, you may never let yourself attain what you want. How? By allowing your subconscious to make choices that prevent you from reaching your goal.

If you can get to the point where you truly believe you deserve something, you will do things, welcome things, invite things, and make choices, that improve your chances of getting what you rightfully feel you deserve.

Write down these words: 'I deserve a baby.' Now write down whatever comes up--do not overthink it or analyze it--just write down your response.

Now do it again. Write: 'I deserve a baby.' Do not analyze what you write, just let whatever is within you bubble up.

Now, what did you find out? Does your subconcsious truly think you deserve a baby?

It is important to know exactly what your subconscious thinks about you deserving a child. Remember--you are a living being and with that, you were born deserving the right to procreate if you choose. It is a right, inherent from the moment you were born.

Here is something to cut out and read daily. Say these words out loud. Shout them, put them deep in your heart, whisper them at your most difficult moments, sing them, visualize them, repeat them over and over, write them, type them, say them over again, hang them in places you can see daily.

- I deserve to have a baby.
- I deserve to be pregnant.
- I am good enough to be pregnant.
- I am ready to receive the gift of a baby.
- I give myself permission to become pregnant.
- I grant myself the power to become pregnant.
- I am worthy of having a baby.
- I deserve to have this work out.
- I deserve to give birth.
- My body deserves to be happy and healthy.
- I deserve to be a mother.

- I deserve to love a baby and be loved in return.
- I deserve good things.
- I am a living being who deserves to able to bring life from my body, just like that tree outside or that flower or an ant.
- My body deserves and wants to have a baby.
- I deserve a child.
- I deserve to be a mother.
- I am good enough to be a mother.
- I am worthy of holding my child in my arms.

Remember--feeling deserving does not mean you are vain, egotistical, selfish, spoiled, or somehow a bad person. Feeling deserving means you understand that as a human being, you are gifted with some basic rights—and that you don't have to be perfect to enjoy some of the pleasures and rewards that come with being a human.

Feeling deserving means that regardless of past mistakes, you sense that as a human being, being happy is something you have a right to. So repeat after me: I deserve to have a baby…I deserve to have a baby…

Chapter 22: Start Living Authentically

An often overlooked part of healing from infertility is living your life through your authentic original self.

Having a baby is a very natural, authentic process, and if you have buttoned up yourself to the point that doing anything real and authentic is absent, you may need to tap back in and welcome your true self.

You need to reunite with your true self so that you can feel completely at home in your body.

Feeling comfortable in your own skin and feeling at home in your body will help release inner reserves of energy, nourishment and peace that could help heal your infertility.

You have the right to embrace and welcome your original authentic self—even if you have ignored her for a very long time.

The authentic self is the 'you' at core of who you really are, not the 'you' people have told you that you are suppose to be.

Due to feeling shamed, judged or rejected, many women live their life through fake, imposter personalities because their true self was never valued or accepted.

The original self is buried—this beautiful, wise, helpful part of ourselves—is left dormant and ignored.

She deserves better. You deserve better.

Starting today, listen to your real self. Let her speak. Pay attention to what she wants and needs.

The false self is stiff. She is not free or real. She lives her life in a defensive position always ready to protect herself from attack, judgment or rejection.

This results in a feeling of constant stress and a tightness that does not allow the body to flow naturally as it was meant to flow.

Starting now, do what comes naturally. Eat, breath, and live in a way that feels natural.

Stop being a robot trying to please others.

Get out of your head and into your heart.

Give yourself the freedom to be yourself.

Say goodbye to the imposter personalities that smother your true self.

Let your true self out! Let her breath! Give her what she wants!

Allow real connection with others. Stop living in a way that only allows artificial forms of connection and disconnects you from the natural world.

Ask yourself: what makes my soul happy and content? What am I truly drawn to?

Do one thing a day that puts you back in touch with your heart. Listen to the little voice in back of your mind. What is she telling you? Be aware of your true likes and dislikes.

Start living in a way that lets you to be comfortable in your own skin.

Let the real you come out and play.

Have you dimmed your inner light because you are afraid for people to see the real you?

Turn on your light! Let it shine!

Think back: who were you before IT happened? The IT being any event, person or experience that withered you a bit, stole your confidence, made you doubt yourself, broke your heart. What were you like?

Are there parts of your personality that are dormant because you are too afraid to let them out again? What were you like as a child? Does your personality today resemble who you were or are you completely different? Are you stuffing the real you to please everyone else? Stop stuffing and stop trying to please. As Anais Nin says, "and the day came when the risk to remain tight in a bud was more painful than the risk it took to blossom."

Take the risk to blossom. Shake off the shame. Let go of the tightness within. Reveal your authentic self. Be 'her' as much as possible. Welcome back the parts of you that were shamed into hiding. Let them talk again! Express again! Let them be themselves again. Welcome back the real you.

Do more of whatever makes you feel alive and joyful. Be aware of your true feelings and preferences. What do you really want to wear? Who do you really want to spend time with?

Start living fully as your real self wants to live.

Stop hiding.

Move to your own rhythm, your own sense of selfhood.

Say yes only when you want to say yes to.

Stop judging yourself. Embrace your authentic ideas, values and personality traits.

Trust your instincts. Define your own values and youw own reality. Follow your intuition.

Your body will feel better and so will you.

Chapter 23: Welcoming Your Mother Within

Within you lies a mother waiting for the moment when she can step forward and assume her rightly role. In many ways, you are probably already stepping forward into the role of a mother by the way you live your life. You have most likely done many things that demonstrate the maternal part of you. It is likely that you already have had the experience of mothering yourself and those around you. So Mom, let it show—you know you are already living and breathing this role that is rightfully yours.

Here are some ways to get in touch with your inner mother:

• Begin today to see yourself as a mother. When you look in the mirror, remind yourself that yes, you are a mother, and it is only a matter of time before your children physically manifest themselves. Say aloud: I am a Mom. Picture being called 'Mom' or write: I am a Mom.

• See yourself surrounded by children. They are smiling. They like you. They like to be with you. Visualize yourself surrounded by children often. Picture yourself enjoying your children, talking with them, playing, and doing things you know come naturally to you. When you picture yourself with your children, visualize it authentically—if you hate to bake, don't try to conjure up an image of yourself baking. Maybe you would rather be racing your children down the beach instead, or teaching them to use a hammer or repairing a fence together. Maybe you love to read, and reading to your children is something you will cherish. Or maybe you want to put on some roller blades and coast down some trails with them. There are a million different ways a million different mothers enjoy their children.

• Write down all the qualities you already have that you associate with being a mother. Examples can include: being responsible, kind, tender, generous, strong, ingenius, creative, courageous, honest, a hard worker, loving, understanding, gentle, funny, fun-loving, responsible, resourceful, directed, nurturing, a leader, active, empathetic, self-sacrificing, playful, self-disciplined, fun.

- Write down all the ways you currently mother yourself and others.

Examples: You bring goodies into work for your co-workers. You write cards to friends and family on a regular basis. You enjoy buying presents for others. You are always ready to help in time of crisis. You enjoy cooking for family and friends. You love planning surprise parties. You are a good listener. You are able to comfort others when needed.
You work very hard. You donate your time, money or energy to charity. You enjoy giving massages or foot rubs. You are a go-getter and not afraid to take on challenges that frighten others. You are dependable, a leader, and very competent, so that your boss and others at work can always rely on you.

You go the extra mile in almost everything you do. You allow others the space and comfort to just be themselves. You are honest with yourself and others. You nurture others and give them the confidence and strength to grow.

- Do you sometimes have a 'motherly instinct'? If so, how do you manifest it? Example: You love your pets and try to keep them safe.

- Make a collage with a picture of yourself and pictures of all the ways you currently mother yourself and others. You can include pictures of yourself with nephews and nieces, cousins, friends and others. Also include pictures of yourself doing things you love that require contributing either at work, toward a charity or in some form in your life.

- Make a list of all the ways you look forward to nurturing your future children.

- Write a letter to your inner mother, and thank her all the ways she is ready to have a baby.

Chapter 24: Hitting Bottom

There are moments in infertility that are so painful, that trying to give advice about how to cope with them almost seems disrespectful.

So I will apologize right now for even attempting to give advice on how to get through moments so devastating that there is really no solace.

The pain of not conceiving is not something to be taken lightly, or something that some best-ten-tips list can cure.

I have suffered that kind of pain. Pain so raw and disappointing, and so completely upsetting to life's balance, that any advice given on how to deal with it can feel trite and disrespectful.

Infertility can attack the core of a woman's intrinsic and basic sense of what is natural and right. When having a baby does not occur naturally, it can rock to the core the way a woman feels about her life in general.

For a woman who desires children, not being able to reproduce can sting like a bloody violation of one of the most basic human rights.

So in your most painful moments, remember this: if you desire to be a mother more than anything, you will find a way to be
a parent, either biologically or through adoption. Your misery will fuel you to do whatever you need to do to become a parent. Your intense pain may be the reason you agree to undergo yet another IVF, and it may be that one more try that wins you the baby of your dreams.

Or that misery may push you to adopt an adorable baby and still try for a biological child.

All I know is no one wants to stay in the stalemate of misery indefinitely, and if you can't stand this feeling, then be glad for a moment, because that horrible feeling will push you to do things, try things, continue things, open yourself up to things, and never give up on things that could very well bring the child of your dreams into your life...as long as you don't give up and get stuck in the misery.

Please understand that anyone so desperately sad about not having a child is desperately needed in this world. You are needed in this world.

A person who is a lover of children is a treasure. This world desperately needs people who want to parent and who love children, and will do anything for that privilege and responsibility. This world needs people who feel that children are a sacred trust, worth all the sacrifices, and not a burden.

And it isn't fair that you have to wait so long for that child you want.

Your attitude toward having children is very different from those who see children as annoying nuisances who do nothing but drop crumbs on the floor, rather than the sacred gift they are.

For that kind of pain, you deserve an applause, a standing ovation, a huge golden trophy, a million hugs.

I have lived through the wretchedness of feeling you are being robbed from the life and family experience you always imagined yourself having.

I have walked that road of bitterness, anger and frustration so intense that nothing I have ever experienced compared to the utter misery of not being able to conceive and bear a child.

Having a child is a right every woman is born with, and to not be able to fulfill this inherited natural human right is beyond painful and grueling. When I reached my lowest points of misery, I sobbed without shame on the steps of an old run down donut shop in an ailing, decrepit town.

On another occasion, after learning I was not pregnant, I cried so much that my neighbors overheard me and were convinced my husband was beating me.

Once, I was so distraught after an IVF that didn't work, I left 12 messages on the voice mail of my nursing team at the clinic asking question after question about what might have gone wrong. So I'm assuming you will be a lot saner in your darkest moments than I was. But if you are not, that is okay and completely understandable too. You will find a way to survive this, thrive and fulfill your need to love and care for children. Just remember a few things:

• **Keep Believing:** Never stop believing that something good is about to happen. The ability to keep hope alive and keep a believing attitude even during the darkest moments can motivate you to keep trying.

Never stop seeing and visualizing that baby you long to hold. Picture it, envision it, talk to it, believe that little sweet human is coming. Hold on to hope even when it looks like you should give up. Act as if it already happened. Each morning, step outside your door, raise your hands to the sky and say, "I am ready to receive a baby" or "thank you. I am ready to receive my baby." When you wake up each morning, whisper, "I am pregnant." When you get out of bed, walk like you are pregnant, act like you are pregnant, and repeat the words, "I am pregnant. I am pregnant."

• **Use Your Anguish To Generate Change:** Nothing motivates a person to action like intense emotional pain. When the pain is so bad you can't stand it, you will also be hitting a powerful emotional point: Stay open. Answers can come when you are in this type of pain. You may be willing to go the extra mile that you were unwilling to go before.

Your pain can be the motor that keeps you going--so as bad as it feels, don't hate it. Great revolutions and profound historical changes have often been propelled by those in so much pain, they had no choice but to force change and make life better. Your pain will force change too.

You will find a way to fill that vacuum inside you--as long as you don't let the pain crush you, stop you, or submerge you into a helpless pit.

When you are in that kind of pain, you will be faced with two choices--either you can fall into a pit of despair and drown, or you can kick and scream and demand that something different happen.

Every day, make one choice that will move you forward and bring you one step closer to your dream. Choose action over inaction. That way you won't be permanently stuck in the pit of despair.

- **When You Have Reached What Seems Like A Dead End, Take An Unexpected Turn in the Road:** Go left. Go right. Start over and do it again. Close your eyes and walk backwards.

Try to think about getting pregnant in new ways, analyzing the situation from various perspectives. Picture yourself sitting at a table with the world's greatest minds: what advice would they give you about your infertility? Be open to the ideas that come. Pretend someone else is in your situation, and ask yourself: what would your inner, say, Oprah Winfrey, do in this instance? Or your inner Eleanor Roosevelt? What advice does your inner Einstein have for you? How about Dr. Phil or Ghandi?

- **Go To A Trauma Release Specialist:** Your body needs to release all the pain and trauma that can result from enduring infertility. Find a chiropractor, kinesiologist or myofascial release expert in your area who specializes in body work or trauma release. Write a list or a paragraph of what you have gone through and give it to the trauma release practitioner. Let them work on releasing whatever traumas are lodged in your body. By doing this, you will be freeing up some energy so you have the stamina it takes to continue infertility treatments.

- **Read Inspirational Books and Listen to Inspiring Music:** Put your mind's focus on what inspires and uplifts you. Bring hopeful music and books into your life. Fertilize your soul with positive words and happy outcomes.

- **Always Remember that During Life's Darkest Moments, The Sun Can Peek Through the Clouds**: Today's heartbreak could end up being the chubby-cheeked twins keeping you up all night next year at this time. One July 4, I was crying at a donut shop in a run down town. A year later on July 4, I was enjoying my new baby girl at the beach surrounded by lots of friends. The same could happen to you.

- **Pain Can Destroy You or Motivate You to Win:** Don't let your pain immobilize or debilitate you. Instead, use your pain to propel you to action.

Let your pain be a motivator—not a destroyer. Use your pain to help you determine what is happening within your body. Then, let the pain of wanting a baby motivate you to make the changes necessary for your body to get stronger and better able to conceive a child.

- **To Cope With The Pain Of Infertility, Keep Seeing the Possibility for Change:** Try to remember that things can unexpectedly and suddenly go right for you. If it seems like things have gone wrong, keep reminding yourself that sometimes, things can take a turn and start going right.

- **Understand that Your Drive to Parent Will Find a Home in This World:** An empty space does not stay empty forever. Voids find a way to be filled. Your fervent desire to be a parent will seek until that desire is filled in some way. You will be a mother. You will make it so. That empty space inside you will be filled. You will find a way.

- **Persist:** When you hit bottom, resolve to try again and try again and yes, try again. Don't let even the most devastating cycle or news prevent you from saying: how about one more try?

- **Change Something or Stick with** Something: Ask yourself: is there something in my journey through infertility that needs to be changed? Am I satisfied with my doctor and the clinic I am going to? Do I need to eat differently?

Or, are you already doing lots of positive things that just need time to work and require that you persistently stick to doing them?

Don't get stuck if change is needed and don't give up and grow impatientif you are already doing something right that will help you get pregnant.

• **Make a List of Every Dream or Goal You Achieved:** Write down every goal you accomplished that required hard work, patience, effort and persistence. List every obstacle you overcame to achieve that dream. Refer to this list often as a reminder that dreams and much sought after goals really do come true.

Remind yourself of how you have won in the past, and how you will win again in the future. Use this list as a reminder that obstacles can be surmounted, and what seems impossible today can become tomorrow's reality.

• **Find Places to Put Your Pain:** Swim, write in a journal, paint. Engage in creative ways to release your pain and disappointment. Give your pain a chance to escape your body. Buy a keyboard and invent original tunes. Sing whenever you can. Write stories about your fertility experience. Create a cartoon or fairy tale about your journey to having a baby—and give it a happy ending! Dance your pain away. Write your pain away. Sing your pain away. Look for ways to physically expulse your stress, frustration and pain.

• **Participate in the Process of Creation So That You Experience That Creating Something is Possible For You:** As you walk this road in creating a baby, allow yourself to experience the creation process that occurs every day in our world.

Let your body feel the relief and joy that comes with creating, whether it is making a sculpture with pie dough or growing a plant in your kitchen. Create a new recipe, create a piece of art, create a garden, create a dollhouse, make something out of fabric.

Do things that remind your inner self that you have the ability to create.

Keep a journal titled: What I Created Today and write about one thing you create each day.

- **Notice the Birth Process in the World Around You Each Day:** Look around and notice the birth process occurring in the world around you each day—and remind yourself that very soon you are going to be part of that beautiful process too.

Visit an animal shelter and spend time with kittens or puppies. Walk through a park and notice the cycle of life happening all around. Observe how weeds grow in the oddest, most difficult places. Watch how bugs and animals can reproduce in your home even when you don't want them too—and then feel your connection to this process as much as you can at this time.

- **Regardless of How Badly You Feel, Keep the Positive Words Flowing:** Even in your darkest moments, continue to speak of hope. Never say: "I'll probably never get pregnant" or "Nothing works out for me" or "This is a big waste of time" or "I hate myself for this." Keep affirming aloud to others and silently to yourself that yes, you will get pregnant….yes, you will have a baby…yes, you will conceive and deliver a beautiful baby.

Even when you are feeling devastated and expressing your sadness to a friend or family member, make sure all your conversations include statements like: "as hard as this is, I know deep in my heart I will have a baby soon" or "I really believe my body is healing and I am about to conceive a child" or "a year from now, I'm going to be holding my baby."

- **Stay Close To Positive People:** Keep close in touch with positive people, and let their positive words sink deep into every part of your consciousness.

- **Become Best Friends With Your Body:** Start enjoying a close, loving friendship with your body. Talk lovingly to your body each day. Let your body know you have complete confidence in its ability to conceive and give birth. Say: "I love you body." Treat your body with kindness. See the efforts your body is making and praise it. Get optimistic with your body! Tell your body that it is strong, it is capable, and all your organs are doing a great job of getting ready to be pregnant.

Let your ovaries know you love them and you have full faith in their ability to create and release healthy eggs. Say I love you to your uterus every day. Let your thyroid gland know you love it and believe it can sustain and nurture you. Treat your body as you would a beloved best friend.

• **Prayer:** For me, the most powerful antedote to my pain was prayer. During my rock bottom moments, it was only through prayer that I was able to find strength and hope.

During my most hopeless moments, it was only my hope that God would help me have the babies I so long for that carried me through and enabled me to keep going.

Without the privilege of being able to pray to God, I would never have been able to endure the painful disappointments I experienced during my infertility treatments.

If not for prayer, I would not have had the strength to continue on.

Sometimes, for me, the greatest and sometimes only antidote to my pain was prayer.

• **Help Others:** When you hit bottom, set out to help another person who is going through a tough time too. Make it your goal to spread hope to someone who needs hope as badly as you do.

Wanting a child is, in part, a desire to give to and love someone outside yourself on a permanent basis. As you await the arrival of your child, keep in mind the other people in this world who need your love.

When I was pregnant with my daughter, so hoping I wouldn't miscarry, a friend from work was in the process of adopting her daughter overseas. She faced many obstacles in her adoption journey, but despite her own challenges, she wrote and told me that she lit a candles at church and prayed for me.

Imagine...she was in the midst of her own crisis and she chose to include me in her prayers. What a generous gesture in the midst of her own pain.

I never forgot this, and marveled at the kindness and strength she showed.

Yes, you deserve a child to love and nothing can replace that, but while you wait, think about where your love is needed in this world and who you can help with all the love inside you.

• **Let Yourself Fall Apart and Then Get Up Again:** When you reach a crisis point and are overwhelmed with grief, let yourself fall apart but then, get up and begin trying again. Infertility can be a wrenching experience and you have the right to mourn...so mourn...but at a certain point, get up and try again.

• **Start A 'Reason to Hope' Journal:** Every day, find reasons to hope and write them down. Be on the lookout for anything in your life, your world, your surroundings that give you a reason to hope. Open your eyes wide and find one hopeful and positive thing to write about. Any time you find a reason to hope, write it down.

• **Read Inspirational True-to-Life Stories of People Who Were Down and Out, but Somehow Managed to Turn Things Around:** Soak your mind in true-to-life stories of miracles, of people who beat impossible odds and managed to overcome the challenges they faced. Read about people who are medical miracles and who somehow defied all the odds.

Put so many impossible-but-came-true tales in your head that soon you won't see having a baby as something out of your reach at all.

• **Watch The Movie Rocky**: Watch all of them. Then watch them again.

- **Make Sure to Eat Well, Sleep Well, and Do Everything in Your Power to Keep the Happy Chemicals in Your Brain Dancing and Ready To Do Their Work:** Work on keeping the chemicals in your body and brain as happy as possible. If you eat badly, the chemicals in your brain will work against you--making an already stressful situation even more stressful.

When you eat healthy and get the rest you need, you are giving your brain and body the power it needs to support your emotional self. Think: lots of greens, some berries, nuts and seeds, early bedtime and light exercise. Make the chemicals in your body your ally.

- **Put Together a Strategy If You Don't Have One:** Creating a step-by-step fertility plan will keep you focused and moving forward when you reach crisis points. Rather than immobilized by disappointment, knowing your next step, and the next step after that, will keep you moving forward towards your goal.

- **Remind Yourself That You Are One Tough Cookie:** Repeat after me: I am one tough cookie, I am one tough cookie...I can do what it takes to get what I want...I can do what it takes to get my baby.

- **Say These Affirmations Each Day:** When you are feeling down, write, type, sing, and speak these affirmations:

I am strong and able to conceive a baby.

My body is love and ready to love my baby.

My ovaries are making lots of healthy eggs!

My baby is on the way to me.

I am a mother. I give birth. I am holding life in my arms.

I receive my baby

I can carry my baby for nine months and then give birth.

Every part of my body is ready to be pregnant.

I am ripe and ready to conceive.

I am receiving my baby right now.

• **Remember, as a Woman on This Planet Earth, You Are Already A Mother--and Are Now Just Waiting to Manifest Your Motherhood in a Physical Sense Differently Than You've Expressed It Before:** If you look after a family member's health, if you buy presents for someone else's children, if you care about the emotional well-being of your friends, if you bring goodies to work for your co-workers…if you give your money or time to a charity…if you care for a pet, if you really, really love someone…then you have already begun your journey as a mother on this planet earth.

One of the definitions of the word 'mother' is 'a creative source' and that, I am willing to bet, you already are. So manifesting a physical child is not a huge stretch for you.

Remind yourself that you are already a mother and will soon give birth to your own baby that will continue your mothering experience.

Another definition of mother is "to watch over, nourish and protect maternally." Your maternal spirit, evidenced by your drive to be a mother, is already in action. Take your power as a maternal being and put it out into the world. Acknowledge that you are, and have always been, a mother. Feel a certain ripeness and centering in your stomach as you acknowledge that you are already a mother, just waiting to physical manifest your already existing motherhood.

• **Start Getting In the Habit of Taking Care** of Living Things: Begin taking care of living things right now, as a way to prepare to care for your babies. Get a pet, plant a garden, commit to feeding the birds, deer or turkeys in your area. Practice nurturing living things. As you do this, say to yourself: "I care for living beings on this earth as I will soon care for my babies."

- **Create Personal Rituals That Strengthen You and Give You Hope:** When I first began infertility treatments, I would play the theme to the movie "Rocky" and march around my living room as the song played, all the while imagining my ovaries churning and babies popping out.

Strange yes, and thankfully no one ever caught me in my marching mode, but this routine strengthened me and by the end of this exercise, I felt strong, ready and the possibility of having children felt very, very real to me. Choose a song to be your personal anthem and dance, march, do whatever your body calls you to do.

- **Spend at Least 15 minutes a Day Outdoors in the Sunshine Looking at Nature:** Let the warmth and light of the sun lift your sadness. Look at greenery whenever you can.

- **Tend to Your Spiritual Self:** Pray, help others, read a book that uplifts your spirit, memorize Bible verses, record your appreciation for even the littlest things in a 'big fat thank you' gratitude journal.

- **Keep Going:** When you hit bottom and feel your worst, keep going--to your appointments, for treatments--just keep going.

- **Act As If There Is No Doubt This Will All Work Out:** Each day, do one thing that demonstrates in a complete and tangible way that you truly believe you will give birth to a baby soon. Start planning your Disney vacation that you will bring your children on in a few years. Sew play clothes, build a toy chest for all the toys that will be in your home soon.

Chapter 25: Remember Who You Are

Even in your darkest moments, it is important to remind yourself of who you are. Your infertility is just a temporary condition that has the potential to be healed. It is not a definitive statement on who you are or what you are capable of experiencing.

You are:

Capable: You are capable. To get through the rigors of infertility, you must remind yourself that you are capable--capable of working hard to get what you most desire, capable of healing, capable of conceiving, capable of carrying a baby full-term. You are capable. Your body is capable. Your reproductive organs are capable. Remind yourself of all the times when you were capable enough to defeat difficult challenges in your life.

Deserving: You deserve a baby. You are VERY deserving of a baby. You deserve this to work out. You deserve to see your dreams come true. Your body deserves the pleasure of conceiving and giving birth to a baby. You deserve to hear 'yes you are pregnant' and nine months later, you deserve to hold your beautiful baby in your arms.

Positive: You are positive. Within you lives a positive voice who has the strength to stay positive even when things are difficult.

Hopeful: You are hopeful. You hope because you know you have many good reasons to hope. You hope because good things happen to millions of people every single day. You hope because the human body is strong and can heal even from the most terrible illnesses. You hope because you've seen others have good results from their efforts. You hope because something deep inside you knows it is okay to hope. You hope because you have faith. You hope because this has worked out for others before you. You hope because you know today's no can turn into tomorrow's yes.

You hope because the birth process goes on millions and millions of times each day, in all kinds of conditions, in millions of places, to all kinds of different people, and one of these days, it very well could include you. You hope because the human body can heal.
You hope because you know infertility is a temporary condition that can be fixed and overcome.

Committed: You are committed. You are committed to your goal of having a baby. You are committed to doing whatever is necessary to bring your baby to life. You are committed to doing the work, asking the questions, putting in the time, and taking this journey step by step to get what you want. Your body is committed to becoming healthy and fertile. Your reproductive organs are committed to giving you a baby. You are so committed that you will do and learn and understand whatever it is you have to do and learn and understand to conceive and give birth to your baby.

Determined: You are determined. You will plow through to get what you want. You are so determined that you refuse to give up until you have what you want. Your dogged determination empowers you to surmount all obstacles. You refuse to listen to the naysayers, the discouragers, the pessimists or anyone else who is not supportive of you. You will try again and try again and try again as many times as you need to try to attain your goal. You realize there will moments of pure discouragement, but you won't let these times stop you you from stepping forward toward your ultimate purpose. Call you stubborn. Call you unstoppable. Call you the most determined mother on earth—a quality your future children will cherish, because the determination that helped you get pregnant will also help you build a great life for your kids.

Curious: You are curious. You ask questions, research, investigate, read, and ask more questions again. You want to know why your body is having trouble getting pregnant and you are not afraid to look for the answers. Your curiosity will move you to search out the reasons behind what is happening to you.

Unstoppable: You are unstoppable. Repeat after me: I am unstoppable! I am unstoppable! I am an unstoppable mother-to-be!

Powerful: You are powerful. You have the power to believe, power to pray, power to persevere, power to heal, power to think positive thoughts, power to visualize.

Ready to Heal: You are ready to heal. Your body is ready to heal. Your hormones are healing and balanced. Everything in your body is healing. Regardless of whatever news you hear from the clinic today, your body is continually walking forward towards healing.

Steady: You are steady. Step by step, inch by inch, day by day: you steadily do the things needed to attain your goal. You keep your 'eye on the ball' and never forget your purpose. Steadily, you are becoming more and more fertile by the day.

Nurturing: You are nurturing to yourself during this time. You give your spirit what it needs to endure this. You do things that uplift and soothe your soul. You put yourself around nurturing people. You engage in nurturing activities. You know how to nurture yourself, and this is going to be very useful because soon you will be called upon to nurture your new baby.

Loving: You are loving. Love gives you an undefeatable power and strength. Fueled by love, nothing can stop you. What force is more potent and unstoppable than love? Absolutely nothing.

Diary Excerpt: Screaming in the Darkness

Today, it came. While I was at work. I had wanted so much...hoped so much...prayed so much...please God, let this be the month. Let this be the month I am pregnant. I especially wanted to be pregnant because then I would not have to have the laparoscopy next week. The idea of going under anesthesia scares me. I so wanted to be pregnant so I wouldn't have to go through this procedure. A procedure that yes, I asked for, but that I still desperately hoped I wouldn't end up needing.

Instead, I went to the bathroom about 1:30 and it was there.

Gushing, spewing and mocking me.

Blood, blood, blood.

My period had, without a doubt, or even a trace of hope, arrived.

I sat in the bathroom stall, feeling like a tiny bomb has just gone off inside me.

Destruction lives.

I have no pride left now that I see it there. I have nothing. I return to the office and don't bother to hide my tears or my disappointment.

"What's wrong?" asks Kevin, a very kindly young co-worker who sits next to me.

"I just found out I'm not pregnant," I blurt out, knowing it was totally inappropriate to say this to a single 20something male co-worker, but not really caring.

You would think I would have some pride, stifle my feelings, shut my mouth, but I am so desperate, I cannot keep my pain locked up inside me.

I have no choice but to let my pain be seen, so somehow I won't feel so alone.

Too much pain to keep inside. I will explode if I don't let it leak out a bit.

"Don't worry. That's not a big deal. You'll get pregnant," said Kevin.

Somehow Kevin's naive words made me feel better--but not for long.

Inside, I feel I'm at the end of a bridge, nowhere left to go, but down. I have been doing IUI's for six months now, and still no baby. Still no baby! Still no baby! Still no baby!!! STILL NO BABY!!!! Why???? Why no baby? Where is my baby? Still no baby! No baby--ever? Is no baby ever coming to me? Why? Will it happen? Please, please, please! Now! When? Why? Will I be old and without a child? Will I? No, no, NOOOOOO! I can't!!!

My friend Chelsea, who is sweet, soulful, sensitive, tries to comfort me the rest of the afternoon. At one point during our conversation, she said, "Paula, for some women, getting pregnant comes easy, even without them trying. For you, it is a long and difficult road, but it doesn't mean you can't arrive at the same destination as those other women. At the end of the road, you can have the same thing these other women have, but your road is going to be a lot harder."

At that moment, Chelsea gave me the hope I needed. She somehow changed how I saw my infertility. Her words did not totally remove my pain, but suddenly I saw my journey ahead differently. Yes, it was going to be a hard road for me and it wasn't fair that other women could get pregnant easily, sometimes even when they didn't want to. But just because my road was difficult didn't mean I couldn't ultimately arrive at the same destination as the most super-fertile woman.

Maybe my road is longer, harder, sadder, but at the end of the road, I could be holding the same prize as all the women who have no trouble getting pregnant at all.

For a few minutes, Chelsea's words gave me a feeling of control and hope.

A new vision of my infertility entered my head: I saw myself walking on a dusty, dirty, rocky road. Big boulders everywhere. I had a hard road to walk, a walk where I get very dirty and tired. But at the end of the road, I see myself joining a group of happy women holding babies. They arrived there via a different road, a nicer smoothly paved road. But, at the end of the road, we all arrive at the same place and we are all holding our babies and we are all happy. Suddenly, my hard walk doesn't seem impossibly hard.

"Tonight, have a cup of tea or some soup. Something warm will make you feel better," Chelsea said.

Chelsea and I leave work at the same time. I thank her for all her kindness. She is a beautiful friend.

It is a hot June day, and on hot days, I feel worse emotionally than I do on cold days. Something about the heat makes my emotions boil over, whereas in the winter, my feelings can safely hide in the cold darkness. Right now, the summer sunshine feels like it is a mocking magnifying glass all over on my negative emotions.

I get in my car and drive home.

At work, surrounded by friends like Chelsea and Kevin, I feel supported, wrapped in the safe, warm blanket of a tribe. As crazy as I felt at work, I feel worse when I leave. The drive home magnifies my frustration.

Traffic.. heat.. trapped..going nowhere, my anger and fury heating up, so much so that by the time I get home, I am an inferno, a raging woman, entangled in frustration. In my heart, a raging fear that perhaps I will never have my own baby to love.

Chelsea's words provided me comfort, but now I am back to feeling cheated and desperate. I have hit an all-time low and every emotion inside me are roaring to be heard. Why did it have to be no this month? Couldn't for once things been easy for me? For once, couldn't this have been a yes?

The laparoscopy next week unnerves me, and I don't want to go through with it.

For once, just once, I wanted it all to work out in my favor.

My husband was sitting in the kitchen when I got home. I hate him right now. I truly hate him. I actually completely hate him. It is his fault I am not pregnant.

His sperm is no good, I just know it. If I had married someone else, with different genes and different sperm, I would be pregnant right now. I tell him this. I tell him how it is his fault I am not pregnant, and instead of being nice to me and accepting the blame and promising to do everything possible to fix his defective sperm, he gets angry, cold and defensive. He is not at all sorry that this is all the fault of his weird genes and his weak sperm.

We start to fight. It is dark now. We are upstairs in our bedroom. I need him to be nice, to hold me, to comfort me, but he doesn't do that. He won't do that. He is mean. I feel so crazy. I want a baby, I need a baby. I need him to listen, to understand, to be as comforting and nice as Chelsea was. He's never nice. He never helps me. He is never there when I need him. Can't he see how sad I am? Doesn't he care? Why is he so mad? Why doesn't he hold me, comfort me, do something to make me feel like we will have a baby someday? He doesn't care, he doesn't try, he's never done the work needed to make this happen. It is always me doing everything. Me! Always me!

I can't stand it anymore! I can't stand him! I can't stand his stubbornness, his stupidity! I start crying.

I jump out of bed, grab a pillow and hit the bed. He is mean!! I hate him! I hate trying to have a baby with him!

"Do you think I will ever have a baby?" I ask pleadingly.

"I don't know," he shrugs. "Probably."

"Why do you say it like that?" I push. "You don't think I will ever have a baby do you?"

"Yah, you probably will," he says blankly.

"A girl? Do you think I'll have a girl? Or a boy? I want a girl first. What do you think?" I am pushing and pushing, feeling angrier and crazier by the minute. He says nothing.

For some reason, I have to know what he thinks. I persist, "Do you think I'll ever have a daughter?"

I ask this, because more than anything in this world, I want a daughter. A daughter...could you imagine the joy of having a daughter?

He answers: "Probably not. You'll probably never get the daughter you want because God hates you. He'll probably give you a son first, if you even get a baby."

Its all over now. I go crazy, ballistic, mad. His cruelty! At my lowest point! I have nothing left to hold on to now. I start throwing things around the bedroom. I knock over the VCR. I am going to kill him. He said out loud every fear that secretly lives inside me.

I am going to kill myself and him. I scream and I scream and I scream and I don't care if my neighbors hear me.

I scream so loud, I have lost my mind. I don't care. I am going to destroy him. I am married to a monster, an unfeeling monster.

My husband, who is suppose to be my support, telling me that God will never give me the daughter I want! How could he!!!!

This is too much, too horrible. I hate him with such intensity, I can barely... I scream again! I pick up all the books on my nightstand and I throw them.

How dare he intrude on my belief that God is going to help me! How dare he invade my brain and try to tear apart my one thread of hope that God is on my side.

Oh God, he is right. HE IS RIGHT! I'm not a good person. I am not good enough for God to help me get a baby. God hates me. He said out loud everything I've always feared, but secretly hoped wasn't true. What if I am not good enough for God to help me get a baby? What if God is punishing me, and will continue to punish me by not giving me a baby? What if God never gives me the daughter?

He knows--my horrible husband knows that the universe would never help a jerk like me.

I am helpless...how dare he steal my faith, my belief that God wants me to be happy and have a baby...how dare he! But... he is right, he is saying the truth: I am a bad person, and bad people don't get what they want.

I cry. I wail. I scream. Nothing but sadness and anger are running through my veins. I am forbidden every good thing in this world. I have no one, nowhere to turn. I am trapped.

It is dark. So dark. I see myself standing by the bed. I am so sad, so enraged. I scream so loud I know the neighbors can hear me. I wish I cared. I don't care. I howl in the night. I howl and I howl, because without God on my side, I cannot dare to ever hope to win this battle.

The night goes on and on and doesn't stop. It is all too much for me.

I can't feel these feelings, take this kind of suffering, to want a baby so badly, to need a child to love so much, and to be told by the person who is suppose to be your life partner that you will probably never get this baby, it is too much for me. The worst part is, he is probably right.

The pain is intense, the longing, looking at my life ahead as blank and lonely, to picture myself 70 or 80 and never having children, to always looking at other people with kids and envying them, wanting so much to love someone this way, and not having it.

The image of myself as old, alone, and hating what my life has become looms stark in my imagination. I get more support at work than in my own home. The night goes on. It never ends. This hell, my hell, never ends.

I am alone in the darkness, in the darkest night, and I am not good enough for anything normal in this world. He took away the only thing sustaining me. How dare he?

He is right! He is right...God hates me.

I can't stop screaming!

Rage is pouring out of me. God hates me!

GOD HATES ME! I prayed and I prayed and I believed, and now I know I'm not good enough for God to help.

I have had sad horrible nights in my life before, but never have I lived a night with such a dark dead end, with no one to turn to and nowhere to go. A like this night that seems to never end. I scream and I scream and I scream. I don't stop screaming, because without God's help, I won't have a chance of this dream coming true.

It is dark and I scream some more. No where to go. No where to go.

At some point, I stop screaming, crawl back into bed, and fall asleep.

To this day, when I'm feeling sad, I remember Chelsea's words and I drink some tea or make some soup. But on that hot July day, I was at my wit's end. I didn't have any hope left inside of me

The Next Day

I woke up this morning raw, angry, stewing in last night's sadness, still feeling the sting of the fight...

My husband and I don't say much too each other. We are all fought out. Nothing left, not even anger to pass to each other. We mumble a few words, apologies, I'm-sorry/I'm sorry too.

Neither one of us are truly the monsters we were last night.

What reaction did I expect from him anyways—after I came home attacking his sperm? Did I expect warmth and kindness after I insulted him? What is wrong with me? Why did I think I could be so mean and disrespectful, and somehow get kindness and tenderness in return?

There is a knock at our door. It is our neighbor Richard, whose condo is attached to ours. He heard all the screaming and wants to know what happened last night. This doesn't feel like an intrusion to us. Our friendship with Richard is open this way: we are neighbors who watch over and take care of each other, and so it is normal that he wants to know what's up. He said his wife thought Chris was hitting me and she wanted him to come over and break up the fight. "I don't like to interfere between husband and wife," he said. "But we were worried." I assured him that Chris didn't hit me, and explained that I was screaming because I was sad over not being pregnant. Richard eyes us, like he doesn't quite believe our story. He is protective of both of us, and we thank him for stopping by.

His visit lightens things between us for a few minutes. His concern is endearing.

Today is Friday. We are suppose to be leaving for a weekend away to Deerfield, Massachusetts with my parents before my surgery on Tuesday. I've accepted that I have to go through this surgery. There will be no last minute surprises saving me from it.

We pack for the weekend trip and head up to my parent's house. We don't talk much on the way there. I feel too exhausted to talk.

I don't know if it because of my period or what, but by the time we get there, my stomach is hurting badly and I feel nauseous.

I lay down at my parents house for awhile, waiting for them to finish packing, and start to feel better, but that reprieve doesn't last long. "Time to leave," my father announces, and we head to the car for our drive to western, Massachusetts.

The back roads are twisty and winding and I feel so nauseous. I ask my husband to please stop the car so I can get some relief. He stops and I tumble out of the car, onto the lawn of a beautiful farmhouse and I vomit, right there on their front lawn. The grass feels so good, I just lay there for awhile, too sick to care.

We continue this way for the rest of the ride down...driving about 10 minutes..my stomach not being able to take it...my husband stopping and me crawling out of the car to vomit. I don't know now how many times he stopped, or how many times I ended up vomiting on someone's front lawn.

Finally, we get to the Main Street area of some sort of sad little run-down town, and my husband pulls into a donut shop that looks like it has seen better days.

At this point, I couldn't stand anymore: the stomach pain, the recurring thought that I will never get pregnant, was like a punch to the gut over and over again. My parents and husband go into the donut shop, but I sit on the front steps of the sad little donut shop and I begin to cry... loudly, and in a way I have never cried in public before.

I hear the song playing inside the donut shop "NECCO Beach" and I cry even louder because I went to a college with the initials NECC that everyone called NECCO, and it was a song popular when I was in college. When I think back to that time in my life, all I remember is sunshine and me wearing a white cotton dress, feeling like life was wonderful and every dream I had was absolutely within my reach.

The song made me sob almost uncontrollably, because I am so far from being that happy girl in the white dress. Here, at this dirty old donut shop, 40 pounds overweight and powerless to have the baby I so want, is who I am now. Hearing that song from my college days seemed like a cruel mockery. I miss my friends from college, especially the ones from WRAZ, the college radio station. They were like a second family to me, and right now, I would give anything to have a place to go where people would accept me like they did. Remembering that feeling of walking into the radio station, filled with friends, was making me feel hysterical and making my stomach pains worse. Why am I not getting pregnant? I don't care anymore who is looking at me, which oddly in this town, no one seems to be doing. No one even seems to notice me crying. People walk by me like they've seen women crying desperately here many, many times before...just a standard for this run-down place. Is there so much sadness in this town that it is normal for a grown women to sit on the steps, clutching her stomach, crying? God knows how many people in this place have had their dreams shattered. Seeing me crying might just look like the norm here...just another loon with a broken heart.

The songs continues to play. Its not fair! I always thought I would have children young, but it doesn't seem like anything I envisioned for my life is coming true. Once, way back when, I naively wrote a list of the goals I wanted to reach by the time I was 30: I wanted to have two children and have won a Pulitzer Prize. Ha! What a complete laugh that turned out to be!

 My life turned out to be one heartbreak after another. I feel crazy inside when I think about it.

So much pain bubbling up inside of me. I long for a child's gentle, soft magic in my life...a little person to love, a love that has nothing to do with romantic love or adult love.

The song continues to play, which makes it all the worse. What happened since college that led me to this moment? Why am I in this place? I can't walk through my life without children. It isn't what I imagined for my life. I always pictured and assumed that my life would include children.

I refuse to stuff it all down anymore. I can do nothing but surrender to my pain at this moment.

My mother, who is probably the only person in this world who actually loves me, tries to get me to come inside. I wish I could be alone with her right now. I feel badly that she has to see me, her daughter, like this, but I feel so tired inside from this quest to have a baby, that I can't stop this gush of despair anymore. My husband is trying to be nice to make up for last night, but I hate him right now and I don't want his kindness.

I finally go inside and lay down in a booth. My husband and father are sitting down, eating donuts like nothing is wrong. They try to cheer me up, the way a negligent dog owner would cheer up a not-so-beloved pain- in- the ass dog. I eat three chocolate donuts. They make me feel better. After awhile, we get back in the car to go to the hotel.

Finally, we arrive at our hotel. Once we check in, I ask for some time alone with my mother. My husband obliges, and goes to my father's room.

My mother comes in and sits on the bed next to me. Talking to my mother, as always, makes me feel better. My mother has a beautiful way of imparting hope, faith and confidence during life's darkest moments. She loves me, understands me like no one else, and says what I need to hear: yes, you will have a baby, she says with confidence.
Even though I know she is probably just saying what she knows I want to hear, her words give me a sense of peace. I relax for the first time in days. The movie "Titanic" is on a cable station. I loved that movie, saw it three times. We stop talking for awhile and just watch the movie.

When it ends, I thank my Mom and tell her I am ready to sleep. I am washed out from the nightmare of the past few days. On Tuesday, I am facing an operation that probably won't change anything at all. But what choice do I have? Giving up is not an option. I can't live in a world without kids. If no children come to me, I will find a way to adopt. I am desperate to love a child.. to care for a child. I am tired of running around, looking to belong somewhere, when belonging never comes in any permanent form. But what if a baby never comes?

What if my life is spent searching? What if I end up being that sad girl on the steps of a dingy old donut shop longing for babies that never come?

I can't bear this. Sleep is a relief.

Weekend Away

This morning, I woke up feeling a bit calmer, washed out from the intense drama of the past few days. We went to breakfast at a nearby hotel this morning. It was delicious. Juice, toast, fruit. I'm trying to eat better (only ate one tiny piece of bacon). I'm beginning to feel a little better about my upcoming operation. I know I have to get it. There is no way around it--the operation will be in three days.

My weekend here in Deerfield turn out to be exactly what I needed: country, quiet, rural, green pastures and Main Streets full of houses with front porches. I wish I could live here...wish I could experience this type of peace in my life. We visit the Yankee Candle Factory, go out to dinner at an Italian restaurant, eat breakfast at a little diner. This is so good for me. I can't imagine what the operation is going to be like. I am scared, but less scared than I was a few days ago. I have no choice but to go ahead and do it. What if I have endometriosis and no one is catching it? What if it is the reason I'm not getting pregnant? Maybe this is the answer to my problem. We drive around a lot. I sit in the back seat, quietly enjoying the scenery of the beautiful mountains, the hills, greenery everywhere. This is exactly the type of landscape I enjoy. I wish I could sink into this landscape and stay forever. Let time stand still. How I wish my baby was here with me.

Will that baby ever come? If I let myself stay on that thought, craziness rises up within me again. But at least my rage and sadness has calmed a bit, and I'm beginning to accept what is going to happen on Tuesday.

Lapascropy

Today, July 5, was my laparoscopy. After the weekend away, I felt a little more ready for it.

I went in expecting it wouldn't be a big deal. I thought that maybe all my fears about the operation was for nothing—that the laparoscopy would end up being a lot like the operation to remove my polyps... a few hours later, I was back home, chomping down dinner and feeling fine.

Once I arrived at the hospital, I went to the outpatient area. Everyone was so nice, from the nurses to the young man who wheeled me to the operating room.

Right before I went in, I asked my doctor: Is everything going to be all right? and being the realist he is, he said, "There are no guarantees."

I prayed a lot. I prayed I would make it through the operation. I prayed, prayed, prayed. If this would bring me a step closer to having my baby, then it was worth it.

A few hours later, I wake up in a small gray recovery room, a curtain pulled around my bed. I have never felt such physical pain in my life. I am not sure what the pain is...

I ask if my husband could come see me. Forty minutes pass.
Finally, I'm sent to the recovery area.

My husband comes in. Oh God, it is so good to see him. The pain is so bad, I am crying. The nurse wants me to go to the bathroom--she says she cannot let me go home until I go to the bathroom. It hurts so much, I cannot imagine going to the bathroom.

Then, my husband kneels at the foot of my bed and starts to rub my feet. He rubs and rubs them, trying to comfort me, and I think to myself that as long as I live, I will never forget the image of him, kneeling down, massaging my feet that day.

I just want to get out of there. I feel like the pain isn't going to stop if I stay here. I just want to go to my parent's house. All I want to do is leave, but because of a weird rule that you can't go home until you go to the bathroom, I'm forced to stay. The nurse is very kind. She sees that I can't stand being there. She keeps trying to call my doctor to ask my for permission to leave, but they can't find him.

I have never felt such pain. I can't even describe the pain. Finally, around 5 o'clock, they let me go. All I want to do is get to my parent's house.

Chris goes and gets the car and the nurse wheels me out. He jumps out of the car to help me. He is so kind. I feel horribly for how I've treated him the past few months.

I just want to be home, in my own bed.

Once we get on Route 128, the traffic is bumper-to-bumper, turtle to turtle, crawling down the highway, slowly and unbearably in the hot July sun. Obviously, I am not getting to my parent's house anytime soon. I am trapped on this forsaken highway. It is hot and we have no air conditioning in the car. I feel like vomiting.

The ride to my parent's home is slow. Slow, slow, slow, slow. The sun magnifies my pain, heats it up until it boils over, me in a steel cage, trapped by traffic every which way, the road feels longer and longer and longer, stretching out so far I feel like I will never get home. The window is down but no breeze blowing. It is such a long ride home.

 I open the window and stick my head out.

I cannot stand it. I am going to throw myself out of the car. I tell my husband I am going to throw myself out of the car so an ambulance will have to come and rush me somewhere and I will have escaped this slow hell home.

Every mile down 128 feels like a victory, a step closer to relief from my pain. Finally....(finally finally what seems like two hours later) we reach Route 3.

The traffic is a bit better, but still so slow. My stomach hurts, everything hurts. It is hot. Hot, hot, hot! I am trapped. I am an impatient child, who cannot bear to wait a second longer. GET ME HOME! GET ME HOME!

Finally, we reach my parents house. I get out of the car as fast as I can, run in the house straight up to bed. I don't even stop to talk to my parents. I am a bit ashamed to be coming here to be cared for, but I can't imagine going home and being alone when Chris is at work.

My mother brings me some tea, and oddly, instead of drinking it, I follow my urge to put the tea bag on my stomach. I don't know why, but the hot tea bag seems to immediately take away some of the pain. Heat. I remember Chelsea's words about the hot tea. I ask for more hot tea bags, and the heat seems to do the trick. I am starting to feel sleepy.

Perhaps I had been dreading this operation for a reason. What a painful experience.

Day After Operation

I cannot believe what pain I'm still in. I wake up feeling terrible.

This is nothing like the polyp operation. This time the pain is sticking.

I am staying in my parent's bedroom. It is comforting here. Although, this bedroom holds some difficult memories for me. About seven years ago, when I was undergoing a severe depression, I got a terrible case of strep throat. I neglected it for so long, that I ended up on the verge of rheumatic fever, and the doctor said I should be quarantined until I was better. So I left the apartment my roommate and I shared, and moved home to recover. I was in bed for three weeks, but I can remember being glad I was sick. Being sick was a relief, because I was in so much emotional pain, that the illness afforded me the chance to zone out, do nothing but watch daytime TV and eat my mother's fantastic Italian cooking. It was a terribly low point in my life.

Being back in this room reminds me of that time. It isn't the bedroom of my childhood--that is the beautiful pink bedroom down the hall.

No, that bedroom holds happy memories for me. That was the bedroom of youth, hope, first love, ease, comfort, lots and lots of phone calls, and little sayings that hung on the wall like: 'when things go wrong like they sometimes will..when the road you are trudging seems all uphill...when the funds are low and the debt is high...when you want to smile, but have to sigh, when caring is pressing you down a bit, rest if you must, but just don't quit. Life is queer with its twists and turns, as all of us sometime learns, and one might have won about, would have won, had they stuck it out. "

Wow--I still remember it. But that was a different bedroom, a different time. That bedroom seems too happy for me to recover in now. Besides, it has no TV and my parents were kind enough to turn over the bedroom with the TV for me to recover in, just as they did seven years ago when I came home to recover from strep throat.

A lot has happened since then. I actually fell in love with a good man and got married. But now, back in this bedroom, I'm reminded of all my failures, and here I am again failing to make the baby I desperately want. Why is everything about creating my own family so difficult for me?

I watch some TV today. It is a pathetic, but daytime TV is a mind-numbing comfort. It zones you out, tricks you into thinking you are engaging in some important learning experience, because a lot of the talk shows deal with the big deal issues women face, like rejection, poor self-esteem, and verbal abuse.

I brought up some stuff to work on my online magazine, Commitment, so I won't feel like I am just lying here going nowhere. Leah is going to come over later. Leah is such a comfort. My husband is back at work now, and he seems very faraway. I still can't believe how loving he was after the operation, how he massaged my feet...

I swear, that no matter what, the image of him at the foot of my bed, massaging my feet, when I was in so much pain, will forever stay with me.

The operation is over. Now what? One foot in front of the other. Inch by inch.

The words from the 'Don't Quit' poem that hanged in my childhood bedroom playing again in my head. Funny how things from childhood can be both a comfort and a foretelling.

Hope Comes

It has been three days since I arrived at my parent's house. I still feel very weak. I pray constantly. Having a baby feels like such a faraway dream, just another thing I'm shooting for that I probably won't get.

Prayer gives me hope, despite these negative feelings. If God could open the Red Sea, if He could save Daniel
from the lion's den, if He could break down the walls of Jericho, I do believe He can help me. From this, I draw strength.

Today Leah and I went out to do a few errands. We ended up at Wal-Mart, where she needed to pick up some film for her upcoming cross-country trip.

While we were in the photo department, I spot a cute little photo album for babies that said on the cover, "Memories of First Summer." Leah caught me looking at it.

"Buy it," she said.

"Why?" I asked.

"Because next summer you will be using it," she said. Leah is always so encouraging, so positive. She is helping me believe that someday I will definitely have a baby.

"Paula, you need to buy this," she said again.

So, diving into her optimism, I bought it.

I will always be grateful to Leah for this moment, when she took my hand and helped me see a brighter moment ahead, when with my own eyes, it was hard to hope.

Leah and I have been here before.

About seven years ago, I was extremely depressed over a bad break-up, an engagement gone wrong. Leah and I were roommates, and one afternoon, we were sitting on the couch talking, surrounded by a bunch of lace and wedding veil that a friend of hers gave her after closing a wedding business. Suddenly, Leah walked over and placed the veil on me and insisted that I stand up and look in the mirror. "No," I kept refusing, wanting that veil off, because seeing myself ever getting married seemed impossible at that point. She persisted. Finally, I stood up and looked in the mirror, "I am going to see a happy ending for you," she said, with such positivity and love in her voice.

I looked in the mirror and saw my eyes that looked dull, haunted, heartbroken, exhausted, "Sure. Nice thought," I thought to myself. "but no happy endings here."

Sure enough, Leah was right: a happy ending did come in the form of my husband.

Dare I believe her again? I left the store holding the book tightly in my hands.

Tonight, I put the little photo album on my nightstand. I am so afraid I will lose it, and that will be a sign that my baby's picture will never be in it.

I check and recheck that the album is still there several times before letting myself fall asleep.

Leah and I have always been each other's cheerleaders when it comes to reaching our dreams. I believe she really does believe I'll have a baby.

Just the way she believed I would find love again way back then.

What better gift can a friend give? Then to bestow upon another hope, a sense of believing that the one thing truly wished for will actually come true.

So I have this photo album, but I don't feel fully convinced that I will ever get to use it. I lift my head off the pillow, one more time, to make sure it is still on the nightstand before heading off to sleep.

Long Week

This has been one long and tedious week. The pain from the lapascropy has continued much longer than I ever imagined.

I didn't feel much like talking this week. Between the pain, the fatigue, and my sadness, I prefer to be quiet right now. So unlike the me from the past, when all I wanted to do was talk.

This time, I feel myself sinking inward to deal with my emotions.

Most of the words coming towards me from the outside world, even from well-meaning people, ring with the tune of: "There goes Paula again, trying for something she will never get." I sometimes feel like they all know the end of my fertility story, and I am the only one stupid enough to believe this can actually work out.

I just can't hear words like, "maybe God doesn't want you to have a baby" or 'maybe you are meant to do something else" or "God knows what we can handle" or "you have to just accept what God gives you." Bah hum bug! That's what I say to all of them. I no longer will talk about this with anyone who even slightly tries to prepare me for failure. They all think I am going to fail, and if I listen to them, I will believe them and my body will never let me produce a baby.

So, for maybe the first time in my life, I don't want to share what I am going through with anyone. I watched a lot of TV this week, and I went on my father's computer about an hour a day to work on my online magazine I enjoy so much. It is called Commitment and I have big dreams for that magazine.. All my big dreams. Sometimes I feel like I am digging and digging a hole that ultimately will go nowhere. For most of my life, there is something inside me that has always believed I should work and work and work, but ultimately get nowhere for all my effort.

A part of me still feels that way, and having a baby seems to fall into that category.

In a few days, I return home and start again on a new cycle. I've decided that if a baby is not here by December, I am going to look into adoption, while still trying for my own biological baby. I so much need a little person to love.

Conference With Dr. P

We met with Dr. P. today to discuss the results of the laparoscopy. I was surprised to hear that I do not have endometriosis. In fact, Dr. P says I was pretty "clean" as he put it. In a way, I am relieved, but in another way it hurts to think the entire operation was a waste. At least if I had endometriosis there would be an explanation as to why I am not getting pregnant.

Well, I did read once about a women who got pregnant after a laparoscopy because it cleared her fallopian tubes or something...so maybe it wasn't a total waste.

Anyways, I am moving past Clomid and on to more powerful medications in the form of shots. Dr. P. asks me again if I can handle the shots. He feels reluctant because of the hard time I've had with some of the tests in the past.

"Are you going to be able to do this?" he asks.

"YES YES YES" I wanted to scream. "GET ME THE SHOTS! I CAN TAKE THE SHOTS IF THEY WILL GIVE ME A BABY!"

My husband and I have to take a class on the shots. I'm nervous, but more than willing to do them. Hell, if this is what I need, I wish they had moved me on to shots a long time ago. What my doctor, and most of the people here. don't realize is, while I may whine and whimper over my tests, I would do 1,000 shots if that is what it will take to get a baby.

What I want to say to Dr. P is: "just because I have a hard time with the tests, and I ask that someone hold my hand during the IUI's doesn't mean I can't endure more pain.

I'll take whatever, maybe whimpering and whining the whole time, but I'll take it, and continue more if that what I have to do.'

One thing this whole infertility mess has taught me is if you want something bad enough, you have to be willing to pay whatever price is asked. I read that in a self-help book recently--if you want something, you have to be willing to throw yourself over the bar, walk through the fire, in order to get what you want.

Would I walk through fire to have a baby? Yes, I would. I think I can honestly say I would do anything asked of me. So, yes Dr. P, I'm ready for the shots. All you can see is the whimpering me, but what you don't know is that I won't stop at anything.

It is odd that if I was quiet and kept my fears locked up inside, maybe so much so that I might destroy myself, they would deem me better able to cope. Don't they understand that it is because I talk about my fears and ask for what I need that I can do this. Go figure.

We scheduled a date for class and get ready for the next cycle. I plan on doing everything I can to make this work.

Chapter 26: What I Did Right…What I Did Wrong…And What You Can Learn From My Stupid Mistakes

Throughout my infertility treatments, I made lots and lots of mistakes. I messed up so much, you might as well learn from all my mistakes. I wish for you a lot less goof-ups than I made, and probably you are going to handle all of this much better than I did. I also learned a few things that helped me a long the way. Here's what I did right and here's what I did wrong:

What I did right:

• **Changed doctors when my doctor would not answer or acknowledge my questions and undermined my faith in my ability to have another child.** When my doctor refused to try a new medication I requested and told me to give up on trying to get pregnant for a second time, I knew it was time to change doctors.

My next doctor was phenomenal, and under his treatment plan, I got pregnant and gave birth to my son.

• **Chose a highly reputable clinic with a great success record:** Always try to go with the best. But be aware: sometimes in a clinic's quest for great statistics, they may try to steer you in a direction you don't feel comfortable with. So aim for a high-quality clinic, but also be aware that sometimes their drive for a high success rate could impact the way they want to treat you.

• **Pursued the latest fertility technologies and medications, and at the same time pursue holistic forms of healing, such as acupuncture and kinesiology:** I combined holistic/alternative medicine with the best of conventional fertility treatments. I delved into holistic/alternative medicine as a way to subtly repair what was going wrong in my body, and at the same time, I took advantage of all the new advances in infertility treatments.

I took vitamins and herbs, went to acupuncture at least twice a week, and went to trauma release specialists to rid my body of emotional pain that was trapped. I also tried homeopathy.

- **Persisted and didn't give up...even after many failed IUIs and IVFs.**

- **Asked for a change in infertility medicine when I didn't see results:** When I first started treatments, I was put on Clomid, but after four cycles of it not working, I scheduled an appointment with my doctor and requested a change in medication. I did that again when I went through infertility for a second time.

- **Researched infertility medications:** I took the time to research and learn about various infertility medications. When a medication didn't seem to be working, I knew enough about the other medications available that I could ask my doctor for one that ended up being more effective for me.

- **Researched the root causes of infertility:** I did research on the root causes of infertility at bookstores, libraries, wherever I could gather information so I began to have a big picture understanding of how the body's reproductive system works and what I could do to improve my fertility. I couldn't afford to buy all the latest books at the bookstore, so I would go to bookstores and take notes--(a big thanks to Borders and Barnes and Noble for allowing me to do this!)

- **I took a vacation and gave my body the chance to relax and de-stress after a key IUI:** During an important IUI, I took a week-long vacation at a local beach. I was at a very low point, having done nine IUIs without success, and I knew I needed to do something different this time. This sweet, non-stressful time of lots of sun, sand and ocean was just what my body needed, because I did got pregnant with my daughter that cycle.

- **I got in touch with my subconscious:** Through journal writing, I dialogued with my subconscious, so that all my feelings about becoming a mother could come to light. This helped me become aware of the ways I might possibly be sabotaging my efforts and working against myself.

By tapping into my subconscious, I also began to see that some of my low self-worth and self-hatred was manifesting itself in the false belief that I did not deserve to succeed at what I most desired.

• **Did emotional release work:** I went to a myofascial release expert and did some very intensive trauma release work. I wrote down almost every major sadness that occurred in my life and worked on releasing these memories. Within a few months, I could feel myself returning to a much younger, happier version of myself.

By releasing some of the hurts inside of me, my body was then able to rise to a new level of energy and health. I believe this dramatically helped me get pregnant.

• **Worked on improving and unblocking my energy:** Through weekly acupuncture treatments, I strengthened the energy paths in my body.

• **Devised a strategy for how I would get my body healthy:** After floundering a long time, I finally realized I needed a plan, a series of steps to follow, a well thought-out strategy for getting my body healthy. At a certain point, after I had done a lot of research, I began to realize that all my organs needed to be working at their maximum capacity and I needed to cleanse and strengthen my body in as many ways as I could. I then did three liver cleanses three months in a row. I set the goal of doing at least one thing every day to improve my health. I completely changed my eating habits and lost weight. I finally began to see the connection between getting healthy and getting pregnant.

• **Asked for tests not initiated by my doctor:** When I did not get pregnant after several IUIs, I requested a laparoscopy to check for endometriosis. I did not passively sit back and let the doctors be the sole drivers in this race.

• **Improved My Environment At Home and Tried to Do Things To Make Myself Happy:** I realized that because of the intensity of what I was going through, I needed to do things to make my home a happier place. I painted my living room a vibrant Tahiti green, put up inspiring pictures and quotes, and tried to make my environment more joyful and authentically me than it had been before.

I chose to stay at a job that offered me less money and less chance for advancement than my previous jobs, but made me incredibly happy and gave me daily contact with a group of extraordinarily loving, intelligent, amazing,and positive people.

• **Got to know the staff at the infertility clinic by name and built relationships with them:** I wrote the nurses, nurses aids, and medical personnel at the clinic thank you notes, brought them flowers, and shared my emotions with them, and thus in turn, received much kind support from a fantastic, talented group of caring medical professionals.

• **Got organized:** After starting out being very disorganized, I got a big notebook and a daily appointment book, and kept all my information in those two places only. At a certain point, I finally got organized.

• **Did homeopathy with a homeopathetic specialist to help bounce the state of my body from one track to another:** I tried new ways of healing, especially if it seemed they could help break negative patterns within my body.

• **Got chiropractic adjustments:** I started paying better attention to my spine and bought good walking shoes to help keep my hips aligned.

• **Started drinking high-quality water and became very aware of the quality of water I allowed into my body.**

• **Cleansed and strengthened my organs:** I cleansed, detoxified and strengthened my liver, adrenals, thyroid, and other organs, because I finally understood how interconnected all the parts of my body are. I did a two-day fast in an attempt to rid my body of gallstones.

• **Took care of my teeth:** Before I got pregnant, I had my teeth cleaned and all my cavities filled to ensure that no infections were festering in my mouth that could weaken my body.

• **Stopped all coffee:** I stopped all coffee while trying to get pregnant and did not drink it during my pregnancies. I also stopped eating or drinking anything that contained caffeine, including chocolate.

- **Stopped talking to people who discouraged me:** I no longer shared information about my desire to have a baby with anyone who didn't understand what I was going through or made statements that hurt me or shook my ability to believe that I could someday have a baby.

- **I started swimming very mildly:** I found water to be a great stress reliever.

- **I saw my infertility as curable and I didn't believe that 'unexplained infertility' was some mysterious diagnosis that had no answers:** I tried to look at my body as having a sickness that could be cured. I didn't interpret 'unexplained infertility' as a label on my head that meant there was no hope for me. I chose to see myself as having a disease that was curable. I made myself see my 'infertility' as something temporary that could be fixed.

- **Lost Weight:** I went on a healthy diet and lost 40 pounds in an attempt to balance my hormones when I was trying to get pregnant for the second time.

- **Went To A Nutritionist:** I went to a nutritionist who did iridology. This nutritionist recommended supplements that specifically helped with fertility.

- **Worked On Improving My Husband's Health:** Although my husband did well on his sperm tests, and according to the fertility clinic, had no problems, I made an appointment for him to also see a nutritionist. She believed that my husband's sperm was being weakened by parasites, and she put him on a parasite cleanse, something hard to detect on standardized tests. His health improved greatly, and soon after I became pregnant.

- **Started eating lots and lots of greens on a daily basis to alkalize my body:** The more I learned about health, the more I realized that keeping the body alkalized was very important. So I began eating bowls of romaine lettuce and parsley daily, along with juicing lots and lots of spinach daily.

Now, I can share with you all the things I did wrong:

- **Stayed With the Wrong Doctor Too Long:** I stayed with the wrong doctor even after she misdiagnosed me, caused me to have an unnecessary surgery and never apologized, and tried to shoot down any hope I had of getting pregnant.

- **Fell Apart A lot Instead of Taking Positive Action:** At first, I didn't realize how many ups and downs were part of the whole infertility process. I would become so devastated when a cycle didn't work that I wasted a lot of time and energy mourning, instead of focusing on the next cycle and moving forward.

- **I Didn't Make the Connection Between the Choices I Made and the State of My Health:** For a long time, I didn't realize the correlation between the choices I made and my health. So I continued to eat badly, not get enough sleep, not reduce my stress, and stay in stress-inducing situations.

- **Took Herbs After an IVF Cycle:** I took herbs after an IVF cycle, which I was warned not to do, because once a cycle begins, there are some herbs that should immediately be stopped because they could harm your child. There are herbs that can be helpful during pregnancy, but in this particular instance, I did not take herbs that were appropriate for pregnancy.

- **Fought With My Husband and Blamed Him For My Sadness:** I fought with my husband and made him the enemy too many times, even when he was trying his best to help. I was so grief-stricken sometimes, I would turn my rage against him and attack. Often, I could not see or feel empathy for the helplessness and fatigue he was also experiencing. Instead of finding ways to manage my pain and stress, I lashed out at him for not being able to fix my problems.

- **Lost Touch With My Subconscious:** I did not always know the conflicting needs and emotions I was sometimes experiencing on my road to becoming a mother. This caused me to sometimes undermine my own efforts and sabotage myself at times.

- **I Had No Strategy for Improving My Health:** I did not pull together a strategy to improve my health for quite awhile. This meant my health did not improve for a long time, and I was spinning my wheels month after month, hoping for a new result when I was stuck doing the same old things.

- **Failed To See That I Had Some Power in the Situation:** At first, I felt very helpless to do anything to change my situation, and this caused a lot of rage and frustration within me. But after many failed attempts at getting pregnant, I started to see that I had the power of choice. I could choose to eat well, try holistic forms of healing, and release my stress in positive ways.

- **I Was Very Disorganized:** At first, I was very disorganized, and was always late for appointments. Eventually, I became more self-disciplined and organized. I showed up to my appointments on time, and began to see that I needed to work along with the clinic as much as possible, not make their life difficult by showing up late or missing appointments.

- **Derailed By the Nos:** I took the no's a bit too seriously and sometimes almost derailed myself through my grief.

I got so discouraged by the nos, I failed to see them as just as "missed shot in the game."

- **Fought With Family and Friends:** I got intensely angry when family members and friends didn't seem to understand what I was going through. I didn't know when to change or lower my expectations of what they were able to understand. I also didn't know when to just overlook a stupid remark or a poorly timed statement.

- **Ate Badly:** At first, I did not see any correlation between nutrition and my body's health. Eventually, I saw the difference when I stopped drinking coffee and started giving my body lots of romaine lettuce, blueberries, sweet potatoes, and other healthy foods. I finally understood that the foods I ate impacted my ability to conceive and give birth. When I was tempted by the candy in the vending machine at work, I would say to myself: 'that candy bar could prevent you from having the baby of my dreams.'

Diary Excerpt: Getting Ready for Next Cycle

I'm now focused on getting ready for the next IUI cycle.

I've decided that I'll take a week off of work right after the IUI and stay with my parents at the beach. Ever since I was 10 years old, my parents have rented at Salisbury Beach, an old-time honky-tonk beach to some, but to my family, the absolutely most beautiful beach in the world.

Maybe some rest and relaxation at the beach will help. I read a lot lately about how reduced stress levels increase the chances of getting pregnant. I'm skeptical, but willing to try it. My boss won't be thrilled. August is pledge month and they need as many callers as possible. I almost don't want the week off, because I like work and I hate displeasing my boss, but I have to put getting pregnant above anything else. I keep picturing myself 80 years old and it is doubtful my friends at work will be with me.

So I'm putting in for the time off. I have to keep the big picture in my head.

Shot Talk

Today, my husband attended a class on how to administer the shots. My husband tells me he is certain he can do this.

We start the shots tonight.

At work, I started feeling so anxious about the shots and what lay ahead of me: will they hurt? Can I handle it? How bad will it be?

I was getting so nervous, I started chatting about the shots today at work. Chatting and talking lightly, almost jovially about it, as if I was talking about an upcoming vacation, or a recent trip to the dentist.

That's how I cope--I open up, spill my guts to the world, make light of my sorrows publicly, put myself on display, like a joke or something, all in an effort to rally the troops around me.

To me, it is easier to open up than keep it inside and carry the burden alone.

Here at work, I feel safe, comfortable, at home and accepted by my work family, a group of people I've come to love, trust, and feel able to share my struggles. Inbetween our phone calls, we talk about everything, from high school crushes, best friends who ditched us, childhood bedrooms, favorite books, worst rejections, biggest disappointments, dolls that we lost, favorite foods, and songs from the 1970s that still make us cry.

I know infertility isn't a light hearted subject--certainly not fodder for slow work day chatter, but that's how I get through the days--talking so much everything starts to seem like no big deal even to myself.

The more I talk about it, the more minor it all seems. The more I hold it up to the light of day, the smaller it becomes. It cannot eat me alive if I spit it out for all to see. If I keep it in, make it too sacred to talk about, then it becomes something more than I can take.

The fact is, talking to my closest friends I've had for years is hard. They've seen me want things before—things that didn't work out. They also know the ugly truth that it ain't pretty when I'm devastated.

So when I voice my incessant longing for a child, they remember me broken, and they don't want to see that again--so they try to prepare and cushion me for disappointment.

I understand where they are coming from. but I can't bear that type of comfort right now. For me to someday give birth, I have to put aside every failure in my life, which have been many, and somehow believe this time will be different. I have to see myself as a person for whom a happy ending is possible.

So I talk to my new friends at work, friends who see a lighter, happier side of me, friends who can believe in my dream, because they do not fear so much for my failure.

Here in our cubicle-filled office with no windows to the outside world, I feel insulated from the realities of my life. I feel so cushioned here, that any sadness and heartbreak I've experienced in my life seems like just another dramatic or funny story to tell.

Suddenly things that shamed me seem like material for tomorrow's good story. I don't hate myself as much anymore, because when I share my stories, I see myself in a different way—I am funny, quirky, creative, original—what was all that self-hatred about? Even the saddest parts of my life don't seem as half as sad when I talk about them at work.

Yet, without knowing it today, I hit upon a subject that was difficult for one of my co-workers and friend. She pulled me into a side room to tell me that she was not at all happy about my chattering about the shots. It turns out, she has been going through infertility treatments for ten years, and the shots are very painful, hard to administer and she ended up never getting pregnant. She told me to ask my doctor about what was in the medication I'm taking, because it could cause cancer.

She had chosen to be very selective about whom she talked to about her infertility, and she didn't appreciate my talking so lightly about a very serious subject.

I feel ashamed, and then I wonder: what if she is right? What if my husband has trouble giving me the shots? What if I do all this and it doesn't work out? What if all this medicine gives me is cancer, instead of a baby?

I thank her, but in that moment, I have no choice but to blank out all the warnings. I want a baby so badly, I have no choice but to take some risks.

Whatever the medicine is, I need it, poison or not.

Why should I have to keep quiet about my infertility? I'm not a bad woman because my body isn't producing a baby. My friend, also, should not have had to feel ashamed about her infertility, as she is an awesome, amazing woman. Why can other people talk about their health challenges but infertility is something best to keep hushed up?

There is still so much shame tied up with this illness. Does infertility mark us as flawed? Bad woman having problems related to sex and marriage, inferior to those fertile lovelies who get pregnant without even trying? Why are we seen as desperate if we say right out loud that we long for a baby and we are devastated because it isn't happening as fast or as naturally as we imagined? Is it because all things pertaining to motherhood and woman in general are disrespected?

There are all sorts of moral parables tied up in not getting pregnant-- that God is denying you a baby, or that you are not up to the job of being a parent, or that you are suppose to adopt or that you are just not good enough to bear a child.

Tonight, my husband has to jab needles into my body. I'm almost too scared to go through with it. Just thinking about the shots makes everything in my life seem hard and heavy.

That's why I can't stay quiet --because once I stay quiet, it all becomes too horrible, too ugly, too awlful to endure. I need people to listen. By talking about it lightly, I am convincing myself that taking the shots is really no big deal.

So I will talk and chatter and make light of what I am facing in a few hours. I'm not ashamed of having a problem making a baby.

I don't need to hang my head in shame over this.

Shot Night

Tonight, for the first time, my husband administered the shots. All day long, I felt a heaviness hanging over me. At 2 p.m. it was five hours away. At 3 p.m. four hours away. At 4 p.m., three hours away.

Finally, it was 7 o'clock. My husband starts by opening the bottles to prepare the medication. I admire his bravery, as I watch him mix the medicines.

Then I sit down in the kitchen. I've learned a few tricks about taking tests:

1) Don't look. Keep your eyes shut. Seeing it only make the pain more intense.

2) Breath out, while blowing, blowing, blowing, kind of like as substitution.

3) Distract yourself with something fun, comforting or sweet.

4) Have a reward waiting.

Here's how I distracted myself tonight: I recently got a cookbook with recipes from bed and breakfast inns.

The book has a beautiful blue and white cover and it is all about cozy, comfortable, romantic places..the delightful stuff bed & breakfast inns are made of.

I opened the book and decide that while I am getting a shot, I will read a recipe--knowing that by the time I get to the end of the recipe, the shot will be over.

We're just about ready. I am praying every moment for the strength to endure this. My husband looks for a spot on my leg. I look away.
I open to a recipe and start reading. The book is comforting and I am transported to a beautiful place.

My husband jabs the needle into my leg, quickly, so quickly, I breath, breath, breath. I pray. I start reading a recipe, and it is over. I've reached the end of my recipe.

Then, like a spring day after a storm, a bit of alcohol to clean it, a bandage and I am free. Tomorrow, I will think about the next shot. But for tonight, it is over and done. It hurt, but not half as bad as I imagined.

Now I can just sit back and enjoy tonight.

Another Shot Night

I'm getting more comfortable with the actual shots, although in the hours leading up to them, I am overcome with a lot of anxiety and dread.

Tonight, some of Chris's friends came over and we went ahead with the shots, despite the fact that they were all standing two feet away in our living room.

Having a bunch of guys standing outside the kitchen, practically watching me get shots, brought an air of humor to this. These guys are mostly single, so completely out-of-touch with this type of stuff, and so it was funny to see them privy to what is normally such an intimate and hush-hush procedure.

They actually seemed scared in a way, and that made the whole thing all the more humorous to me.

Back to the Pool

In preparing for my next IUI, I am eager to start my morning swim routine. After reading about the link between stress and infertility, I realized that I needed to find a way to release my stress.
Since swimming has always relaxed me, and I chose swimming as one of the ways I am going to release the stress in my life.

At first, my husband was skeptical. "Are you really going to get up early every morning and go swimming before work?" he asked.

"Yeeees," I replied with great irritation. "Just watch me."

So every morning (well, almost every morning) between 5:30 and 6 o'clock, I wake up, creep quietly out of bed, put my towel in the bag, check to make sure I have my club ID, and then I head down to the door, hoping it won't wake my husband.

I like the whole rhythm of going for a swim in the early morning.

I like the way the sun cocks its head and shines that time of morning, as if to say hello and welcome to your day. I like the early morning drive, with so few cars on the road, lots good music on the radio, and the sense that by getting out the door early, I am part of the early mornings' rock and roll.

The first day I went to swim, I was terrified, like the shy awkward kid on the first day of junior high. There is always a moment of fear right before I go in the water: Can I actually do this? Actually go in the pool? What if the water is cold? What if the water is too cold for me to take? I throw my body in anyways, and it feels like a moment of triumph.

One day, something odd happened. I swam 40 minutes straight. Being 40 pounds overweight and out of shape, this was a lot longer than normal for me. Afterwards, I felt limp and floppy. When I got in the car to drive home, I suddenly burst out crying—but it was an odd type of crying, because I didn't feel any emotion. It was more of a physical releasing cry than an emotional cry. I wasn't thinking of anything particularly sad. It was as if my body was just releasing. I sat in my car, just crying and crying. By the time I got home, I had stopped crying and a crazy massive feeling of joy had overtook me. Joy as I went in the house! Joy as I ran up the stairs to my bedroom! Joy ! Joy! Joy!

Something bad left my body that day and it was replaced by a light-heartedness I had not felt in a long, long time.

My husband immediately noticed the change in me. "you seem so relaxed," he said.

When I swim, I am proving to myself that I can do what it takes to win this battle with infertility.

Getting Ready

I feel a momentum building towards the IUI coming up next week. I've gone to Dr. Kim for acupuncture treatments three times so far. I know it is a lot, and that we can't really afford it, but I need to do everything up my chances.

I made Chris go twice, as it can't hurt if his body is operating better too. Between the swimming, acupuncture and eating better, I feel my health is changing I took next week off so I can stay with my parents at the beach. Doing the IUI and then having a week to relax at the beach should help this whole getting-pregnant-process. Lots of praying daily too.

The Night Before The IUI

It is Saturday and I'm here at the beach with my parents. They are renting a house for three weeks. It is the same beach we have stayed at since I was a kid and so my family has loads of wonderful memories tied up at this beach. Things have been going well in preparation for tomorrow's IUI. I feel oddly happy and optimistic even. I took the week out of work so I could stay here at the beach and rest after the IUI. The water, the sunshine, the chance to sit and do nothing, should up my chances of getting pregnant. I took the week off during my department's busiest time, but all my choices right now have to be for my baby. Work and everything else cannot matter right now.

Tonight, we are taking it easy. I had a nice meal.
I ate lots of plums, because I've been reading about the blood type diet and plums are suppose to be good for O blood types.

All my hard work has paid off in one way so far: I feel much better than I used to feel.

I had three acupuncture treatments in the past six days, and I made Chris go twice. Even though we can't really afford it, I pushed Chris and begged for this. I know the more acupuncture I have, the better. It will clear my energy, enhance my life force, make me stronger. Dr. Kim is marvelous.

Tomorrow, a new life begins...it has to...I beg God for this.

Day of IUI

Today is Sunday, August 2. I felt happy on the ride to the clinic this morning, the sun shining with a big grin, and a week at the beach I love ahead of me. Thank God there was no traffic this morning.

Driving to the clinic is normally so hard, scary, stressful and frantic. Today, on an early Sunday morning, a piece of cake. From the beach, we took a different route than we usually go and everything just felt easier, safer and more joyous than usual. No 128 traffic!

I did something a bit different than usual too--I brought along a bottle of red wine!

Last week at work, Judy told me she thought that a glass of wine can sometimes help a person relax and have a better chance of getting pregnant. I listened and decided I would drink some wine before the procedure.

Once we were inside the waiting room, I realized that I had forgotten the wine in the car.

"Go get it," I whispered to my husband.

"Really? You want it?" he hemmed and hawed.

'Yes, please," I said, feeling an urgency to try something different this time.

"You can't drink it here," he said.

"I'll go in the bathroom," I whispered.

Kooky, yes, but what the heck. I needed to relax.

He went to the car, came back in with the wine bottle hidden under his shirt. He passed it to me discreetly, I put it under my shirt, went into the bathroom, and slugged a bit down.

Well, at the very least, I immediately feel more relaxed—and it felt pretty good to do something so forbidden at the clinic.

My husband went first, as he always does, to give his sperm. I have no idea what this is like for him. We never talk about it. Awhile later, they called me in.

I hate the whole IUI process. I hate the speculum they put inside me, that is so tight when they screw it in. Every moment the speculum is inside me is difficult and painful, and when they finally start to unscrew it, a huge relief passes through me. Thankfully, the nurses hold my hand and talk to me during the IUI. They ask me questions, like what movies I saw recently and what I do for work. They are so kind.

Today, the IUI is done by Melissa and it is quick. She always does a good job. Then, my husband comes in and I continue laying on the table. I put my legs high up in the air, against the wall, hoping this will help the sperm get to where it needs to go. I do this for 40 minutes, even though they say you can leave in 10 minutes. We decide to wait as long as we can. Give that sperm some help swimming up! Will it happen this time? Hope lives in my heart. I pray fervently, night and day, for my baby to come alive. Oh God, please. I know that the only hope I have is that God hears my prayer, and because of that hope, I do feel hope despite everything. Oh God, please.

We return to the beach, and enjoy a quiet evening sitting by the ocean. I eat lots of dark purple plums. Did the IUI work? Two weeks from now, we'll know the answer.

In Waiting Mode

Now that the IUI is done, I am in a waiting mode. It is very relaxing being at the beach. I am enjoying just sitting by the ocean day after day, feet in the water, head in the clouds, the womb-like thrash of the ocean waves in my ears.

My uncle and his family came to the beach one day, and I swam in the water like a giddy eight year old.

There have been hard moments this week too. A neighbor we recently met dropped by, and when I confided to her that I was trying with great difficulty to have children, she told me that maybe God didn't intend me to have children. At that moment, I felt slapped down by her proclamation.

But right at that moment, an odd thing happened that seemed to save me: three little girls with dark curly hair walked by, looking much the way I envision my future daughter will look. I grabbed the sight of those little girls as a sign that maybe I am intended to have kids--dare I hope, maybe even a daughter--and I should ignore my neighbor's careless comment. I stayed focused on the girls and slapped her words out of my head.

My young cousin Chuck slept over. One night, Chris and Chuck all went down to the amusement center. Once we got there, we all started acting like kids, running, skipping, acting crazy. In that moment, a snapshot of the three of us running to the center imprints on my memory. I think: if it turns out I am pregnant, this night marks the beginning of something new and different in my life.

The next day, at about 1 in the afternoon, I was hit with a wave of tiredness like a tiredness I have never felt before. I laid down and actually slept for three hours.
Since I never nap, this was quite different for me. My body was so exhausted. Could it be???? I dare not analyze this too much, but I pray and keep up my optimism.

The waiting is hard. When people say that maybe God doesn't want me to have children, I want to scream. 'Why???? Why do you say that? Why do you think that God would not want me to have children?'

Why is it so easy to automatically think God is all about denying and withholding, when the Bible speaks mostly about God's great love and how if we have faith, we can move mountains? It is a disgrace that people are so quick to think of God as a chiding schoolmaster, who would rather rap you on the knuckles and deny any and all requests, rather than being the loving kind merciful God He is.

This whole process of trying to get pregnant sometimes reminds me of a time when I was younger, and deeply in love with a man who didn't love me back, or who loved me sometimes, and didn't love me other times. Back then, friends would say things like, "I don't think you two were meant to be" and I bucked it.

They ended up being right. I still sometimes wonder why. Why wasn't that relationship meant to be? How could I love someone so much and him not feel the same way in return? Is having children going to end up being just like that episode in my life--something I desperately want and yearn for, only to have the answer be no?

I feel so alone right now. What will I do if I'm not pregnant? Get sperm from someone other than my husband? Someone whose sperm is more compatible with mine? A guy with stronger sperm? At this point, I just want a child and I'm beginning not to care how I get it. Should I adopt a child? I can hardly bear another month to pass.

For now, I sit by the ocean, and wait. My 96 year old grandmother Maria teases me, and tells me to sit down and let the ocean water float into my vagina. She knows I'm trying to get pregnant (she doesn't know about the infertility treatments--how in the world would I explain them to a 94 year old woman from Italy.).

She says the water will help my body be strong and will help me get pregnant. I do what she says, laughing, but secretly hoping that my wise beautiful grandmother is right, and that the strength of the ocean strengthens my tired body enough to get pregnant.

For The Love of My Mother

I am sitting on the beach late this afternoon, wondering (as usual..so what's new) if I am pregnant or not.

If I think about it, I have to admit that a part of me doesn't think I deserve to have a baby. In fact, most of the time, I don't feel like I deserve even the smallest of things, never mind the one thing in this world I want most.

I realized, as I was sitting by the ocean, that for me to help my body get pregnant, I need to trick my body into thinking it is doing this for my mother, and not myself.

From now on, in an attempt to trick my body into giving me what I want, I am going to tell my body that it must rise up and produce a baby for my mother.

Body, we must do this for my mother.

I need a motivation outside of myself for this to work.

I know my mother would love to be a grandmother. Recently, my mother ran into the mother of one of my childhood friends. This woman, who has three grandchildren, announced to my mother, "Sally, you don't know how wonderful it is to have a grandchild. Just think, you are the only one (out of this group of friends) who isn't a grandmother."

Talk about insensitive. Maybe this lady meant no harm, but I know it hurt my mother to think that most of my childhood friends have babies and I do not.

I have to have children, so this will be the last time some petty, mean-spirited, or just plain clueless person will have ammunition to hurt my mother again.

I will not allow my mother to arrive at her old age without grandchildren.

Never do I want my mother to feel that because of my failures, she ended up missing out on one of life's grand last-minute surprises.

I don't want my mother to pity me, or herself, because we are babyless people.

As I focus my thoughts on my mother, I can actually feel my body getting stronger.

For myself, I probably won't allow my body to be strong enough to make a baby.

For my mother, I can put aside my own self-loathing long enough to let my body do its natural thing and make a baby.

I saw how sad my mother was when this woman alluded to the fact that all my friends from childhood have been successful enough to make a baby, and I, the only freak in the group, still does not have a baby.

Nope, I'm sick of being a freak who causes my mother pain. I have to do something normal her sake.

Why should she look at other women and feel they are rewarded in some way that she is not?

To make this happen, I need to keep focusing on my mother and not myself.

For myself, my body will say: "You are too bad of a person to ever get what you want."

But for my mother, my body will be better than it naturally is.

When I think of my mother, the uneasiness in my stomach disappears and is replaced by something much clearer I can't fully explain.

I feel stronger.

My body wants to do right by my mother. I sit on the beach, inhaling the sun and air, and hope and strength return to the self-hating me.

Because I love my mother so much, I will create a grandchild for her.

I'm tired of being the freaky, quirky, odd daughter she always has to apologize for.

I'm hoping that my body will agree that even if I don't deserve a baby, my mother certainly deserves a grandchild.

Friday Came

Chris left for work early this morning. Since there is no phone here at the beach cottage, I will have to use the pay phone at the convenience store down the street to call my answering machine at home later today to hear the nurse's message. I could go home and wait for the message, but since we have only one car, I would be stuck there all day today and tomorrow, and I don't want to be sitting at home waiting to hear no.

Most of the day, I sat by the ocean. The waves crashing and diving up and down the beach massage the weary part of me. Being here has been more relaxing than I ever imagined.

There have even been moments I almost forget about my desperation to have a baby. Well, not really moments, but maybe a minute or two of peace, here and there. The ocean can do that, give even the saddest most desperate person, a few moments of peace.

Today, I am fidgety all day. The nurse will call by 4 o'clock, as they always do. I wish 4 o'clock would just come and be over with. I know what it coming. I want it done.

Four o'clock comes. I borrow some change from my mother and I walk down the concrete sidewalk to the convenience store. This is the same convenience store where my cousin Sheri and I used to hang out at as budding teenagers. We would stand in the store's parking lot, preening, flirting, enjoying the teenage world of cute boys and shy smiles.

It is the same store where as a 12-year old girl, I stood outside the door and asked customers to sign a petition to bring back the 100-year old merry-go-round that developers sold to an amusement park in San Diego that had graced Salisbury center since the.

I loved that carousel as a child. I can still see myself trying to grab the gold ring. I felt so powerful back then, so naively powerful as to think a silly petition would make the owners of the carousel give up whatever profits they seized from the sale and return the carousel back to its rightly place at the center.

How odd that now I walk to this store feeling anything but powerful--
did my 12 year old self ever imagine that life would return me to this
store, on this day, in this way, to do this task, to hear this news,
to feel this way?

Thank God we cannot see the future. The spirited little entrepreneur
with the petition! What has become of her? A shadow self enters the
parking lot, a pathetic desperate woman bearing no trace to the hardy
girl with the petition that once came here.

I go to the pay phone and there is someone on it. I wait. Finally it is free.

I put in the coins, and begin to dial the number that will tell me whether
I am pregnant or not.

I stop. I cannot do it. I cannot bear to hear the news. Not here, not
surrounded by all the memories of this place. I hang up, press the return
button, get my change, and head back down the concrete sidewalk to the
beach cottage. Better that I don't know. Better that I stay wondering a
little longer. Better that I allow a tiny bit of hope in me to stay alive a bit
longer, because I might go completely crazy here in this parking lot if
the answer is no. One more day of not knowing is okay, a reprieve from
all the hard choices facing me.

I walk back to the cottage. I did the right thing. I could not bear to hear
that no over the phone, in the old
parking lot where I hung out as a teenager, with people coming and
going, buying beer, candy, chips.

I will go home tomorrow and listen to the message alone, with no one
around to see me fall apart. I don't think my parents, or the store's
patrons, could take seeing the rage that is inside me if the answer is no.

A little girl that once had hope in everything used to hang out here, and
she didn't deserve to have her heartbroken in a place where she once
felt so strong.

Friday Night Longing

It is a beautiful dark starry summer night and I feel anything but carefree.

Tomorrow I will go home to listen to my answering machine and find out the news. Bad news, I am pretty sure. The answer is going to be no. I know it. The answer for me is always no. I have learned that whenever I really want something, ultimately the answer always turns out to be no. I have come to understand that when I really want something, or someone, truly love this person, this thing, this whatever, the answer is no. So I already know the answer to the question I am waiting to hear answered. How else could it be?

I can barely stand to think of my future right now.

It is Friday night and my cousin Susan has come to visit us. Susan is one of my favorite persons on this earth, and yet tonight, even her visit isn't cheering me up. Susan had her children young in the most beautiful and normal way people are suppose to have children. She is surrounded by children, grandchildren, and right now, in her presence, I feel woefully inadequate.

On my father's side of the family, it seems the tree bears fruit, in the normal way the cycle of life is suppose to work. Childbearing, getting pregnant, having children, comes easily, naturally, the family growing and multiplying. No one is alone or freakish. Life blossoms beautifully. They are part of the normal life continuum.

Susan doesn't know I'm going to an infertility clinic. She might vaguely suspect I want children, but she has no idea that tonight I feel like the biggest failure in the world in her presence. She was a grandmother at 36. Here I am, 33 years old and still no children. I once thought waiting until you were older to have children was the thing to do, and now I realize that the tables have turned and actually I am the unnatural freak who missed the biological boat.

Susan, my parents and myself go down to the center to get some fried dough and pizza.

The "center" as we call this part of the beach is to an outsider nothing but a honky tonk bunch of neon signs, fried food, men in tattoos wearing leather jackets and girls with store bought bleached hair and too little clothes. But to my family, the center is a place of beautiful, never-to-be forgotten memories, of amusement park rides and favorite ice creams, the bright lights thrilling us in the darkness. It is the place where me and my cousins Sheri and Tina roamed around as teenagers, enjoying the tiny element of danger the night held, along with the ice cream and moon pies at Willy's, and most of all, the camaraderie of family.

Usually, staying at my favorite beach in the world, one laden with such glorious childhood memories, and having my beloved cousin Susan sleep over, would feel like a great and grand treat.

But tonight, the world feels ugly and sad to me. I am too old to be longing for the past. I should be over wanting and yearning for what used to be by now. Everywhere I look tonight, the past feels so much better than the present or even the future. It seems that at 12 years old, I had more than I have now--more connection, more family, more love, more fun. A child would bring it all back, change the life I have now. In the presence of my cousin who had four children by the time she was my age, I feel dull, barren, like a wrinkled fruit that never fully ripened. I live my life missing the past, and I'm tired of that...Tired of looking back all the time. I want a reason, a someone, to look forward for. I need someone to create new memories for, rather than yearning for people and memories long gone in my life.

I want a child to introduce me to a new way of being, and reconnect with an old way of being that I have lost.

I want to be part of the club. That's it...I want to be a member in the natural process of life. I want to do what people, animals, bugs, birds, and all living beings have been doing since the earth came into existence. Trees have leaves, squirrels have baby squirrels, from dirt comes weeds, plants and flowers, the sky gives out rain and ants breed more ants, and even old trees find a way to resurrect themselves in the spring to heave out a few more twigs and a few more leaves. Then, why is having a baby so hard for me?

Why, from the beginning, has everything about creating my own family been hard for me, from getting married to now having a baby? Why is this natural part of life such a struggle for me? My cousins seem to get married and have children without barely a thought, they so fit in the natural cycle of life, and yet for me, having my own family is a grueling, frustrating, nearly impossible dream.

I sat in the car while my parents and Susan went to get pizza at a place we've been going for years. I feel too sad to enjoy pizza or even get my body to move out of the car.

I stay in the car while they get in line for the pizza--I cannot bring myself to participate in the buzz of life going on around me tonight, when there is no buzz in my life that even remotely mirrors what is happening in the center tonight or what has happened here for generations.

I cannot help but thinking that by the time Susan was my age, she had given birth four times. I remember her at my age--she was all mother, all grown-up, a part of life's process. She had a family, a definite somewhere to belong in this world.

I sit in the car, watching all the life around me, the life I used to believe I would have long ago when I came here as a child. I feel like such a failure right now.

The drizzle starts to fall and my heart is slowly and dully breaking.

News Arrives

Today I woke up with one thought in my mind: get out of here before you get the news. I'm am a raging volcano ready to explode. If I call my house, check my answering machine, and hear' no, sorry-you-are-not-pregnant, I am going to flip out'. No, I am going to die. I am going to blame everyone around me for my life, for my lonely existence in a childless world. So this morning, I made some excuse about needing to go home to do some work on my online magazine, and I borrowed my mother's red Toyota Camry.

The drive home was fast, as I live only about 35 minutes from the beach. The Toyota ran so smoothly I felt like I was flying. I drive a clunky old Volvo, and I'm not used to this feeling of gliding down the highway. The ride home, so mockingly free, gave me a reprieve from my pain.

When I got home, I went straight up to our office where the answering machine lives. The red button was not blinking. I pressed play. Nothing. No message.

What happened is clear: my husband came home, played out the sad message of no, and decided not to save it, so as to spare me the pain. He wants to tell me himself.

He is right. I feel better not hearing it. I like the silence. I've heard enough no's loud and clear in my life. I don't want to hear no again. My husband is kind, and I feel a dull sense of relief, although I know this means terrible choices wait ahead for me.

We've done seven IUIs now, and I'm growing more convinced that the reason I can't get pregnant is that my eggs and my husband's sperm don't want to mate. What next? Look for somebody else's sperm? A pretty immoral idea, but not one I haven't toyed with. My husband says fine, go do what you want, and a part of me screams yes, I deserve to be able to find a better biological choice, because above all else, I want children. Terrible. Horrible thoughts. I would never actually do something so immoral, but this is where sadness can lead: to desperate ideas that are wrong and that I would never do.

I get on my computer, one of the few places in this world where serenity comes over me. I am working on my online magazine, and I have met an amazing web designer named Ann Sowers who is going to redesign the site. When I'm working on Commitment, I become enraptured, in flow, and my thoughts of bearing children are replaced with creative thrill for a short time.

When I work on my magazine, I escape, if just for a few minutes, from being the washed out failure I am. I am dashing out West in my covered wagon, towards a new life.

Working on Commitment always calms me down. A few hours pass and it is almost time to get back to the beach.

I'm going to hear no tonight. Right out loud tonight I will hear no.

But at least it will be from my husband, and not from the voice of a nurse doing her routine calls, who says 'no, you are not pregnant' with the same kind of faux sympathy of a salesgirl who tells you, no, that blouse is no longer on sale, but try back next week.

I need to get back to the beach.

The Answer Comes

I am sitting in the kitchen at the beach cottage. Early evening has come and a light darkness sprinkles the world. We have plans tonight with our friends Melanie and Darren. I am waiting for everyone to arrive. It is getting dark and my husband walks in.

"Did you hear the news?" he says casually.

"No," I answered, immediately starting to hate him. It is easy to blame him, hate him, consider it all is his fault that I have to endure this.

"You are pregnant," he says, almost matter-of-factly.

I stop. "You are lying," I blurt out.

"I'm not," he says. "I thought you knew. The nurse called. She said you are pregnant."

I am stunned. Happy. Disbelieving. Shocked. Not sure I'm ready to believe it.

"Then why didn't you save the message for me?" I retort, challenging this notion.

"Because I thought you heard it Friday night. So when I got home I didn't save it. I thought you knew," he explained.

I sat stunned for a few moments, still not fully comprehending this. Then the world changes hue and a different color comes over everything. The universe has shifted, in the way I had begged and pleaded and waited for. A new and different door has opened for me and something that resembles calm, gratitude, and quiet jubilance enters my soul.

Yes, there was optimism this cycle. Momentum was definitely building. I even felt joy during certain moments. Hadn't I prayed constantly? I know God hears prayers and maybe He heard my prayer.

Still I couldn't let myself believe that yes had finally arrived.

My husband then told me the nurse said I had to go for three more pregnancy tests to be sure.

Always more tests...Three more tests.

Only in the world of infertility does 'yes you are pregnant' also mean you need three more tests to ABSOLUTELY BE SURE you are pregnant.

I am shocked and happy. Maybe I was even expecting this. I had begged God so much, perhaps He heard me. Perhaps he saw me last month throwing myself on the side of the road crying, and He wanted to help me.

Melanie and Darren arrive. We sort of blurt out the news to everyone-- my parents, Melanie, my grandmother. Everyone is happy, but they seem dazed and shocked too.

You would imagine this would be a big night of celebration. I suppose now you expect a few pages about the glorious night I enjoyed with family and friends, celebrating the fact that I was finally pregnant.

But instead fear rose up in me. Fear rose up in my husband. After months and months of stress, we were not accustomed to hearing yes.

We were so accustom to disappointment and anger, it didn't feel quite natural yet to sit back and enjoy.

We all went out to dinner, and the problem started with a bowl of soup.

At first, I ordered a bowl of soup, but then I saw the steak, and decided to get that instead. We were on a tight budget and so I asked the waitress to cancel the soup. Well, the order came, and she brought the steak and the soup. I told her I didn't want the soup, and she said it was too late to send it back.

If I had the money, I would have simply paid for the soup--but I didn't have the money for both, (going to acupuncture so many times depleted our budget) and I proceeded to get into an argument with her over the bill. No, I told her, I am not paying for the soup. She was snappy back at me. We went back and forth, until finally she took the soup off the bill, but not before saying something nasty about me.

Now, instead of backing me, my husband got really angry at me. He was (boo hoo) embarrassed. I wanted to say, is it not my fault we don't have the money for both. And so a big fight between us began. He thought I was rude and immature. I thought he was a wimp for not standing up for me. How could he not defend me, when I was carrying his child?

On the way home, all our pent-up rage and exhaustion from the past few weeks exploded into a rip-roaring fight. He wished he wasn't having a baby with me! I wished I wasn't having a baby with him!

All the fight in us burst open and tumbled out and we said some horrible things.

I think the fact that we had been walking on pins and needles around this IUI for so long wore us out.

We got back to the beach cottage and went to bed.

Looking back, I don't think I felt comfortable allowing myself to feel the joy that was rightfully mine that night.

I expected to hear no and had gotten so used to hearing no, that a very destructive part of me needed to make trouble because pain and trouble was what I was accustomed to.

You would think that now that I finally had what I wanted for so long I would be happy, but that is the beauty of being a human--the paradoxical feelings that can exist within one person. Just a month ago, I was throwing myself on the side of a road, crying with agony, because no baby had arrived for me yet. Now, a month later, I am pregnant and I'm scared of having a baby with my husband, and I'm not sure I'm ready. I want it, the baby, so much, and yet I am scared.

This whole infertility process up to this point made us both a bit insane--the whole trying/not getting/trying/not getting/ and now finally, when we didn't expect it, getting. We had both been so hurt and so disappointed for so long, and now a yes. Did we deserve this yes? Were we ready for this change?

But when I woke up the next day, everything was already feeling very different.

Yes, Its True

I am pregnant. Let me say again those three long-awaited magic words: I am pregnant.

Yahoo! Yipee! Who cares about last night's fight? Who cares about anything? I, me, the person I am, is actually and really pregnant.

I need to go for three more tests, but that doesn't matter. I am truly pregnant. Thank you God. I am going to be a Mom!

The world looks like a different place today. The sun shines differently, the breeze blows differently, I look in the mirror and see myself differently...I am pregnant! I am pregnant! I am pregnant!

I Am A Pregnant Lady

I still can't believe I am pregnant!

It is a week after we got the good news. I am walking around dazed and happy.
I have to get two more tests to confirm that officially I am pregnant, but once I have those tests, I am officially on the way to having my baby!

I never felt more important and more wonderfully ordinary in my entire life.

I am finally part of humanity's drumbeat, a note heard in the universal rhythm of life, life going on, life beating heart.

Let me shout it from the roof top--I AM PREGNANT!

We returned home from the beach after we got the good news. My parents are still there on vacation and we went for a visit today. When we get there, my mother's best friend Lydia was visiting. It felt so exciting to share the news with her. I could tell my parents felt so proud too...so proud to be part of something so normal. My mother already bought me a baby name book. I immediately start flipping through it admiring all the beautiful baby names.

I feel like I'm finally part of life's parade, one of the marchers, no longer forced to sit on the sidelines cheering for all the others passing me by with a march of their own.

 I am going to have a place in this world, a starring role, and that will be of a mother.

A Third Yes!

   Today was the third test to determine if I am pregnant. The day started out beautiful and sunny, and I had a good feeling.

I drove to the clinic about 6 a.m. It felt good to be there, and in a strange way, I've come to really enjoy this place and the people.

Carol did my blood test and was excited for me. As I was walking out to the elevator, I thought that if I am pregnant, I will miss this place.

Then I came home, did some chores, and decided to watch, "All My Children" before I had to leave for work—something I almost never do.

Oddly enough a character on the show, Liza, found out she was pregnant today. I started to cry, and felt that maybe this was a good sign, if not a very odd coincidence.

If I am pregnant, I will always remember that Liza found out she was pregnant the same day I did.

I left for work, and knew that by the time I got to work around 4 o'clock, the answer would be waiting on my answering machine.

I got into work, went to my desk, dialed my home number to check my messages, and yes, the nurse said, all my numbers were right: I am pregnant.

Three tests and all confirm: I am most definitely and completely pregnant.

A loud hooray is going off in my brain. Louder than probably any hooray I've ever experienced in my life before.

I'm not sure quite why the first test was not enough, but in the world of infertility…everything is slightly different.

I immediately logged off my computer, went into the conference area, and wrote my baby a letter, with the exact time and date on it.

Then I called Chris at work. I could hear all his friends at the salon congratulating him.

My friend Bonnie overheard me and gave me a big congratulations hug in the bathroom. Then I told my boss George, and asked if they had shields to protect me from radioactive waves from the computer. He said no, so I'll try to find out to buy to protect me.

What a great day!

But tonight, as usual after hearing good news, Chris and I fought.

We should have been so close tonight, but instead, after a long day at work, we sat at the kitchen table and bickered over this and that.

Strange, because we tried so hard to get pregnant and now we are fighting and stressed because we got what we worked so hard for. We are happy and angry, excited and scared out of our minds. The infertility treatments have made us tired and in some ways, we see one another as the enemy now. I blamed his sperm. He blamed me for being so driven to have a baby that I ignored our relationship.

I don't care, however--because bottom line is I want a baby more than I want anything else in this world and I'm actually pregnant!!!! He is not the issue right now. Little by little, the agitation left, the fight ended, and I went to bed thanking God.

I Am Pregnant!

The first few months of my pregnancy have been about being cautious. I am on a bed rest to ensure a healthy delivery, meaning I have to take it easy. I have taken a leave from work.

The first obstetrician I had was a difficult personality for me, but it wasn't until my best friend Cindy told me, "if you leave someone's presence feeling afraid, that is a signal to get away from that person." So I listened, followed my gut instinct, and somehow found the exactly right doctor for my personality. He agreed to do all the tests I needed, and immediately gave me the documentation I needed to continue on bed rest. He even scheduled weekly ultrasounds at the hospital to monitor my baby's progress. No more wondering if my baby is okay!

Wow, I am relieved. This is the kind of doctor I have needed for a long time. I'm glad Cindy forced me to listen to my feelings about my ob/gyn- -if you walk away feeling bad about an experience, that is usually a sign that something is wrong and the warning should be heeded. Thank you Cindy!

It's A Girl!

My doctor wants to ease my worries over my baby, so he scheduled a high resolution ultrasound this morning at a local hospital. A technician from the Boston area came to do it.

It was thrilling, a relief, and totally mind-boggling all at once to learn that my baby's heart had formed correctly, that the spine was formed and aligned properly, that the kidneys looked good, and that it appears that there is no sign of down syndrome. Not that it would matter, but it was a relief to learn that as far as the technician could see, my baby was healthy.

My baby is healthy! I say a quick prayer of thanks to God.

Then the technician asked me, "Do you want to know the sex?"

I hesitated, and asked my husband if he thought we should find out. "It is up to you," he said kindly.

"Yes," I whispered. I was convinced I was having a boy. I don't know why, but I assumed my baby was a boy. Maybe because, in my heart, I desperately want my first child to be a girl, so I assume that whenever I desperately want something, I'll get something else.

I also am reminded of what my husband said, that God would probably never give me a girl, and even though that nasty fight is behind us, his words stay with me. On some level, I too believe that I probably don't deserve a girl...

"It's a girl!" the technician blurted out.

"Are you sure?" I asked, not daring to believe it.

"I am absolutely sure," she said.

Oh my God, a girl! A girl! A girl! A girl! A girl! A GIRL! A GIRL! I want to shout it from the rooftops! Have it announced on the evening news! Ring every bell in every city!

A daughter...can you imagine me, me-- actually having a daughter? My daughter...has there ever been two more beautiful words in the English language or any language? Have two words in the history of humankind ever been more significant? More beautiful? More life-changing? More profound? I am in a daze. A cozy, warm haze forms around me. I am in a cocoon, as I began the transformation into a new life as mother of a daughter! MY DAUGHTER! Me? Can I really have this? A confirmation from God that He doesn't hate me. A divine high-five that He allowed me to actually conceive a daughter. My husband was wrong...God wasn't going to punish me by never giving me the daughter of my dreams...I am actually receiving what I wanted the most.

A son would be amazing someday, but first, I need a girl, a daughter, to share my life journey with. Someday I will be ready and anxious for a son. But for now, all I have ever wanted was a daughter.

A daughter...a daughter! my daughter...my daughter...I can't say the words enough. I feel a ticklish thrill! I keep a journal about my pregnancy and tonight I started my entry with, "To my daughter:"

My daughter....two words more profound than all the works of Shakespeare.

My baby...my daughter...my daughter is healthy! MY DAUGHTER! HOORAY! THANK YOU GOD! Her heart is strong! Her spine is okay! Her head is the right size! I am basking in the glow of this new life that I am walking towards and who is coming towards me. God is not denying me what I have wanted more than anything else in this world. Maybe I am not such a rotten person after all. Maybe I will actually get what I want for once.

My daughter...no words have ever been spoken on this planet that could be more beautiful to me.

My Routine

There is a comfortable and joyful quietness to the rhythm of my life right now. I go few places. I mostly stay home, work on my online magazine, welcome occasional visits from friends and watch TV.

I haven't felt this protected since I was a child. I've never had a time in my adulthood where so little was expected of me and where I am the recipient of so much love and goodwill. My husband massages my feet every night. Chelsea mails me homemade cards and gifts to cheer me up. Roz, who is overseas in Armenia waiting to adopt her little girl, wrote and said she is praying for me. This is a happy, happy time for me. I still worry at times. I am very, very careful. I don't eat anything that could possibly harm my baby. I juice spinach every day, and when I don't feel like drinking it, I say to myself, "good for my baby girl...good for my baby girl...good for my baby girl" and it goes right down.

My husband and I, after living here a few years, have a group of friends who come over our house a lot. I usually retire to bed early, but my husband stays up playing cards with Lenny and Matthew. We have wonderful neighbors, like Richard, Janice and Helene, who are the perfect neighbors for me.

Infertility was so hard and long. Having this baby is the culmination of so many dreams. Now I wait, and try to enjoy the wait. It is a blissful, peaceful, quiet time.

Fourth Month

I have reached the four month mark of my pregnancy. Now that I've successfully reached the three month mark, I am feeling more comfortable. Knowing I am having a girl, and seeing the high resolution ultrasound and learning that somehow, miraculously, she has a heart and a spine that has formed correctly, is giving me comfort. I am also feeling a lot less anxious, since I have a doctor I like and he is checking on the baby with weekly ultrasounds

Life has taken on a different, warmer, rosier glow.

Now that we are at the four month mark, my daughter's ears have grown enough that she has developed the ability to hear. So I tape recorded a message to her that I play every night. I put the earphones on my stomach, and play 30 minutes of Mozart to her, and then I change the tape and play my message to her.

When I play the tape to her, an amazing sense of contentment, unlike anything I've ever experienced before, envelopes me. In my message, I tell her about all the wonderful things we are going to do together...Honey, we are going to bake cookies together. We are going to spend lots of time at the beach jumping waves and building sand castles. We are going to build a tree house, read wonderful children's stories, have sunny Friday afternoon picnics, and fall completely in love with each other.

Corny, I know. Sappy as anything. Over-the-top sentimental. God, I love her so much.

Then I play her the message my husband taped to her, where he talks about how much he loves her and is excited to see her.

Usually I fall asleep by 8 p.m.

This routine appears so mundane, but for me it is pure excitement--a new door opening that had been closed for such a long time.
It is not only the beginning of my daughter's life, but also the start of my life as a mother.

I still feel afraid at times. There are still moments when I worry a lot.

I am very careful. I don't eat restaurant-cooked meats.
I stay away from cheese. I juice spinach every day, and I take chlorophyll because I read somewhere that it is healthy for pregnant women. I take three folic acid vitamins a day, plus a prenatal vitamin. And I pray, and I pray. I pray constantly that my baby lives and grows.

A daughter is coming to me. Praise God. Somehow the heavens have opened to me. How did this happen?
How did I actually get pregnant and conceive a daughter who has a heart that is working properly, and a head and a spine that formed exactly as they should? How did I get to this place, where I sleep and relax in a bedroom with the prettiest green color walls on earth, with my baby growing inside me listening to my voice, her father's voice and Mozart's majestic music, every night?

Getting pregnant was so hard for me. Wrenching. A continuation of many years of disappointments, but the bitterest denial of all. So I take nothing for granted. Not a day do I complain. I have never felt happier, more content, than I do now.

Ever since I was pregnant, it seems the world around me has opened their arms with support and comfort from all directions.

A year ago, this life would not have seemed possible.
How did this happen to me? Could it be true? After a long bloody nightmare, I am living a dream. At night, when I'm playing this tape, I feel like I am beginning a new chapter in my life that is the start of a happy-ever-after fairy tale, not a blighted tragedy.

Gray Day in Pregnancy

It is a gray day in every sort of way. My pregnancy these past few months has been wonderful. My new doctor, Dr. Michel Lirrette, is the best doctor in absolutely every way.

Because he knows of my nervousness, he ordered weekly ultrasounds at a nearby hospital for me. It is a routine I have come to love. I leave the house by 7:30 a.m. and drive about seven minutes to the hospital on the hill where I will deliver my baby. I park not far from the door, enter the cheerful hospital lobby, and go up to the third floor. Ah--the maternity floor. I love when the elevator doors swing open and I enter the maternity zone. Babies! Babies in the nursery window!

I can hardly believe that my baby will someday be in that nursery. The nurses are always so nice. I am brought into a room and lie down on a comfortable bed where I am hooked up to monitors that chart my baby's heart. The nurses are always so reassuring.

Yes, she is doing great. Yes, look how strong her heart is. Yes, yes, yes-- your baby is okay. I leave each Wednesday morning feeling relief and joy. And for a little while, all my fears and insecurities disappear. Every week, things get easier. Until today.

Usually, my baby girl is quite active. She kicks a lot, and I do what the nurse recommended in always trying to make sure I feel ten kicks a day. Normally, that is pretty easy.

But today, she is still. So very still. Eerily still. I keep hoping and thinking that at any minute she will start kicking like she always does, but there is nothing--no kicks, no movement at all.

 I cannot shake the feeling that something is wrong.

I tell myself that by lunch she will kick. By 2 p.m. she will kick. By 3 p.m. Still nothing. No movement at all. I am getting scared. It is 5 o'clock and she still hasn't kicked all day. I can't get the idea out of my head that maybe something is wrong. Why isn't she moving?

I am far enough along in my pregnancy that if something is wrong, they could take her out and she would survive. Oh God, is she dying inside of me? I've heard too many horror stories to take anything for granted. Ever since I got pregnant, there have been so many times, like today, that I wish I had given birth when I was a naive 18 year old who knew little about the whole birth-and-babies process. At that age, you don't know enough to be scared, and you are young enough that most of the time, not a whole lot goes wrong. I think of one of my neighbors who was 18 and didn't know she was pregnant until almost four months into her pregnancy. Four months of no ultrasounds, no folic acid vitamins, no juicing spinach, and with just 30 minutes of labor, she delivered a beautiful, healthy strong baby boy. At one time, I felt bad for girls who had their babies young. Not so much anymore.

As the day wore on, the sky is looking grayer and grayer, I am getting more and more nervous. Is my daughter hanging on for dear life? Is the umbilical cord wound around her neck? My imagination has begun to take me places I don't want to go.

I decide to ask my next door neighbors Richard and Janice for a ride to the hospital, since we only have one car and Chris has taken it to work. I need to have my baby checked, just in case. By now I've learned that better safe than sorry. Sure, they say. I can tell they think I am being paranoid, but still they are ready to help. Please God, please God, please. I pray fervently. At moments like this, I realize that all the tests in the world and all the best doctors in the world cannot compare to believing God is there to listen. Please God, I pray, please save my baby.

Please save my baby...these words have echoed in my heart and soul and traveled right up to heaven perhaps ten thousand times since I became pregnant. And now today again, these same words pour out of me.

Right as Richard and Janice come out to drive me to the hospital, my husband pulls in the driveway. Thank you God.

"What is going on?" he asks concerned.

I tell him how I haven't felt the baby move all day, and how the hospital is waiting for us to come. He doesn't hesitate for a minute. "Let's go," he says seriously.

It is moments like this that I am so grateful for my husband. Another man,
perhaps a more logical, man, would put aside my fears and worries and convince me not to run off to the hospital. But my husband didn't blink. If his unborn child has not moved all day, to the hospital we go without a moment's hesitation.

At the hospital, I am immediately hooked up to the fetal monitor. What if my baby has died? I let myself think that for a moment and a feeling so completely dreadful washes over me I have to stop.

I pray and pray, and if not for the comfort of prayer, I might completely loose my mind, especially as the ultrasound begins and the nurse says nothing. Why is the nurse saying nothing?

"What is happening?" I ask the nurse.

"I can't tell yet," she says.

I begin to cry, "Tell me please, is my daughter okay? Did you get a heartbeat?"

I am impatient, demanding, ready to scream.

Finally, after a long minute of silence that seemed like a century, the nurse says, "Your baby is fine."

"We wish all babies that come in here have hearts that beat so strong," she says.

"Is her heart really strong?" I ask, beaming, relieved that yes, my daughter's heart is beating strong.

"Very strong. We would wish that all babies were that healthy," she repeats.

Thank you God! Thank you God. Thank you God. My husband and I leave the hospital beaming, relieved, and happy. This short scare made me vow to be all the more vigiliant in getting the rest I need and eating healthy. .

Thank God I have a doctor like Dr. Lirrette, who immediately upon receiving my phone call told me to go to the hospital to be checked. Thank God for my neighbors Richard and Janice who were so willing to drive me to the hospital.

Thank God for my husband, who didn't make me feel like an idiot for wanting to have my baby checked. Thank God for the nurse who reassured me so completely by saying my daughter's heart was strong.

To imagine how this night might have gone, it is too much. I know there are women who have faced the unimaginable.

I crawl into bed tonight, exhausted but happy. The gray day is over.

Beautiful April 10 Baby Shower

The months before my baby's birth now seem shrouded by a warm fuzzy sunshine glow. The quiet joys of this pregnancy and the intense love I have received from those around me culminated into a baby shower that turned out to be one of the best days of my life.

On April 10, my mother threw me the most perfect and beautiful baby shower in the clubhouse at my grandmother's apartment complex. My grandmother Maria and I are very close, and having this shower at her place meant a lot to me.

It turned out to be one of the most perfect days of my life--so perfect, it was like I wrote a script detailing what a perfect day in my life would be like. Lots of balloons, a big pink cake, relatives and friends from the various parts of my life and of course, presents.
Lots and lots of wonderful presents: little pink dresses, a child size wicker rocking chair, a jumper with cherries on it, hand-crochet afghans. I wore a beautiful yellow dress with flowers, thanks to a gift certificate given to Chris and I by our friend Matthew. This dress was so joyful and beautiful, it seemed to embody the day we experienced.

The day started early that morning with my next door neighbor Helene bringing me flowers, and ended that night, with me lying in bed, with all the beautiful little dresses and outfits given to me at the shower hanging in my closet.

Leah arrived at my house with candies for me. My cousin Susan gave me a beautiful little white wicker rocking chair, and balloons. Her daughters, my cousins Sheri, Dina, Johnna and Bethany, gave me a beautiful white bassinet. Judy sent an afghan made by her mother.

My mother prepared stuffed shells and bought a huge beautiful cake with pink and white icing. So many friends and family were there...Aunt Betty, cousin Denise, Aunt Angie, Aunt Sandra, Aunt Rose, Leslie, Elaine, Judy, Leslie, on and on it went. My mother went all out with this shower and did so much work to make it spectacular for me. She made so much food. I love my Mom so much.

I looked so big that at the shower, my Aunt Angie thought I might be giving birth soon.

Sitting at the table with Chris, my mother, Aunt Betty and Aunt Angie, was a feeling of closeness I have not felt in such a long time.

The sun shined in the most spectacular spring way all day.

My little girl was coming soon!

That night, Chris went out with our friends Melanie and Darren, Tyrone and Lenny, and I stayed home. Every few minutes, I would jump up from my bed, run to my closet and look at all the pretty clothes that were given to my daughter that day.

 I did this for hours.

Every few minutes, I would get up from bed and run to the closet to look at all the cute little dresses and adorable outfits. I kept pinching myself figuratively--my little girl would soon wear those dresses! Then, I'd get out of bed again, run over to the closet, touch the dresses and all the outfits, and feel almost giddy with glee. I knew from that night on that never again would my life be as lonely as it had been before. A little girl--my little girl—was going to wear those dresses! She is almost here!

A new life was beginning for me...Then out of the bed I'd pop again, run over to the closet to touch and look one more time.

I went to bed with prayers of thanks on my lips and a feeling that this beautiful day was one I will never forget.

My Baby Is Born

On May 17, 1999, the most miraculous thing ever to happen in my life actually occurred: my 8 pound, 11 ounce little girl was born.

"Beautiful like Mommy," Dr. Lirrette declared at 7:30 a.m. on that glorious Monday morning when he pulled her from my stomach and there for the first time ever, I laid my eyes upon the loveliest little creature imaginable to have ever come to the earth.

It happened. I gave birth to a baby. Me! She made it through the pregnancy!

Yes, I actually conceived and gave birth to a baby. Me! Yes-- actually me. To describe it as wonderful would be a terrible understatement.

The night before, my grandmother Maria prepared a beautiful meal for me, my husband, parents and cousin Susan.
Then, at 5 o'clock the next morning, we went to the hospital.

My Dad, Mom and cousin Susan were all there, waiting for us. They had come to be there for my daughter's birth.

While I was getting my epidural, a very wonderful nurse named Mary held me and asked, 'do you want to say a prayer?' I nodded. Her kindness got me through a rough moment.

Then, I laid there waiting to feel some pain. Friends had told me to expect a lot of tugging during the caesarean, so I waited for the tug.

Suddenly, there was Dr. Lirrette, swinging around saying, "she's beautiful like Mommy" and my daughter had arrived without barely a blink of pain.

She was covered in blood and oh so beautiful. They took her to be cleaned up and I was sent back to my room.

While I waited, my parents, grandmother, and aunts came in. My father was beaming, "she looks so strong," he said.

Then, the most amazing thing happened. When they brought her to me for the first time, I held her and suddenly she held my finger. I could feel a connection between us, sort of like, 'Hi Mom! I know you." She actually was holding my finger! She was connecting to me!

The rest of the day, I was on such a high that despite all the pain medicine I was on, I didn't stop talking, I talked and talked to whomever would listen. I was so happy that all I wanted to do was talk!

My daughter is here! She made it!

My life has never felt sweeter or more complete.

Chapter 25: Advice and Ideas for Fertility Clinics

Here are my suggestions for infertility clinics:

• I would love to see a Room of Hope near the waiting room, where infertility patients could go for comfort, support and validation.

During those minutes waiting for their appointments, rather than feeling alone and stressed, women could be guided in activities that relax and soothe them. This could include sing-a-longs to songs about getting pregnant and art tables where patients create art about their body's ability to get and stay pregnant.

A positive affirmations group, led by a life coach or therapist, could be held once an hour throughout the day in this room. Rather than patients waiting alone before procedures, they could join others in saying positive affirmations about getting pregnant. The coach could lead groups of women in brief five or ten minute affirmations, such as "My body is strong" "I am ready to conceive" "My body can conceive." Relaxation exercises, deep breathing and positive visualization exercises could be part of the support available in this "room of hope."

At the clinic I went to, they offered infertility support groups that met at night, but after getting up for 6 a.m. blood work and then working all day, I wasn't up for driving again at night for 40 minutes to attend a support group. But many times, as I sat in the waiting room, I wished I could have talked to other patients, and shared experiences and emotions, even just for a few minutes.

No signing up ahead should be required for participation in these ongoing activities. It should be open and available to whoever needs it throughout the day.

This room of hope could also have a book where women who have already gone through infertility could share advice and write encouraging letters and well-wishes for those undergoing infertility treatments.

In this "room of hope" there could be a wall called
The Wall of Hope with pictures of infertility patients who successfully had babies.

Along with pictures of themselves and their babies, there could be information on how many cycles and procedures they experienced, along with advice and information on the challenges they faced.

Seeing pictures of women who endured a lot, perhaps even suffering miscarriages and months where their infertility treatments didn't work out, would have given me hope during my most difficult times. These women, as veterans of infertility, would probably have had a lot of valuable advice to share with me.

- It is long overdue that infertility clinics incorporate
elements of holistic medicine into their protocol. Acupuncture should be available at clinics, perhaps in the weeks preceding an IUI or IVF as a way to help get the body ready for conception. Perhaps group acupuncture could be made available to patients as a way to lower the. Big, soft comfortable chairs, warm blankets, soft lighting, could be provided in the group acupunture room, along with soothing sounds of nature or music, as a way to enhance the treatment.

I also recommend that massage therapists be available, perhaps to give 15 to 20 minute massages before IUIs and IVFS to relax the patients. Again, perhaps this could be done in a group setting, as a way to lower the cost for the clinic.

Studies could be done to see if the rates of conception and live birth go up with the addition of acupuncture and massage to the infertility clinics.

A nutritionist should also be available to help patients evaluate, monitor and keep track of their food choices. When a patient begins infertility, she would meet with this nutritionist to go over information on foods that can help a woman conceive and maintain a pregnancy. Perhaps this nutritionist could be a food coach of sorts, helping patients keep a log of everything they eat as a way to track how many healthy foods they are putting in their body each day.

- I also recommend that infertility clinics take the time to negotiate with local holistic and alternative health practitioners in securing discounted rates for their patients. Acupuncture, massage, trauma release, kinesiology, homeopathy, and other modalities can be very expensive, but perhaps alternative health practitioners would lower their rates for infertility patients.

- How about the addition of a hope coach to infertility clinics? This hope coach could be available talk to patients before IUIs or IVFs.

As I laid on the table for several IUIs and then IVFS, I would have loved someone to come in and say to me: "Paula, you are strong. Your body is strong. You are capable of getting pregnant" or "I believe you will get pregnant today. I can picture you holding a baby. You deserve a baby."

Words this incredibly positive may very well have bolstered my body's ability to conceive. Instead, most of the time, everyone in the medical profession is so nervous to give false hope, and rightly so, because they could be sued by patients who felt their hopes were raised only to be devastated later.

The clinics could offer this service only to patients who are willing to sign a waiver saying the clinic is not in any way liable if the treatment fails.

This hope coach would not be a medical personnel, and patients could opt whether or not to have this service. I would have chosen it, as I believe that the body hears and believes the positive messages it is given, and it would have been a great form of support to my body.

I don't think a hope coach can replace great fertility medications and aggressive medical techniques, and I am not in any way advocating abandoning any of the medicines, testing or procedures available in infertility clinics. What I am advocating is adding the subtle element of positive thinking to the mix, to raise the odds of conception.

- Infertility clinics should also be sure they are teaching and guiding all staff in giving kindness, comfort and courage to patients.

Training in how to emotionally help patients should be an absolute must for every clinic.

Fortunately, I am very thankful that the clinic I went to had an incredible, loving, kind staff that held my hand, both literally and figuratively, through the entire process. Literally, if I was coming in for a procedure or test, they would go and get someone I knew and felt comfortable with to hold my hand! I was fortunate to have the kindest, most patient ultrasound technician named Christine working with me, and nurses like Carol who were willing to hold my hand and talk to me during the tests.

It got the point that when I came in for a test, Carol would see me, alert the other nurses that she would be with me during this test, and would come in to hold my hand and talk to me through the test. These women are heroes in my book, the top in their fields, and every clinic should train nurses and aides to be that kind and understanding. The support staff at the clinic I went to was superb and a part of the reason I didn't give up.

Every clinic should give workshops to all staff members, from the technicians to the receptionists, on the various emotions experienced by infertility patients and the type of support they might need during their visits to the clinic.

• For patients having a particularly hard time getting pregnant, clinics should consider introducing a two month prep program. This program could include an evaluation of eating habits, stresses,
lifestyle, and various modalities available to strengthen and cleanse the body. Based on individual needs, a plan could be put into affect, linking the patient with resources and healthcare providers in the area that could assist them in becoming more healthy during this prep period.

• It might be helpful for clinics to hold an informational workshops on how infertility medications chemically impact the emotions and how marriages can be impacted by infertility. I'd also love to see a workshop for husbands on what they can do to help their wives through the ups and downs of infertility.

This workshop could also be a place where men would be able to freely express their own stresses and fears about infertility treatments.

• Clinics should consider making available to patients a library of books on infertility, nutrition, and alternative/holistic medicine, so that patients would have easy access to information right at the clinic.

• Since coffee can adversely impact a women's fertility, I would love to see all clinics stop serving coffee and caffeinated beverages in their waiting rooms. Instead, it would be helpful if they served fresh fruits and vegetables as an example of how patients should be eating.

Part II: Secondary Infertility

Having a baby was everything I dreamed it would be and more. To say that my daughter changed my life and gave me a sense of happiness, purpose and belonging that I have always longed for would be an understatement.

All the pain, frustration and difficulty I endured to have her was absolutely and completely worth it. And looking back, it all now seems like a rather beautiful memory because it culminated into the birth of my daughter.

Now I begin another chapter in my book, and it is about the pain and frustration of secondary infertility.

I will acknowledge right now that I am very lucky to have one biological child. I know many people would be overjoyed and content with that. On many levels, I was too. If I had only her, my life would be complete.

Yet, once I had her, I was fueled with an intense and driving desire to have more children. Why? Well, ever since I was young, when I pictured my family, it always included more than one child. I was an only child, and as happy as my childhood was, I wanted to create a different family structure than the exact same one I had. Perhaps I
felt that way because I never had siblings, and what we don't have as children, we always want to give our children. Whatever the reason, I desperately wanted my daughter to have a brother or sister.

I also wanted the chance to love more than one child. I wanted four, five, six or more people living in my home. I have always craved hustle, bustle, and noise in my home.

I naively thought that because I had finally conceived and given birth to my daughter that I would easily get pregnant a second time. A friend asked me, 'are you going to try to get pregnant again?' '

Yes,' I answered.

'How long do you think it will take?' she asked.

And very cavalierly I said, "maybe three or four months."

How wrong I was.

This is the irony of secondary infertility. Just because you had a baby the first time, doesn't mean it is going to happen easily the next time.

When my daughter neared a year and a half, my husband and I decided it was time to begin trying for a second child. I saw how outgoing she was, how much she loved other children, and how sometimes she was lonely and needed companionship.

Every week, when I went to story time at a local library with my mother. I saw up close how the children with brothers and sisters enjoyed a sense of security and belonging that my daughter lacked. They didn't seem as desperate or as lonely as she was. They weren't trying to become part of other people's parade, because they had children in their world who belonged to them. Each week, a mother and her three daughters all about a year apart came to story time. I saw how happy they were and how they didn't want for anything or anyone, and I ached for my daughter to have that serene sense of belonging and permanence of a sibling in her life.

Whenever we went to the park, my daughter would get so excited seeing the other children. Sometimes the children were friendly and eager playmates, and sometimes they weren't. That burned. I couldn't stand to see her at the mercy of these kids.

I wanted my daughter to have loving relationships, with a foundation based on family, not on the fickle ups and downs of childhood friendships.

Thus began my uphill battle to give my daughter a sibling, and myself a second child to love.

Secondary infertility can seem trivial, especially to a person going through infertility treatments for the first time. I understand that completely. Before I had my daughter, I would have scoffed at anyone who pitied themselves for being unable to have a second baby.

When you have no child, there is little room for pitying anyone who has one child.

But once I had a child, I felt compelled to create a family structure that included the sibling relationship. I need to add a side note on this: I was an only child, and truthfully, I probably had one of the best and happiest childhoods a kid could wish for.

So if you have one child, don't for a moment be misled into thinking only children are unhappy children—I was an only child and I wouldn't trade my childhood memories and life with anyone, including those with siblings.

The next part of my book will talk about the challenges of secondary infertility. Not being able to have a second child puts you into a certain family structure, and if that family structure is not one you chose, it can be hard to accept.

Secondary infertility is more heart wrenching than imagined. There is less validation for the pain involved. If people tell you God doesn't want you to have a baby the first time, they can't wait to tell you that maybe you were meant to have only one child the second time. Some people, think were already given enough with one baby--who are you to push it and think you deserve two babies. Friends who also suffered with infertility the first time, and are understandably content with their one baby, aren't always keen to give you the encouragement needed to try again.

Here is my experience with secondary infertility. I hope it can help you in some way. My experiences reflect what many of you have gone through, whether you are trying for your first or second baby. I hope it can help or comfort you in some way.

Diary Excerpt: Baby Making With Husband Nowhere In Sight

Today was my third IUI trying for a second child. Today was different than any of the other IUIs I've done before my husband and I were not even together during the IUI. We went to the clinic at different times, in separate cars. Because he had to work all day, and there was an ice cream festival at my work that my mother and I were bringing my daughter to, my husband drove to the clinic at 7 a.m., gave his sperm, and went off to work. An hour later, I arrived for my IUI.

How odd, I thought as I was driving to the clinic, I am now going to make a baby with my mother and my daughter, with my husband nowhere in sight. I felt sorry for myself, because as a young teenage girl, I would have never imagined that my baby making experience would include my mother, a nurse, and a speculum that really, really hurt.

Not that the other IUIs have ever felt natural to me, but having my husband at the clinic with me felt at least more normal--at least, I reasoned, we were doing this together.

Imagine how far science had come--that two people can make a baby separated by a few hours and several miles.

Nothing at all romantic about this baby-making exchange.

When I was young, and imagined having children, I never could have imagined that this would my future. Thank God I didn't know it would turn out this way. Thank God no one at 17 ever showed me a crystal ball into my baby-making future. My heart would have been broken. But I want another baby so much, that most of the time I dismiss these sentimental yearnings, I can't let anything interfere with my fertility treatments.

But today the yearnings got me good, and I feel a heavy load of melancholy.

I am so far away from the original way people usually create a family.

Once the IUI was over, my Mom and I drove to the ice cream festival at my workplace, a PBS station in Boston. Some of my co-workers got to meet my daughter for the first time.

As we drove home, my mother turned to me said, "Maybe you are pregnant."

Her hopefulness was sweet.

It must have been weird for my mother to go with me to the clinic, while I went into a room to be impregnated with my husband's sperm.

I can only imagine what my mother was thinking. But my Mom, always brave and tactful, didn't say anything mean or negative.

That night, I told my husband how sad I was that we were not together for today's IUI. He said he felt the same way.

He doesn't take things as passionately as I do, or get as worked up when things don't work out. I think because I had such high expectations for love and romance, that times like this put a spotlight on how far I've travelled from the original dream for my life.

I have to let it go. I know I am so lucky to have my first baby. I could feel it today when I walked into that waiting room with my beautiful daughter and I saw the expressions on the faces of some of the women, and even men, when my daughter and I began to play with some toys. Their eyes lit up--a baby! Their eyes looked sad--a baby!...Someone else's as usual. I remember how I used to feel when someone would come into the waiting room with a baby. I felt excited, resentful, frustrated all at the same time. Sometimes seeing their success in having a baby made me hopeful. Sometimes their success made me jealous. Sometimes I felt all goopy to see a baby and to dare to imagine what it must feel like to have little hands to hold and cheeks to kiss.

I saw in the faces of the couples in the waiting room that same longing, mixed with hopefulness. So I know I shouldn't complain.

Tonight, I want to just snuggle up with my husband, and imagine that I am 17 and still allowed to believe that babies are made in bed by two people madly in love.

Chapter 27: Coping With Shots and Injections

Enduring injections is part of the infertility process. The first time I did it, I worried about it all day. As the time came closer to the 'shot', I felt like I was trapped in some type of dreaded countdown. It never really became easy, I found ways that made it bearable and sometimes relatively painless.

Here are my best tips for coping with injections:

• **If your husband or someone else is giving you the injection, have something interesting that you can read sitting in front of you.** For me, I put a beautiful book on bed and breakfast inns in front of me. The lovely blue cover on the book soothed my soul. It was pretty and sweet, and represented everything that getting an injection wasn't. Looking at it was an escape: I'm not about to get a shot…I am visiting a lovely bed and breakfast inn and about to have homemade blueberry muffins, jam and a cup of tea. Right before my husband would insert the needle, I would turn to a recipe in this book and start reading it. Somehow, doing this helped me get through the many nights (and years) of shots.

• **Put on a favorite song, some comforting music, or a real party song.** Close your eyes and sing-along.

• **My opinion: Don't look.** Especially if the shots scare you, it is best not to look. Close your eyes and look away.

• **I am an expulsive person.** I like to talk and expulse my feelings. For me, it helped to exhale through my mouth a few breaths during the shot. Using my breathing as a release always helped me.

• **Open a candy bar or some favorite food and smell it, take a bite.** Distraction works. A delicious chocolate, a song, a book—get your senses engaged in something else during the injection.

• **Remind yourself that the discomfort you might experience is going to be worth it.** Give yourself something to look forward to when it is over.

Chapter 28: How To Protect A Cherished Pregnancy

If you have had recurrent miscarriages, you might want to:

• Ask to have an infection screen of your vagina.

• Ask for a Vitamin D deficiency test.

• Ask for a mineral deficiency test.

• Get tested for antiphospholipid syndrome (APS) which causes blood clots to form. A doctor can treat this condition with a low dose of baby aspirin or injections of heparin, which is a blood thinner.

• Visit your dentist and make sure there are no infections in your teeth or gums.

• Let your doctor know if you have any chronic conditions, such as thyroid disease, epilepsy, lupus, or a family history of clotting disorders.

Ways To Protect Your Baby and Prevent A Miscarriage Once You Are Pregnant

First off, it needs to be said: sometimes you can prevent a miscarriage and sometimes you can't. Most of the time, you can't. If you do miscarry, please know it is not your fault. Nature does this more often than we realize. Even in past generations, many women suffered miscarriages, they knew nothing about. There are some things you can do to protect your growing baby, but please be aware that it is not your fault in any way if a pregnancy does not continue. The pain, of course, is immeasurable and intense, and there are no words to gloss over the immense sense of injustice and sadness this awful loss brings. Please, if possible, do not give up in trying again if you have endured this great loss.

Here are some things you can do to help maintain a healthy pregnancy:

• Boost Your Progesterone Levels

Maintaining adequate progesterone levels is absolutely key when you are pregnant. Ask your doctor if progesterone is something you should take to reduce the risk of miscarriage. If you have miscarried before, you might want to request progesterone from your doctor. Progesterone plays a role in maintaining the uterine lining, and because of this, some researchers have theorized that low progesterone plays a role in causing miscarriage.

Taking Vitamins C and B, and minerals such as zinc and magnesium, can help the body produce progesterone.

Foods that help raise progesterone levels include: walnuts, bananas, wild yams, spinach and kale. Pumpkin, watermelon, chickpeas and squash seeds, which are high in zinc.

Try to avoid getting yourself in a stressful 'fight of flight' situation, which tends to reduce progesterone levels. Avoid all foods and herbs that can increase levels of estrogen, such as dong quai, hops, lavender, licorice, tea tree oil, and red clover blossom.

• Keep Your Thyroid Healthy

If you have had recurrent miscarriages, you may want to have your thyroid tested to be sure you are maintaining a TSH above 2.0. Foods that encourage a healthy thyroid include artichokes and pineapple, which offer natural sources of iodine. Other foods to help the thyroid include garlic, sunflower seeds and turkey, which are high in selenium, and flaxseed, that contain high levels of Omega 3. Copper and iron rich foods are also very important to thyroid function. These include cashews, leafy greens,and lean red meats. Avoid Bromide, a chemical found in fluoride and chlorine, that disrupts the endocrine system. Bromide can also be found in soft drinks, plastics and some hair dyes. Also avoid soy, which some health practitioners believe can weaken the thyroid.

- **Nurture Your Kidneys**

In Chinese medicine, it is believed that if a woman has suffered a miscarriage, she needs to work on her strengthening her kidney Qi. Start by drinking lots of water. Try to avoid situations that bring up feelings of fear. Eating deep red foods like red bell peppers, red grapes, cranberries and beets, that can help rebuild and replenish the kidneys. Blueberries and apples are also good for the kidney. Avoid fluoride, artificial sweeteners and fructose. Avoid root canals and exposure to toxic mold, along with pesticides and toxic cleaning products.

- **Be Aware Of Your Homocysteine Levels**

High levels of homocysteine can be a threat to your growing baby. Homocysteine is a sulfar-containing amino acid that can cause your blood to clot more easily. Be sure your prenatal vitamin has adequate levels of B6, B12, and folic acid, because this combination of B vitamins has been shown to prevent miscarriages that are caused by high homocysteine levels.

- **Avoid Excessively Stressful and Sad Situations**

As much as possible, try not put yourself in situations that bring up extreme and intense feelings of fear, stress or sadness.. Stress tremendously affects the hormonal stability within the body. Let yourself sleep more, relax and say no to increased responsibilities and work at this time.

Avoid people, situations and activities that bring up a strong 'fight or flight' response. Limit time spent in situations where you feel nervous, anxious and uncomfortable. Do not listen to sad music or watch movies that bring up feelings of grief. Deep breath and give yourself permission to relax.

Never underestimate how powerfully grief, sadness and toxic connections with others can impact your hormones.

- **Keep Your Hormones Stable**

Keep your blood sugar levels stable, eat lots of leafy greens, don't exhaust your adrenal glands through stress or lack of rest. Foods that help balance hormones include olive oil and berries. Avoid white flour products, sugar, caffeine and alcohol.

- **Make Spinach Your Best Friend**

Eat lots of spinach, it offers a rich form of iron that is needed for healthy **cellular division.**

- **Find Out If You Have Celiac Disease or Are Gluten Intolerant**

Gluten, found in rye, wheat or barley, has been known to cause miscarriage in those who are allergic.

- **Take Your Minerals**

One study linked a history of miscarriage to low levels of magnesium. Symptoms of magnesium deficiency can include agitation and anxiety, restless leg syndrome, sleep disorders, irritability, nausea, vomiting, abnormal heart rhythms, low blood pressure, confusion, muscle spasm and weakness, hyperventilation, insomnia, and even seizures. Foods high in magnesium include spinach, brown rice and pumpkin seeds.

- **Make Sure You Are Getting Enough Iron**

Lack of iron has been reported to cause miscarriages. You may want to talk with your your doctor or nutritionist about taking an iron supplement. Food sources of iron include red meat, turkey, chicken, kidney beans and chick peas. Be sure you are taking Vitamin C to help iron absorption.

- **Take Baby Aspirin**

Some studies have shown that taking one baby aspirin a day can reduce the risk of miscarriage. Ask your doctor about this. One of the benefits of baby aspirin is that it prevents blood clots that can cut off nutrients to the baby and prevents preeclampsia.

- **Be Alert To High Or Low Blood Pressure**

Be sure you are aware of your blood pressure levels. Avoid fried or processed foods, deep breath and get plenty of rest. Repeat the word 'relax' several times a day.

- **Keep Blood Sugar Levels Stabile**

Avoid sugar and do not let your blood sugar levels fluctuate. Your goal while pregnant is to maintain stable blood sugar levels. Avoid white flour, carbohydrates and sugar products that spike blood sugar levels.

- **Consider Taking Coenzyme Q10 Supplement**

Research has shown that women with low levels of coenzyme q10 are at an increased risk of miscarriage.

- **Zinc**

In some studies, zinc deficiency has been linked to miscarriage. Be sure your prenatal vitamin contains zinc. Symptoms of a zinc deficiency include frequent colds and infections, white spots on fingernails, mental exhaustion, poor appetite, dry skin and hair, poor sense of taste and smell. Natural sources of zinc include pumpkin seeds, lean meat, whole grains and oysters.

- **Folic Acid**

Some studies have shown that women deficient in folic acid have up to three times the risk of miscarriage compared to women who have adequate levels of folic acid in their system. Folic acid reduces homocysteine levels.

Be sure you are taking a high-quality folic acid supplement.

- **High-Quality Prenatal Vitamin**

Be sure to take a high-quality prenatal vitamin with minerals such selenium. Selenium is a powerful antioxidant that can prevent chromosome breakage and DNA damage. Natural sources of selenium include brazil nuts and sunflower seeds.

- **Eat Lots of Grapes and Cherries**

These foods contain the flavonoid quercertin, which keeps particles in the blood from sticking together and forming microscopic clumps, which can reduce or sometimes even block, blood flow from mother-to-baby.

- **Get Lots and Lots of Rest**

This is no time to play superwoman. Nor it is the time to try to prove something. Be generous with the amount of rest and sleep you give yourself. Don't for a moment feel guilty that you are not running around doing what you used to do. Your developing fetus is the priority right now. You have nothing to prove. Listen to what your body needs and relax. Don't push yourself when you are tired. Yes, that invitation to go out sounds great and you don't want to be a spoil sport and say no—but you are feeling run-down. Guess what? This is the time to assert your right to say no—for your own good and your baby's good. This is not the time to try to prove something and if someone insinuates that a pregnant women shouldn't be babying themselves, ignore them and stay home.

Be careful of late night social engagements, and trips where you might become exhausted from traveling or not sleeping well in a strange bed or new location. Before you book a cruise or a trip to Europe, you might want to consider the stress flying and being in a new place might have on your pregnancy. If you feel that commuting to work or working at all is too much, talk to your ob/gyn about getting a note that you are in need of some bed rest.

You might also want to delay taking on big home projects, like moving, remodeling, or painting. Your new kitchen floor can wait until after the baby is born. This is not the time to do anything too emotionally or physically demanding.

Reduce the hours you work, ask to work from home, hire someone to clean your house and stop doing most of the chores. Guilt be gone—this is the time in your life to allow yourself rest so your baby can develop and grow. Ignore anyone who tries to make you feel guilty or goes on and on about how they did everything they normally did while they were pregnant. You deserve rest and you need to do whatever possible to get it.

- **Drink Lots of Water**

It can help flush toxins from your body and away from your baby. Be sure to drink pure, filtered water.

- **Do You Have A Mineral Deficiency?**

If you've had a miscarriage or recurrent miscarriage, you might want to have a mineral deficiency test. Be sure you are taking minerals in the form of a prenatal vitamin or a mineral supplement. Ask your doctor about this.

- **Talk To Your Doctor About Vitex**

Agnus Castus, also known as Vitex, has been known to help women who have experienced a miscarriage because of a luteal phase defect. Vitex stimulates the function of the pituitary gland which controls and balances hormones. It also increases progesterone production.

- **Stay Away From Toxic Metals and Toxic Chemicals**

Reduce radiation exposure, by reducing time spent on laptops, hair dryers, cell phones, iPads. Do not use hair dyes or deodorants.

Avoid exposure to insect repellants, disinfectants, cleaning products, paints and anything with gaseous fumes. Do not use plastic utensils or Styrofoam cups at this time.

- **Avoid Heavy Lifting or Vacuuming**

Avoid any type of exercise that strains your lower back or could impact your abdomen.

- **Exercise Lightly and In Moderation**

Nothing strenuous or aerobic at this time. Avoid any excessive physical activity that could elevate body temperature and reduce blood flow to the fetus. Avoid activities like skiing, horseback riding, and surfing, that may cause you to lose your balance and lead to an abdominal area injury.

- **Less Sex Please**

If possible, engage in gentle intercourse, and avoid putting too much pressure on your abdominal area. In Chinese medicine, it is often recommended that a couple abstain from sex during the entire nine months of pregnancy.

- **Avoid Vaccinations of Any Kind While Pregnant**

There are some reports that flu shots have been linked to miscarriage. It is best to avoid vaccines while pregnant.

- **Herbs to Help Maintain Pregnancy**

It is best to check with your doctor or a nutritionist before taking herbs.

- **Reduce Your Work Load**

If possible, can you take a leave from work? Reduce your commute and work from home? If you feel you need to reduce your work hours, talk to your doctor about obtaining medical permission to go on bed rest. If you have miscarried in the past, or are concerned about a possible miscarriage, your ob/gyn may be able to help you obtain legitimate medical documentation for a leave from work or a request for a reduction in hours or a work-from-home situation.

- **Eat or Juice Garlic**

Garlic can boost immunity, reduce inflammation in the body, reduce infections and cut the risk of pre-eclampsia. It reduces harmful bacteria, fungi and viruses, as well as improves blood circulation.

Do not, however, take large or excessive amounts of garlic, as it can interact negativity with certain medications, lower blood sugar levels and reduce iodine absorption, which could lead to hypothyroidism.

- **Eat Foods High In Antioxidants**

These include blueberries, cranberries, artichokes, Red Delicious and Granny Smith apples.

- **Be Careful What You Eat At Restaurants**

If there is any chance you are pregnant, stop eating all meats, salads, fruits and vegetables at restaurants. You don't want to take a chance on foods that could be contaminated, dirty or undercooked. No tacos, hamburgers, hot dogs, or sausage subs either.

• Sit in The Sunshine

Make sure you have adequate levels of Vitamin D. Women with low levels of Vitamin D are at a higher risk of developing preeclampsia.

• Avoid Infections

Infections to be aware of and try to avoid include chicken pox, bacterial vaginosis, Chlamydia, fifth disease, toxoplasmosis, trichomoniasis, rubella, herpes, group B strep, and listeriosis. Wash your hands often with soap and warm water, especially after you have touched raw meat, eggs, unwashed vegetables, dirt or soil, or have been in contact with someone who is ill, gotten saliva on your hands, changed a diaper, played with children, or handled pets, including hamsters and guinea pigs. Do not share eating or drinking utensils. Avoid situations where you will be exposed to flus and other illnesses. Do not touch or change cat litter. Avoid contact with rodents or hire a professional to get them out of your house. Have someone clean your refrigerator, as juices from packages of hot dogs or deli meat can sometimes leak.

Foods To Avoid Or Be Very Careful Of While Pregnant

- No Chinese food

- No uncooked sausages, salami and only pepperoni if it has been heated until steaming hot.

- No prepared salads from a deli, especially if they contain eggs, chicken, ham or seafood.

- Avoid buffet or picnic food that has been sitting out in the heat.

- No stuffing inside a chicken, turkey or other bird.

- No unpasteurized fresh squeezed juice

- Avoid transfats.

- Do not drink the water if you have a water softener in your home.

- Be careful for toxoplasmosis, that is catchable from unwashed vegetables and cat feces.

- No blue cheese

- No raw cookie dough

- Do not drink raw milk, goat's milk or goat's cheese

- Even if you buy hot dogs that have been pre-cooked, you want to reheat until steaming hot, as they could contain listeria

- In Chinese medicine, it is believed that you should not eat pineapple or papaya in early pregnancy, as they can heat up the body and cause uterine contractions.

- **No Raw Meat:** Undercooked beef or poultry should be avoided completely when pregnant. Be very careful about this. I would recommend that while pregnant, do not eat any beef or poultry you did not cook yourself. Do not order meat at restaurants and if eating at the home of a friend or family member, be very sure they cook their meat well. Avoid rare meat or uncooked meat. Undercooked meat should be avoided because of the risk of contamination with coliform bacteria, toxoplasmosis, and salmonella. Even if you like your meat raw, cook all meats very, very well.

- **No Deli Meat:** Deli meats have been known to be contaminated with listeria, which can cause miscarriage. It may be best to entirely avoid deli meat while pregnant. Listeria has the ability to cross the placenta and infect the baby, leading to infection or blood poisoning, which may be life-threatening.

If you feel it absolutely necessary to eat deli meats, reheat or microwave them until they are steaming hot. Do not eat deli meat rare.

- **Avoid sushi.**

- **Avoid Smoked Seafood:** Refrigerated, smoked seafood often labeled as lox, nova style, kippered, or jerky should be avoided because it could be contaminated with listeria.

- **Avoid Fish Exposed to Industrial Pollutants:** Fish that might contain high levels of mercury should be avoided. Mercury consumed during pregnancy has been linked to developmental delays and brain damage. Some of these fish can include: shark, swordfish, king mackerel, and tilefish. Tuna should be eaten in moderation. It is recommended not more than six ounces a week.

Do not eat fish from contaminated lakes and rivers that may be exposed to high levels of polychlorinated biphenyls, which is primarily fish that comes from local lakes and streams. So if someone you know is a fishermen and brings you something they caught, say no thank you. These fish can include: bluefish, striped bass, salmon, pike, trout, and walleye. Contact the local health department or Environmental Protection Agency to determine which fish are safe to eat in your area.

- **Avoid Raw Shellfish:** If you eat seafood, it should be cooked well. The majority of seafood-borne illnesses are caused by undercooked shellfish, which includes oysters, clams, and mussels. Cooking helps prevent some types of infection, but it does not prevent the algae-related infections that are associated with red tides. Raw shellfish pose a concern for everybody, and should be avoided altogether during pregnancy.

- **Avoid Soft Cheeses:** Imported soft cheeses may contain the bacteria listeria, which can cause miscarriage.

Avoid soft cheeses such as:

-Brie

-Camembert

-Roquefort

-No feta cheese, which means avoiding Greek salads, spinach pie, and other foods made with feta.

-Gorgonzola and Mexican style cheeses that include queso blanco and queso fresco.

If you are eating at a restaurant or a friend's home, be sure to inquire as to what cheeses are in the food. It might be best to avoid Mexican restaurants at this time.

- **Avoid Unpasteurized Milk:** Unpasteurized milk may contain a bacteria called listeria. Make sure that any milk you drink is pasteurized.

- **No Pate:** Refrigerated pate or meat spreads should be avoided because they may contain the bacteria listeria.

- **No Caffeine:** Several studies have reported that caffeine can cause miscarriages. This is, of course, a personal choice, but it might be best to stop all coffee at this time. Many experts recommend avoiding coffee during the first trimester of a pregnancy to avoid miscarriage. You'll need to get your energy boost from natural sources, such as drinking green juices and eating lots of vegetables. If you need coffee for work or a long commute to work, you might want to consider taking time off or taking a leave from work if possible.

Your ob/gyn may be able to give you the documentation needed to obtain this. Overall, it is best to stop all coffee during your pregnant.

- **No Alcohol:** There is NO amount of alcohol that is known to be safe during pregnancy, and therefore alcohol should be avoided during pregnancy.

- **Avoid Vegetables Or Salads At Restaurants:** Make sure all vegetables you eat are washed very well to avoid potential exposure to toxoplasmosis. At this time, it might be best not to eat vegetables or salads from restaurants. If you are eating at the home of a friend or family member, be sure that all salads and vegetables have been washed thoroughly.

- **Avoid Undercooked Eggs:** Make sure any eggs you eat are well-cooked. The egg yolks and whites should be firm. Raw eggs or any foods that contain raw eggs should be avoided because of the potential exposure to salmonella.

Foods containing eggs should be refrigerated. Be sure all utensils and pans that contained eggs are washed very, very well before you use them again. Consider putting them twice through the dishwasher to be safe.

If you eat well-cooked eggs, they should be eaten immediately after cooking—do not eat if they were left out for any length of time.

If you are baking at this time, remember that the eggs in a recipe are not yet cooked, so do not lick the spoon!

Do not eat foods made with raw or partially-cooked eggs, such as:

-Hollandaise sauce

-Caesar salad dressing

-Some frostings, both store bought and homemade

-Eggnog

-Homemade ice cream

-Custards

• **Avoid fast-foods:** This is not the time to be ordering a hamburger at the local fast food restaurant.

• **Make Sure All Poultry is Well-Cooked:** Do not buy raw poultry that has been pre-stuffed, because the raw juice can mix with the stuffing.

• **Avoid Unpasteurized Foods:** This can include mozzarella cheese, cottage cheese or skim milk.

• **Be Careful of Herbal Tea.** Some herbal teas can induce labor and be dangerous for pregnant woman. It is best to consult with a physician or a very-experienced nutritionist on herbal teas.

• **Avoid Soda**

• **No Liver:** Avoid or eat very little liver. It contains high levels of Vitamin A which have been known to cause birth defects.

• **Do Not Eat Artificial Sweeteners While Pregnant.**

• **No Raw Sprouts:** Avoid raw sprouts, as they have been linked to salmonella outbreaks.

• **Avoid Prepared Meals that Include Deli Meat, Turkey, Beef, Hot Dogs, or Chicken from a Restaurant, Supermarket.**

• **Avoid ordering sandwiches at restaurants, supermarkets, delis or take-out while pregnant.**

Diary Excerpt: Third Try and You're Out?

This month marked my third IUI try, and the answer has been, every single month, has been no.

No.

No.

No.

I'm tired of hearing no.

I thought after my daughter was born that trying for a second baby would be easy, quick and fast.

I thought once I decided it was time for another baby, it would be simple: an IUI, some medication, acupuncture every week, and kazam--a baby!

Now I'm getting nervous. Three IUI tries and no baby? What if I never get pregnant again? It has been three years since my daughter was conceived and two years since she was born.

Every year that goes by means my eggs are older. Maybe I should have tried for another baby when she was six months old. But I was so tired. Too tired to even imagine another baby. Now I'm wondering: did I wait too long? Are all my eggs gone? My periods are weirder too--lighter, no cramps anymore since my daughter was born. At first, I thought that was a sign of health. Now, I'm guessing it means that my body isn't producing much to give me cramps anymore.

Oh, for the pain of cramps I enjoyed during youth.

How could I have known that those cramps were a sign that my body was toasty and ripe for baby-making?

Sometimes, I see young girls who got pregnant a bit too early and I think: wow, do they know how lucky they are?

By the time they are my age, their children will be 10, 15, sometimes 17 years old. If I had given birth at 18, my child would now be 16 years old.

Imagine...living most of my adulthood with a child to love.

That's how being infertile turns everything on its head. Teenage pregnancy is nothing to envy, but when baby-making becomes the hardest thing in the world to achieve, the ease of a teenager's stroll into babymaking can seem oddly be enviable.

At one time, the idea of having a baby very young seemed like a living prison, a trap to avoid at all costs.

Now it seems ideal.

Had I known what I know now maybe I wouldn't have been so determined to wait.

Wait.

I'm always waiting. I feel like I'm always waiting for something. I'm tired of waiting. I want another baby. Now! I know I am
lucky to have my daughter. Without her, I would be in a constant mourning. Because of her, I can bear this.

But as she grows older, I see a certain neediness within her that reminds me of myself. She loves people and when we go out, she immediately wants to connect to other children. The hard part is sometimes other children want to connect and sometimes they don't.

Some children are very friendly, warm and open, and some children are so completely content with their brothers and sisters, they don't want outsiders crashing in and disrupting the status quo.

The bottom line is: I don't feel capable of raising her as an only child, because I don't want to experience a redo of the issues I faced. I loved my childhood, but I want a different experience for her.

It is the same reason that adults from large families who never had their own bedroom or clothes that weren't hand-me-downs have only children: the grass is always greener and we want our children to have what we didn't have.

I want more babies. I need another baby so my daughter won't be lonely. I need a baby so my family will be larger, fuller, noisier. I am craving the commotion that comes with lots of children. I am sad that because of my age, it is unlikely I will ever have the three or four children I once thought I would have.

If I even have one more baby, I am doing well.

Starting Down IVF Road

I had a consultation with Dr. P. today. He says the IUIs don't seem to be working and its time to take the treatments up a notch and move on to IVF. Add to that my age, which is now 37, and the difficulties I encountered getting pregnant the first time, he explained.

So this cycle I will start my first IVF.

Physical Manifestation of My Internal Self

This IVF has been harder than I imagined. It is a dull January. Usually I love winter, but there is nothing cozy-and-hot-chocolately about this winter. I drive constantly to the clinic. I take blood test after blood test. Ultrasound after ultrasound. I'm sick of tests. I'm sick of driving.

Today I went for a routine blood test, and on the way home, a blizzard started. It was snowing wildly, when suddenly, my windshield wipers broke. Just like that, they broke, right on Route 128. I couldn't see a thing. I couldn't even see the road, or the breakdown lane, or anything.

I started praying out loud.

Every few feet, I would roll down the window and put my hand or some object out the window in an attempt to clear the windshield.

The snow was coming down in heaping buckets and most of the drive, I couldn't see a thing.

The whole time I prayed out loud. Please God, let me get home to my daughter. I felt if I could just get home to my daughter, I wouldn't care so much about anything else. Why did I put myself in this danger? Maybe this is a sign that I shouldn't keep trying for a second baby. Maybe I should have been thankful for what I had. Did this happen because I am greedy for trying for another child, when maybe I should just be thankful for what I had?

In two days they remove my eggs. This is not what I need right now--to be on 128 in the middle of a storm and have my windshield wipers break. God, this is so hard right now. I feel desperate, crazy. It is all too much for me.

Finally, I get to an exit and pull off the highway. I had to keep driving to find help, because I don't have a cell phone.

God, I need a cell phone.

The snow falls heavily. I kept driving, until finally I reached a convenience store where I called for help. By the time I reached the store, I was frantic.

I phoned triple AAA and they came and got me.

The whole time, I kept thinking, 'maybe this is what I get for wanting more children--maybe wanting too much is going to be the end of me. Maybe I should have been grateful for what I have."

This incident was a perfect physical manifestation of how alone and in danger I feel lately. If the physical world can mirror one's inner world, that snapshot of me today, driving down the highway in a blinding snowstorm with no windshield wipers, would be the perfect physical manifestation of my life right now.

This drive seemed like a literal translation of walking by faith, not by sight. I prayed so hard today, as prayer seemed like the only thing I could do.

I remember once a long time ago telling Leah that if I couldn't have babies the natural way, I would just do IVF "they put the egg with the sperm in a dish, and wham, a baby." Wow, was I naive.

Nothing feels fun anymore. I don't like this IVF. It is hard and overwhelming.

First IVF

It is gray today. Everything feels gray. I enter the clinic, and for the first time, I am ushered into the part of the clinic where the IVF patients are sent before they go to the operating room to have their eggs retrieved.

This area in the clinic is deceptively pretty. The wallpaper is a lovely pastel. Once inside, the wallpaper's softness dissolves into an eerie color. This part of the clinic is oddly deserted, compared to the busyness of the rest of the clinic. No one is here, except for one nurse at the check-in.

Since I have done about 17 IUIs, I always imagined that doing an IVF would be no big deal, just another step in my goal to have children. But this is harder than I imagined. I can't say why exactly. Maybe because at this point, I know way too much about baby-making.

I hate waiting in this room, laying so high in this bed, as my daughter runs around.

As sad as the IUIs were, they did not feel quite as heavy as this.

It is scary to be here. Scary to be doing this.

I don't know why I feel so depressed today.

Maybe because the weather is cold and gray and I feel as cold and gray as the weather.

I am the only patient here today, today's sole exhibit in this warped science show.

I need someone to tell me it is going to be all right. It is frightening to think that this seems to be the only way I am going to get a second baby.

The level of stress I am feeling is way too high. No matter how badly I feel right now, it would feel worse not to have the hope of a second baby. So I will endure this gray hell pastel wallpaper and the doctor coming in to tell me that my eggs are poor quality, but that "even poor quality eggs can make a baby" (gee, thanks for the comfort.) Then, later, I will endure learning that out of the ten eggs retrieved today, only three lived. Yikes! What happened to the other seven? I needed those seven. Why did they die? Are my eggs dying because I am too old? Will they all die? Will my other eggs live to make a baby?

I don't like knowing this stuff. I don't like knowing "the quality" of my eggs--or the fact that out of the ten eggs all that medication produced, only three lived to be transferred back into me. Why did those seven eggs die? I was so excited when I learned they retrieved ten eggs. Good for you ovaries, I thought, good job! Man, I thought: seven eggs, of course I'll get a baby out of this. Maybe two or three babies. I kept imagining myself happily exhausted by triplets. My daughter suddenly blessed with three brothers and sisters. Me instantly having the large family of my dreams. Now I know seven eggs have died. I am so sad for those seven eggs. I wanted them to live. Then I'm told my egg quality isn't great. Why isn't my egg quality great? What have I done to make my egg quality so bad? Is it pollution?
Bad eating habits? Being fat?

In this part of the hospital, I feel so lonely. It is as if I am being escorted into a life I never wanted. I wanted children younger. I wasn't a CEO of a corporation who chose to wait because I was enjoying some grand career.

Life made me wait, and now I am in this gray zone where baby making isn't a night of lovemaking, but a stilted series of strategic steps that demand I stay on course, disciplined, a pilot at the cockpit during a dangerous storm where one error is not allowed. One misstep..crash..game over.

Will I ever feel light again? Will anything ever feel easy again?

I am glad science has given me this chance, but I am also sad that I needed science to give me this chance. I am thankful this is not 100 years ago...hell, even 30 years ago, because this chance would not have existed for me. I wish I never had to know the ins and outs of babymaking in the way I know it now—egg quality? Can you imagine anyone in my family ever worrying about their egg quality before? I am the first woman ever in my family, for as far back as time goes, to ever get a baby this way. Ever! In the history of both sides of my family! Thinking about this makes this all seem too serious, too sad and makes me feel too flawed. I want to be 21, in love, in bed, making a baby without thought or strategy or a list of what I need to do today to get pregnant.

I think of women in past generations, trapped because no one could tell them why a baby wasn't coming. I can only imagine the frustration they felt when month after month, no baby came, and there was no ultrasound machines or medications or IVF procedures to give them a chance. At least, despite all this, I have hope and I have options.

After the retrieval, I return to this room, feeling sore and hoping my ovaries were not damaged as they probed me for my eggs. My parents are here to watch my daughter, probably wondering how we all ended up here.

Wasn't I suppose to be a normal girl, who got married and had kids, without all this drama? Somewhere along the way, things in my life got really screwy, and normal things stopped happening. Now, I have to have my Mom and Dad here to watch my daughter while my husband goes to put his sperm in a cup.

My poor eggs.

My poor, poor eggs.

Please God, please. I know that without prayer, I could not get through this--only my hope that God is helping me enabled me to keep going today.

Now I have to wait two weeks for the results of this IVF. It has been a hard few weeks.. all culminating into this one big icky day.

Oops! Pee Pee Problem

The hardest part of the IVF was something I did not expect at all.

It was not the myriad of shots I had to endure every night, or the insane number of times I had to drive Route 128 during the height of the morning commute.

It was having to hold my urine after the IVF.

After the eggs and sperm were mixed together and planted back into me, I was wheeled back to the room and told to hold my urine for a half an hour.

I did not know that to help the eggs and sperm take hold, they have you drink an enormous glass of water and hold it.

This sounds simple, right?

Wrong.

It was hard.

So, so hard.

I laid there, dying to just get to a toilet and let it all flow out.

Holding one's pee pee has to be one of the hardest things to do on this earth.

Every part of me was screaming, "Let me go! Let me go! Let me go!"

Nothing in this whole process felt as horrible as being forced to hold an enormous amount of pee. I am expulsive by nature and inherently holding things in--feelings, anything--is grueling and painful.

"How many minutes?" I kept saying to my husband. I'd look at the clock. Five minutes had passed... I wanted to get up and disobey them, but I want this baby so bad...

I stared at the clock: one minute down, five minutes down..ten minutes down. It went so slow.

I hoped that by staring down the clock, the minutes would pass quicker.

Finally, I hit the thirty minute mark. I vaulted out of the bed into the bathroom.

Relief....it never felt so good.

Now I head home and wait for the results to find out if the IVF worked and I am pregnant.

Try, Try Again

I woke up the other morning and knew it had happened.

"I think I got it," I whispered to my husband.

"Oh no," he said softly, in a heavy tone full of sadness.

I tip-toed quietly to the bathroom.

"Yes," I confirmed a few minutes later. "I got it."

The red hot signal that I am not pregnant had arrived.

Inside me, walls came crashing down and others went up.

I should be pregnant. I should be, should be, should be!

"We'll keep trying for a baby," my husband said kindly.

Try? How dare he! Try was not a word I wanted to hear. The very word 'try' enraged me. Try? Trying isn't an option....we'll make this happen! We'll will it to happen, force it to happen, bend its arm backwards and make it happen.

"What do you mean 'trying'?" I asked him, frustrated that he would relegate having our second child to simply an act of trying and not an act of will.

"I said we'll keep trying," he repeated, not at all understanding why I was getting so mad at him.

The rest of the day was a fuzzy blur. I ended up with a razor sharp headache and a stomache. The next day, I find out that two of my friends are pregnant. They are certainly not specimens of health and yet they are pregnant.

Why is it so easy for some people? Why is it so hard for me?

I need a plan and came up with this:

• My husband will see a nutritionist to strengthen and improve his sperm.

• I will see the same nutritionist.

• I will also go to a person who specializes in emotional release. Sounds flaky, I know, but a friend highly recommends it and for $35 I figure why not try it.

The premise is that trapped emotion in the body can cause illness and dysfunction, and that once negative emotion is released, the body can return to health and normalcy.

My guess is that deep inside me, some sadness is trapped, and perhaps it needs to be released in order for everything in my body to work properly--kind of like an old clock with a big piece of dust preventing the hands from turning.

- I will go to acupuncture once, sometimes twice, a week.

- I will begin eating an extremely healthy diet. I started eating healthier a few months ago, and recently I have seen a big increase in the number of eggs I am producing.

- I will also swim everyday, or every other day. Swimming for me is a great stress reliever.

- I will pray more, although I already pray about 1,000 times a day. Prayer is a privilege that I cannot imagine living without. Thank God that He gave us the ability to talk to Him and go to Him for help. I will ask God to show me what I need to do in order to heal my body and conceive a second child.

Getting Happier

Today I had an appointment with Dr. Deutsch and Eileen. I started going to them to help me clear out past traumas and bad memories, as a way to free up energy in my body to get pregnant. Leah goes to them and recommended I start going, just to clear out anything from my past that might still be lodged in my body. Thankfully, I listened to her and they have turned out to be more than amazing.

I see them every Tuesday. It is an hour and a half trip, but so worth it.

Dr. Deutsch is a chiropractor and an expert in kinesiology. Eileen does myofascial release. Eileen has been working on helping me release sad memories from the past that have been weighing me for years.

Sometimes, it is small things—a hurt from a childhood friend that happened 20+ years ago. A teenage break-up. The body seems to hold everything. I give her a list of names, and it is surprising to find who has smudged their emotional fingerprint on me and who hasn't.

She explained that she is preparing my body to receive.

Sometimes during the treatments I cry a little. Afterward, I feel relief. I feel lighter and lighter, like the joyous 18 year old girl I once was is being resurrected.

After Eileen works on me, Dr. Deutsch follows up. Today, I released so much emotion, when Dr. Deutsch came into the room, he started waving his hand and fanning himself, as if, wow a lot of emotional energy has been released today.

On the way home, I felt overcome with a rush of pure happiness. The sun was shining, a Maine country radio station was playing, and I was feeling lighter than I've felt in years

I am spending a load of money on this right now--about $140 every time I go to them. I'm not buying any clothes. We don't have a second car, and the $400 our tenant Lenny pays us is primarily used for these treatments.

I am lucky to have found this new way of healing.

With Eileen and Dr. Deutsch, I am experiencing a transformation I never imagined possible. Things that hurt or bothered me for 20 years all of a sudden don't bother me anymore.

I never imagined that much of the emotional pain living inside me could be erased, like an eraser on a chalkboard. I never understood that the body stores emotional pain in a physical way…and it can be removed!

That is why something that happened at age 5 can feel as fresh and raw as the day it happened 40 years later.

It can sound hocus-pocus when you learn about this for the first time, but it isn't.

When I see Eileen, it is as if she is vacuuming my body clean of all emotional pain.

Driving home today, I felt like I used to feel back in college--light, hopeful, full of optimism.

I have not felt like this for a very long time.

Truthfully, it is a feeling I thought would never return.

Sometimes in life, you experience things that are so painful, you enter a place so dark, that even when you finally escape the darkness, parts of you stay prisoner of that darkness—and the light never shines through to you as fully as it once did.

Now, because of Eileen and Dr. Deutsch, I won't have to live my entire life filled with long-ago wounds.

A ride home on 95 South, sun-a-shining/radio-a-blaring/the new-me-old-me-new-me emerging. Times are a changing.

Writing My Life Story and Seeing Patterns

Next week is my appointment with Begbetti, a homeopathic expert in Cambridge, MA.

She mailed me a questionnaire and asked me to write my life story, that will help her determine what patterns in my life need to be unblocked.

Writing this life story has been revealing. It seems my life has two themes running simultaneously: one is about joy, happiness, friendship, achievement and faith. The other theme is loss and rejection.

I wrote about losing my best friend in seventh grade to the 'cool kids' and this pattern of loss, followed by great mourning and sadness, seems to be a reoccurring theme in my life.

There seems to be a lot of dramatic endings in my relationships. It was hard to write this and see in black-and-white all my failures.

I'm bringing a copy of my life story to Eileen so she can work on helping me to release some these memories. I know all these painful losses live inside me and are sapping physical strength from me.

How can I successfully carry a baby for nine months, when I carry around so many lost people in my heart?

First Homeopathy Appointment

Today was my first appointment with Beghbetti. It started snowing on my way there and of course, (no surprise) my windshield wipers broke. Why do they only break when I am doing something to help me get pregnant?

I couldn't drive without wipers, but I was not about to miss this appointment, so I called Triple AAA and had them tow me and my car to a parking spot near her office.

I'll deal with getting home later.

Beghbetti's office hip, warm earthy, and welcoming.

She asked me lots of questions, like: do I like to sleep with the window closed or open? What type of things am I afraid of. Then she prescribed a remedy for me.

Tonight, I took the remedy for the first time. The moment I finished swallowing it, I felt a sharp pain jump out of my left breast and a throbbing pain leave my right buttock.

I have no idea why that happened, but I'm hoping something is changing in my body.

I'm glad I didn't let the broken wiper stop me from getting to my appointment.

Needing People to Talk To

Every day, no matter what I am doing, all I think about is whether or not I will ever be able to give my daughter a brother or a sister.

No matter where we are or how much fun we are having, the thought of getting pregnant is always scampering around my head.

Infertility is a part of everything I do, twining itself around every experience I have, whether I like it or not.

For example, on Monday, my mother and I went to the mall for ice cream and a friend who also went to the same fertility clinic as I did works in the food court.

I saw him and his wife at the clinic the day I had my laparoscopy and was being wheeled down to the operating room, when the elevator doors opened and Tom and his wife walked in.

It was a pretty incredible coincidence. Neither one of us knew that the other was going through infertility treatments.

Then, today we found out Tom is one of the managers at the ice cream place at the mall where we get my daughter her Monday cup of vanilla ice cream as part of our routine.

Now every Monday, I get to see Tom and guess what I talk about?

It feels so good to talk to someone who knows the same doctors I do, whose has sat with his wife through the same tests I've endured, and who even can talk about which medications worked best for them.

It is a wonderful part of my week, because with Tom, I am comfortable enough to burp up my worries, even if just for a few minutes.

I usually ask Tom questions, but really what I'm looking for is hope, reassurance, words from someone who believes it will all work out for me.

Tom is very comforting. Not only is he a nice person who offers simple but positive comments like "it will all work out. Don't worry," but he has experienced the success of having infertility treatments culminate into the birth of his daughter last year.

He is the only person I know, other than my husband, who can understand the world I inhabit when I walk in that clinic.

We've exchanged opinions about which doctors have the best bedside manner, which ones answer questions the best, and which ones administer tests with the least amount of pain.

Overall, I don't talk much about my infertility this second-time around. Sharing my feelings with most people is not very comforting, but usually makes me just panic more. I see in the faces of those around me fear and an expectation of disappointment. They are afraid to see me hurt again. They think by not giving me hope they are shielding me from falling too far down if this doesn't work out. I feel more and more like I am cast off on a lonely island. I have to live inside my own head right now. I can't face hearing out loud from another person the possibility that my daughter will never have a biological sibling. As I write these words, I almost fall apart. It can't happen. I won't let it.

I'm not asking for a lot--just one more sibling--not five, not four, not even three, just one right now. As much as I enjoy every minute with my daughter, there is a constant gray cloud hanging over me, a threat that our family will never be larger than it is right now, a family with two adults and one child.

Sometimes when we go to the park, and there are siblings playing together, and my daughter is trying to break in, my heart tumbles in defeat.

What she doesn't understand is that she can't break in to what they have, no matter how much she tries.

When I see her so wanting to be friends with every child she meets, there is nothing I desire more than to give her a sibling who will be her friend, and who will shield her from at the mercy of childhood friendships' that can be fickle in nature.

There are a few people I still talk to: my mother, Leah, Tom and Judy. If I see even a glimmer of fear or anxiety on their face, I fall apart. It is better I keep this all in my own head right now. I can lie to myself very well. I can keep hope alive. I can ignore even the most basic tenets of reality when I have to.

I'm relying on my faith in God right now, on my belief in miracles and the body's ability to heal. I believe the impossible is possible. Alone without other voices, I can hold on to this way of thinking without interruption.

 I believe God opened the Red Sea when all looked hopeless.
 I believe he heard the cries of Hannah who desperately wanted a child. I believe that scripture that says if you have faith, you can say to a mountain move this way or move that way, and it will move. If I didn't believe this way, I would give up right now, because a lot of evidence is against me and the physical world does not seem to be supporting my dream. Instead, I have entered a reality of believing without physical evidence. Faith is all I have.

So I just keep praying and staying silent.

 I am anxious for it all to work out.

NOT MUCH IMPROVEMENT! Are you kidding me?

   Today I felt lousy all the way around. I went to Dr. Kim for acupuncture and asked him how my body was doing. I expected to hear some glowing report on how much progress I made. Instead, he felt my pulse, frowned a bit, and said frankly, my life force was still weak.

Still weak?

I have been going to acupuncture every week for almost three months and I am still weak?

'Not much improvement," he repeated.

Come on! I didn't need to hear that!

After that comment, I felt pretty lousy the rest of the day. All day at work, I kept thinking: why isn't my body getting better? I have to shake what he said out of my head. Isn't even a bit of an improvement still an improvement? I can't help but worry.

Praying Hard

Prayer is an integral part of my infertility treatments. God is my partner in this infertility quest.

I don't pray expecting that if I make all the wrong choices, I'll still get a baby. I pray that He gives me the strength to keep trying when I want to give up. I pray that He helps me find the right doctors and do the right things to heal my body.

I don't naively think if I pray for a baby, but drink sugary soda, miss important appointments, keep on this extra weight, and guzzle coffee that my body is going to produce the baby of my dreams. I know God hears my prayers and I know He wants good things for me, but I also believe He has gifted me with power over my life to some degree. I have the power to make choices, to investigate information and pursue treatments that will help me.

So I don't just pray to have a baby, but I also pray to find the right treatments to heal my infertility.

I read that when you have a goal, you have to be ready to walk through fire to attain the goal.

Well, I'm ready. I would cut off my foot if it guaranteed that I would have a baby. I will go anywhere, spend any amount of money I have, try just about anything to make my body able to conceive and give birth.

I have to work along with my prayers, and if my prayer is for a baby, I have to be doing things to get myself healthy enough to have a baby.

I think the biggest lie told about God is that He wants to deny humans and say no to their requests whenever possible. I can't say how many people have said right out loud, or insinuated, that God may not want me to have a second baby. Why do so many people naturally and easily assume that if I want a second baby, God doesn't want me to have one? Why do they find it so easy to think God wants to deny me what I most want? Why can't they think that God wants good things for me--and why wouldn't a second baby be good for me? Why is everyone so ready to attribute everything bad or denied in their life to God saying no, when really it could be their own choices, their own lack of initiative and willpower, or their own choice to stay a victim rather than work hard to improve the situation?

If I give up now, should I blame God if I never have a second child--or blame myself for giving up?

Maybe God wants me to have a baby, but He is leaving it up to me to keep trying.

I do not blame God for my infertility. I blame human imperfection. I am sick. I am not ashamed that I have infertility problems. I am tired of people insinuating there is something shameful about my condition.

I am not ashamed.

I am not a bad person because I have problems getting pregnant.

I am not a weak person, a morally bad person, a cursed person, or a woman punished by God.

I am not weird and do not deserved to be whispered about because of my problem.

I am a person with a health problem, who is seeking to get healthier and who is asking God to help me.

I do not pray and eat Twinkies.

I do not pray and do nothing. That would be an insult to the power God has given me over my life.

I have choices. I have the ability to seek out answers to the questions in my life, and right now, the question is: why is my body having trouble getting pregnant?

I think God wants me to have another baby. I think He wants my daughter to have a sibling to love. I think He will help me. I think He also expects me to work hard for this myself. I do not assume He will say no just because I want to hear a yes.

On Track Like Never Before

I don't think there has ever been a time in my life when I have been more focused, more with my eye on the ball, than I am right now.

When I wake up every day, the first question on my mind is: what can I do today to get one step closer to being pregnant? Then I write in my daily appointment book what I can do to help me reach my goal.

I can't do an IVF for another two months, and so during that time, I'll whatever I can to get healthy. I eat bowls of romaine lettuce, chicory and parsley, which everyone at work jokes as being my "rabbit food." I juice spinach, snack on walnuts, and have cut out most white flour and sugar products. When I think of how I used to eat--lots of cheese and meat, so much bread and white flour, I am amazed that my body was able to take it. My head actually feels like it is clearing a bit on this new diet.

I sometimes joke that I'm taking a kamikaze approach to healing. Or maybe it's a 'if-you-throw-enough-darts-you'll-eventually-hit-the-target' approach. Basically, I'll try anything that seems remotely reasonable to get my body strong enough to have a baby.

Every day, I vascillate wildly on the hope meter. I'm up! I'm down.... I'm optimistic! I crash....

One moment, I am having fun with my daughter and loving my life. A moment later, I see her bored, lonely, wanting to play with other children, and a fingernail-on-the-chalkboard desperation to get pregnant hits me.

For the first time in my life, I understand the power of looking at a problem from every angle, and the power of making good choices. Maybe, for the first time, I see clearly my role in how this will all turn out.

As sad as I sometimes feel, I don't think I've ever been more on top of a situation than I am right now.

Does Loss of Authentic Personality Equals Loss of Fertility?

Today was my first appointment with Dr. Zhu, an acupuncturist and master herbalist, who I wanted to try because I've heard a lot of wonderful things about Chinese herbs helping infertility.

I have to say that driving to his office was among the worst driving experiences I've had lately. But then, driving to the clinic is pretty harrowing too. I have no choice but to drive this highway, but sometimes I feel like the drive down Route 128 is a metaphor for my infertility: you must do what you have to do to get to your destination, regardless of how frightening and horrifying it feels.

Dr. Zhu's office was so peaceful, in contrast to my drive over. He felt my pulse, which acupuncturists and Chinese herbalists do to determine what is wrong. He then had me read a paragraph from a book on what he considered to be some of my problems. The paragraph described me perfectly.

Then he put together a bag of herbs for me to boil and make into a tea.

Before I left, he gave me a short, but very powerful, acupuncture treatment. During Dr. Khu's treatment, I could actually feel parts of my brain opening that had been closed off for a long time.

After he inserted the needles, I sat reading a 'People' magazine article about the problem of bullying in the school systems, and how one young boy even committed suicide because he was so tormented by bullies. I was overwhelmed with inspiration, got out my notebook and started jotting down ideas how to curb the bullying problem. In all, I wrote nine pages on how to stop bullying and while I wrote, I felt different than I had in a long time: powerful and capable of changing things, unblocked by the usual shame, fear, embarrassment or failure I often feel when I imagine that I can change things. It was like an old part of me resurfaced that wasn't ashamed or burdened down with memories of failures.

Charging forward with solutions and fighting for causes was a part of who I was long time ago. Over time, and with lots of failures, I lost this part of me who believed I could change things or make things better for others. When I was a child, I was always coming up with ideas to fix things and right wrongs. I ran a Jerry Lewis carnival for muscular dystrophy, got signatures for a Save the Whales petition, and in college organized a two-week Feed the World weeks festival, where the governor of Massachusetts declared April 25 Feed the World Day.

'Feed the World' weeks turned out to be a big disaster. I was 19 and not really ready to undertake a fundraising operation of this size. We raised $5,000, but I made a million mistakes. The experience shrank me. After that, I never had the confidence to spearhead anything again. When I heard about this crisis or that crisis, I no longer imagined that I could do something about it. Maybe I lost the belief that I was competent enough to make positive change. I never consciously realized, or even acknowledged, that this change had come over me, but my life slowly became more about protecting, hiding and defending myself, rather than reaching out to help and make a difference.

Yet, all of a sudden during this treatment, I felt that activist part of me come back to life. I felt angrily energized about the problem of bullying in America and I somehow felt capable of coming up with solutions to the problem, much the way I used to feel when I was young.

Is it possible that this acupuncture treatment resurrected a dead part of me that was once a pillar of my personality? And how did losing this part of me relate to my infertility?

Is my infertility related to an inability to manifest my will and power in this world?

What is the correlation between my infertility and this loss in my personality?

I can't speculate too much about this--as I don't really know what this treatment did to me exactly, but I wonder if the disappearance of who I am also weakened my body's ability to manifest things I care about in general.

I left very contented to have added yet another layer to my healing.

Second Homeopathic Treatment

Today, I had my second visit with Begbetti.

What a sharp contrast to my first visit. The first time I went there, I felt very stressed—like the elements were against me and yet another snow storm was trying to block me from getting the treatments I needed.

This time, it was a beautiful spring day. As I walked up the Cambridge side street to her office, I felt an old buoyancy return that I haven't felt in years. I felt light-hearted, dare I say happy even, in a way I haven't felt since college.

Way back in college, before I had my heart broken about 100 times, before I had lost jobs at places I thought I would work at forever, before I failed at so many things, I walked around with a kind of happy, confident, naive girl-in-white optimism.

Youth, some people would call it.

I have always longed to regain that feeling--a feeling that life is beautiful and great things were within my reach.

I struggled many times to get back to the me that was capable of enjoying the quiet of nature on a beautiful day. As hard as I tried, I could not get back to that whole, happy me.

Beauty in nature made me sad, uncomfortable, because my insides no longer matched the beauty of the outdoor world.

Today, surrounded by the dizzying beauty of spring, I felt the old me return.

Beghbetti's receptionist, Paris, noticed the change in me right away. "You seem so much happier than you did the first time you came here," she said. "You look so alive."

Perhaps everything I am doing to heal: going to Eileen, Dr. Deutsch, Dr. Kim and Dr. Zhu, is healing something deep inside me and restoring parts of me that I thought were lost forever.

At today's appointment, Beghbetti asked me more questions, like what type of weather conditions I feel most comfortable in. I told her I like the winter a lot, but hot summer weather seems to bring up anger and a sense of helplessness in me. She prescribed a remedy.

I left feeling full of hope. This healing process to get pregnant has turned out to be exactly what I needed on many levels, aside from just the infertility aspect. I have been in emotional pain for a long time. So many heavy hurts were trapped inside me, and now I have been given a chance to heal and remove them permanently.

My Diet Is Actually Working

My diet is actually working and I am actually losing weight. People are noticing. For the first time in ten years, a diet has worked.

My motivation to look better is about stabilizing my hormones to increase my chance of getting pregnant.

I hit my highest weight about a year after my daughter was born. I went on this pepper-steak-onion-cheddar-cheese-in-a-wrap binge, and one can imagine how I looked after eating those night after night.

Now I eat foods I once wouldn't have dreamed of eating and it is amazing how much more energy I have.

When I got married nine years ago, I was tired by 1 in the afternoon and would sometimes spend the rest of the day in bed watching TV. Now, I can go all day, and still have energy left at night.

This whole infertility ordeal has changed all sorts of patterns in my life. It has forced me to become a disciplined soldier in this war I'm waging against all the forces conspiring to keep me without the family I long for. This includes my own self-destructive habits and my own self-hatred that often thinks that I should end up alone and with nothing.

Sometimes, when I listen to the theme from Rocky, I envision myself in a jungle, climbing and swinging through trees with my daughter strapped to my back. It is for her I am trudging through this jungle of infertility. For her, I will climb trees and fight lions and paddle down raging rivers.

For every nasty, uncomfortable, painful test I have to endure, the image of my daughter enjoying a sibling keeps me going.

It is amazing what one a person can do when there is enough desire. I have not been able to lose weight in years, but now when I am tempted to buy a candy bar in the vending machine at work, I say to myself: 'that candy bar could prevent you from ever having another baby' and suddenly I can reject even chocolate! I lived for a long time through a weaker version of myself, a version that wanted to hide, and didn't want to try too hard for anything because she was too sad and scared. I was tired all the time and just wanted to rest from all the sad experiences I had. Now I will do whatever it takes. My family will not be complete until we have another child. He or she has to come to us—or our family will have a gaping hole in it.

Infertility is testing me and pushing me, and I like the person I am becoming because of it.

Back to the Clinic

Awhile back, I decided to change doctors. I left Dr. P and switched to Dr. M, a female doctor, because I need a change. I am so worn out emotionally right now, that I need some kind of a change. I need a doctor with more of a bedside manner. Each time I had to see Dr. P after hearing some bad or disappointing news, he acts like it is the most inconsequential of events. I realize he must deal with hundreds of people every month, and he has a basic kindness that comes through, but I don't have the strength for so much logic and rational right now. I need a bit more babying, and since Dr. M was so kind during some of the tests she administered, I wanted to try her.

Good thing I did.

She immediately discovered from an ultrasound taken this morning that I have a large fibroid that needs to be removed.

A fibroid! That explains everything! I am thrilled at this news!

Finally, I know why I am not getting pregnant.

I feel so relieved right now. Once the fibroid is out, I'll be able to get pregnant and have another baby in no time!

Maybe this has been my problem all along. When did this fibroid start? Before my daughter was born? After my daughter was born? Thank God this fibroid didn't hurt my daughter. I hate it intensely. And how did it get so big?

I am so glad that at least now, I have a clear and true explanation for my fertililty problems.

Fibroid Operation

Good thing Chris set the alarm this morning or I might have overslept. My friend Katherine is driving me to the clinic.

When we got to the hospital, Katherine dropped me off at the curb, and wished me well. It all felt so normal, I almost forgot I was on my way to an operation.

Then, the automatic doors to the hospital whooshed open and I went in.

One thing I have to say about this clinic is that the staff is always so on the ball, organized, caring and kind. This morning was no different. As always when I am going to have some type of procedure done here, I feel very taken care of. I was proud of myself for being able to so casually arrive at the hospital alone for the operation. That is what years of dealing with infertility treatments have done to me--I'm braver than I once was, and what would have once been a big deal isn't a big deal anymore.

I prayed a lot as they got me ready for surgery. I pray they don't make any big mistakes during my operation.

For a few moments, I felt utter panic. Alone in that room waiting I missed my husband. I wish he was here.

Then, all the usual stuff happened. I was put on a stretcher and wheeled to an area near the operating room, next to another woman also waiting for surgery. She has been trying to get pregnant for more than a year (I will listen to anyone's story looking for a glimmer of hope). Then it was time. She and I wished each other well, and it helped to have someone sending me off with good wishes.

I remember little after that. I'm so accustomed now to those last few moments before...wham...lights out.

When I woke up later, I was once again in that horrible recovery room.

Man, I hate this room. It has to be the ugliest, most cheerless, uninteresting recovery room in the world. It looks like it should be in a prison or something (isn't infertility like being in a prison sort of?) Can't they just throw some paint on it? Its like I'm stuck having the same bad dream over and over again.

A nurse asks me how bad my pain is on a scale of 1 to 10 and I always say 10 because I like getting the highest dose of pain medicine possible. The more pain medication, the better.

They say I have to stay 40 minutes, or something like that, before going on to the other waiting room. Every few minutes, I ask if I can go. I can't stand being here. I want to go now. I can't stand waiting here. Now I know how people stuck in nursing homes feel. There is no comfort in this setting. I'm in a lot of pain and I JUST WANT TO GO HOME!

Finally, I am brought to the other waiting room and my husband comes in to see me. Finally, I am allowed to go home. Thank God!

I can't wait to be home and get comfortable in my own bed.

Once in the car, I suddenly feel nauseous.

Everything hurts.

We get on Route 128, and the traffic is thick, slow, unbearable. Why couldn't they let me out before the commuter traffic started? (MOVE THIS BACK)

Cars, cars, cars...rows of cars crammed together.

I start throwing up all over myself.
I don't care. Why so much traffic? I need to throw up again. I open the window and stick my head out. I can barely stand this. The pain, the car.. moving so slow. I want to get home. I need to be home.

My stomach has never hurt this much in my whole life. This is worse than a caesarean. I can't take this snail-like drive that seems to never end.

Was it not two years ago this month I was on the same road, feeling the same type of sickness, trapped in the same overheated afternoon traffic just like I am now? God help me.

My husband tries to comfort me. "Do you want….?" he asks. No. No! No! I just want to go home. Get me home!

The pain is getting worse. I hate July heat! Will this ride ever end?.I have no patience for it. I need to be home. They said this would be painful, but this is more than I imagined. Why is it so hot? What is making the traffic go so slow? I need the windows down. No, I need air-conditioning. Put on the air conditioning. Oops, I forgot: we don't have air-conditioning. Please God, kill me right now. Just kill me. No--I take it back. I can't die. I have a daughter. She needs me.

Forget safety--speed, crash into another car and make the cars move. Stop. I have a daughter. The window looks so good wide open. I am going to jump out. I can't be sentenced to this heat a minute longer. But if I jump, the cars will run over me. ...I can't jump. I am stuck. I am stuck in this heated highway hell forever. I will never escape. God help me. Oh God, please help me. Why is the traffic so bad right now? Why is it so hot? The sun is too bright and too hot. We will never get home. How far to Route 495? How far? Are we almost there? We are starting to go faster. I feel a breeze on my face. I am going to stick my head out the window. I am going to throw my whole ugly fat head out the window. I am going to jump out the window and feel the breeze. No. No. Be patient. When will I feel some relief? I hate the month of July. Every July is bad for me. It is like the heat magnifies whatever pain I am enduring.

God help me. Please God, help me. Be with me. Heal me. Stop this pain. Somebody, please, stop this pain. Chris, drive faster. Get me home. Oh my husband, I love you/Ihate you/this is your fault/it is their fault/it is the doctor's fault/why did they keep me so long and let me get stuck in this?

We are now on Route 495. The Andover exit. God help me, please, faster, let the exits come faster. The Middleton exit. I am closer. Oh God, it is our exit. We have to drive through a few streets.

We are almost at my house.

Finally...we pull in the driveway, and I throw open the door and run out, not even stopping to shut the door. I'm home! God, I am home. It feels so good to be home, but the pain doesn't stop. I lie down on the couch.. my beautiful green couch...

My father sits at my feet. He has brought some Young Living Essential Oils to help me. I am dying. Daddy, I am dying. My stomach is on fire. Why am I dying? My daughter is looking at me frightened. I have to be quiet. I need to be quiet. Why can't I shut up? My father starts rubbing my stomach and my feet. It isn't going to help. Nothing is going to help. Chris, call the doctor. Somebody get my doctor. My mother is crying.

My daughter is crying. I am making her scared. I need to stop, be brave, be silent. Oh please...My father keeps rubbing my feet and my stomach.

Could his oils actually be working? I am starting to feel better. He has an oil for stomach pain. He has me drink something. I trust my father. He is smart and kind, and he knows a lot. Please God, let my father help me. Let somebody help me. I am in such pain. My daughter is running around and seems confused. She is scared and I can't help her. Chris, take her upstairs to watch TV. I can't be needed right now. I can't be anything right now. I need to be taken care of. I can't be a good brave mother now. My father keeps rubbing the oils and some of the pain is leaving. Relief. I am actually getting some relief.

I start to feel better.

Being so tenderly cared for by my father was a gift I'll never forget. My father has a healing nature, and a true healing ability. I am so grateful he used this on me today. He could have been a doctor, that's how good he is with helping others.

The oils helped stop the terrible pain in my stomach.

My mother tells me that the doctor called while we were driving home to see how I was.

She told my mother everything went well and that she is on the way to vacation, but will talk with me more when she gets back. Thank God—that monster fibroid is gone! Good riddance you terrifying fibroid!

Soon, it is time for my husband to leave for a concert in Boston. Jerk. Complete and utter jerk. I'm sorry to say that, but that is how I feel right now. How could he leave me tonight--for a Monkey's concert? It doesn't matter. I can't flip about this. I have to be cool and just let him think it is fine. His behavior won't matter when I'm 80 years and on my death bed. Then, I want to see at least two children around my bed in those final moments. He probably won't be there anyways and so what he does today won't matter much then. I can't let him be the focus. I can't flip out at him, because he is so sick of this infertility stuff, he'll leave me if I get too difficult, or he'll just stop agreeing to help me have another baby. He deserves some fun. He puts up with a lot. It is fine for him to have fun. Oh God, why is he leaving? I need him. Get a grip. Don't make him suffer for what you want. This is your baby, your project, your obsession, not his. He picked you up and was kind to you on the way home. I have my mother and father here, how much more do I want?

Hopefully he'll remember how nice I was about this.

Plus, we are introducing a friend of ours to a guy tonight. If I have to be without my husband for a night for an old friend to find love, I guess that's okay.

Hey, I can even walk a bit. Everyone said after the fibroid operation I wouldn't be able to walk, but I actually can walk. Now I want to go to bed and sleep. I am so tired.

Day After Fibroid Operation

Today I did not feel half as badly as I expected to feel. First, my husband reported that the friends we were trying to 'fix up' at last night's concert really hit it off.

I thought I wouldn't be able to walk today, but I can walk. Yesterday was harsher than expected, but today I hardly feel any traces of it.

Today, I am going to rest, while my husband takes care of our daughter.

It feels so good to have that fibroid gone. I have an appointment in two weeks for a check-up, and then it is on to the IVF.

Now that the fibroid is gone, I should be able to get pregnant soon.

Thank God!

And A Fibroid Would Have Been So Easy.....

A ton of bricks. Falling on me. Right now.

I went for my first check-up since the fibroid operation.

My doctor very calmly and with no apology whatsoever, told me I did not have a fibroid after all.

Oops.

That explains my amazing recovery. It also explains why I could walk so well after supposedly having a large fibroid removed. It explains why all the pain I was told I was suppose to feel after the operation never came.

And here I was thinking I was some kind of medical marvel.

I'm very confused right now.

The doctor didn't seem upset by her findings.

Or embarrassed.

Or even slightly apologetic.

She told me as if it was no big deal. So I reacted like it was no big deal, because I didn't want to make her feel bad for making such a stupid mistake.

If no fibroid existed, then why am I having so many problems getting pregnant a second time? Now I have no easy answers. The fibroid gave me a way to understand everything.

I am back to square one.

Does this mean I went through all that worry, nausea, and postponement of my IVF for absolutely nothing?

I had thought that changing doctors was a good idea, especially when she discovered a baby-eating fibroid. I thought, 'finally, someone has found the root of all my infertility problems."

As it turns out, she diagnosed me incorrectly.

Now I have to wait until September to do another IVF. Every month that passes means my eggs are one month older.

Having a fibroid made it all so black-and-white.

When I told friends I had a fibroid, many reacted with 'oh yes' 'ah ha' and 'that explains it' and I was told story after story of their sisters, best friends, and co-workers, who had trouble getting pregnant, discovered they had a fibroid, had it removed, and soon had babies born without a hitch. There wasn't something deeply wrong with me on some unexplainable cellular level! It was all the fibroid's fault.

Simple.

Nope. As usual, nothing is that simple.
I have no fibroid. No easy explanation to hang on to. An apology, or an oops, I led you down the wrong path these past few months, would have been nice.

When I thought a fibroid was at the root of all my problems, I sometimes felt slightly carefree. I thought my infertility problems were now going to be simple and straightforward: I have a fibroid. It is killing my babies. It needs to be taken out. Once it is gone, all will be well.

Now I'm left to think that maybe our daughter was a one-in-a-million chance that won't happen again. I feel an almost overwhelming grief.

I want to think this doctor knows what she is doing. She was named by a magazine in our area as one of the best infertility doctors in New England. I like her personality and I trust her.

I just hate that because of this operation my IVF was postponed. I also hate that I had to go through all that pain. For what? For nothing? I told everyone I had a fibroid, even the alternative practitioners I was working with, which might have impacted the treatments they chose to use on me.

And a fibroid would have been so easy...

Preparing for IVF

Lately, everything I do is centered around preparing for the next IVF.

I am stuck in a waiting zone right now. I can't plan ahead for anything, because my plan is to be pregnant, and once I am pregnant, I will quietly nest at home and not do anything else.

Normally, I am an extrovert and I love being with friends. Now I prefer to retreat within myself. I hide more than I ever did before.

Besides, when I come out from my shell, everything feels too real and I am at the mercy of how other people view my chances of becoming pregnant. I can't look at this through anybody's eyes but my own right now. Only in my eyes do I see hope for myself.

God is really the only one I want to talk to about this. He will help me. I believe that. If I didn't believe that, I might just go insane.

I walk around pretending to be part of life's normal routine, when nothing is normal or will be normal until my daughter has a sibling. My husband says I have a one-track mind. But what else am I suppose to focus on? What is more important than this right now? Not much, at least to me.

When I talk out loud about this, I actually feel power leaving my body.

I went up to see Eileen and Dr. Deutsch twice this month. I brought lists of almost every person and memory that might be weighing down my body. It is surprising that old emotional pain, as far back as 1976, can still live in my kidneys, liver, and heart.

Every time I leave their office, I feel joy like I haven't felt in years.

At the same time, one of my best friends and one of the persons I am closest to in this world, Leah, is moving to Portland, Oregan. I could easily be devastated about this, but right now I have to push out all feelings about mostly everything because I have to leave room for this baby to come.

Imagine

I feel so nothing today.

Like I am a bad, flawed person. How could anything good ever happen for me? Nothing I ever do is good. I make so many mistakes. I can't imagine this will ever work out. I'll probably make some big mistake and screw it all up. Other people do this almost without thinking.

I need to stop thinking like this. Today just feels lousy.

Somebody like me doesn't get things. I am not the type...

No, stop. That all changed when my daughter was born. My rotten pattern was permanently altered. I can't think like that anymore. I am good enough. I deserve a baby.

No I don't. I am a bad person.

Yes, I do.

No I don't.

Shut up!

Transition Time

This must be a time of transitions, of doors opening and closing and I'm not sure what it all means.

I've been at this type of intersection before, where one road closes and an alternative route opens up.

Right now, movement seems to be going on in my life to an extreme. My 98 year old grandmother Maria, who lived on 133 Amesbury St. for the past 29 years, has moved out of her lovely apartment and in with my aunt.
The apartment where I slept about a million times and felt so safe in, the one I spent so many happy times visiting, is no longer my grandmother's home.

The white hairbrush on the pretty rose-colored hamper that I always loved to brush my hair with since I was a little girl is not there anymore. How can that be? Shouldn't that brush be in that spot forever?

Suddenly, I can't joke around about 'to grandmother's house we go' since grandma doesn't have a house to go to anymore.

Then, my best friend Leah, who is really more than a best friend, but also a soul mate, a kindred spirit, the kind of friend who sat with you moments after one of the saddest goodbyes of your life, took you by the hands, and somehow made you believe you could survive and go on, is moving to Oregon.

And I start the preparations for my IVF treatments next week.

Beginnings and endings. People leaving, and hopefully, new people arriving.

I've don't like change. One part of me wants to yell at Leah for moving so faraway, "where the hell do you think you are going?"

A part of me wants to say to my grandmother, "Grandma, why did you have to get old? Why can't you stay in your apartment? I miss visiting you. I miss sitting in your kitchen talking to you.

I miss watching TV in the living room with you. I miss showing up at your apartment at 7 a.m. for a cup of coffee. I miss the quiet content times we spent together that that lovely place." Pause. The sobs are coming. Hold on. "Grandma, please don't keep moving away from me like this."

I'm pissed off. Scared. Nostalgic. Teetering on the brink of something.

A part of me wants to run back, hold tight one last time, before life inevitably moves us all on.

Who is coming to replace them? I've found in life that usually when lots of changes occur like this, other things blessedly arrive in their place.

I'm hoping for a little 8 pound somebody.

The Second IVF Begins Now

I am entering a climatic, exciting, and frantic zone.

So much build-up...now reaching a crescendo.

I went this morning for a blood test and I found out that Sunday will be the day of my egg retrieval, Wednesday the implantation, and it all starts tonight
with my HCG shot between 7 and 8 p.m.

I've waited since last February for this moment—and it ends up happening on the same weekend as Leah's going away party and my cousin Lori's wedding.

Because the shot needs to be taken by 8 p.m. tonight, I can only stay an hour at Leah's going away party. That is how infertility is--it butts into your life and demands priority regardless of what else is going on.

I built this party up so much to my daughter, talked on and on about "the fun we were going to have at Aunt Leah's party" and now we will basically walk in to the party, say hi, give a few hugs and leave.

I could easily start screaming.

Why is this happening at the same time I have to say goodbye to one the most important people in my life?

A part of me wants to hide out until my baby is born and not deal with anything but baby making. God, I have to get pregnant soon. How many more IVFs will they let me do? How many chances do I get? I can't delve into that murky place right now. This time has got to work.

After all this waiting, it boils down to now. Tonight, finally.

Leah will leave for Portland in a few days. I won't see her after the party tonight. She has been there beside me through everything the past 10 years. How am I going to do without her?

The pain of her leaving is starting to make me physically ache. I can't focus on this or I will fall apart.

I've waited so long for this IVF and now finally it is here. I think I am ready.. I just didn't think it would all start tonight.

We were one of the first ones to arrive at Leah's going away party. I couldn't really explain to her mother why we couldn't stay long. As usual, I feel like I am walking around keeping secrets. Ssh--don't tell anyone. I'm taking my shot tonight. Always, always secrets. Then tomorrow is my cousin's wedding. Chris is stressing about money again because I'm going to see Eileen on Tuesday so she can prepare my body for the implantation Wednesday. Between her and Dr. Deutsch, it will cost about $140. Chris is cranky about this, but I told him I need to go. Good God, to come so far and not do everything possible to make this happen--that would be crazy.

I'm trying not to show Leah how sad I am right now and I'm trying to tell myself that we will always stay close and in touch.

My gut tells me that she will return, but another part of me wonders: will she end up living across the country for the next 20 years? Is one of the most important persons in my life permanently leaving.

I made an attempt to act brave and casual with Leah, talking excitedly about Portland and the wonderful people she is going to meet. I told her how proud I was of her for making this daring move.

I am just feeling very sad for myself.

Around 6:45 p.m., we say goodbye. I feel selfish leaving the party so early, but the shot has to be priority right now. Leah and I stood at the door of the old Grange hall, hugging tightly. Leah starts to cry, and I am starting to be overwhelmed by a tidal wave of grief. I try to hold it back. I can't let myself despair over her departure. She is doing what she needs to do to create the life she wants, and I am doing what I need to do to create the life I want.

Oh, if only it was all so cut and dry. My dear beloved, best friend Leah is leaving.

We got home, and at exactly 8 o'clock, Chris gave me the shot.

Now, my ovaries are cooking with eggs. Oh God, please let me get pregnant. Please God, make this work. I've done so much, prepared and waited so long, please God don't let me be disappointed

Cousin Lori's Wedding and the IVF

Today was my cousin Lori's wedding. It was absolutely beautiful and I was thrilled to be there. Amber looked so pretty in her dress. Bringing her to the wedding meant so much to me. Everything takes on a different hue when I'm with her. She loved the cake. She loved the outdoor wedding. She loved Lori's dress. She loved seeing Lori dance with her husband Bob. She loved dancing and twirling with me and Chris, and really, there is nothing I love better than dancing and twirling with my little girl.

Despite all this happiness, I felt like I was walking around with a big ticking time-bomb of a secret, as if people looked at me closely enough, they could see that I am a walking mound of infertility drugs.

I didn't eat a piece of wedding cake because I want to make sure my body is in optimum condition for the retrievel tomorrow.

There is a eerie stress level that accompanies an IVF. It is so completely unnatural in one way, and yet so natural in another way to be doing whatever is needed to expand our family. I wonder what it must be like for people who can simply make love and then discover—surprise!-- they are pregnant. Something that happens so naturally for millions of people is a faraway reality for me.

Today, surrounded by the normalcy of a man and woman getting married, I felt like a big fake because there is nothing even near normal in my reality right now. Doing an IVF is like walking into a steel metal futuristic world, where all the old comforts are gone and in their place are new technologies that in order to work cannot allow in even a trace of the old softness. Imagine the comfort, safety, and casual joys of quilts, puppies, old-fashioned porches and children playing outside on a spring day. Then imagine the opposite of all that. That is what an IVF is like.

While dancing with my daughter, I thought: Am I the first person in my family who ever got a baby this way? I looked around at all my cousins and their babies and their babies' babies, and my aunts and my grandmother and my mother, and I thought: all these women had babies the good, old-fashioned way, and me, always so odd, had my baby come to life through heavy infertility medications and weird scientific procedures.

And you know what? I didn't care. As I danced with my beautiful daughter, I thought, 'she is here, and if my road was different to get her here, so be it.' Thank God I was born now, and not 100 years ago.

As strange, weird and oddball as I am, I was not a childless woman at this wedding today, but like all my aunts and cousins and their babies and their babies' babies and my aunts and my grandmother and my mother, I am a mother now too.

Regardless of how I am making a family, I am making one. Ultimately, that is what matters most.

9/11

The day started out sunny. A bright, beautiful sunny. The kind of sunny that gives you a wink and a nod that it is going to be a great day.

I am driving down Route 95 heading to Portland, Maine to see Eileen and Dr. Deutsch. I am in high spirits.

Two days ago, they retrieved ten eggs from me. Ten! Tomorrow they will implant them. With God's help, I could be pregnant soon.

I am thankful as I drive that today the weather is beautiful. So beautiful. Alone, on a highway that is a joy to drive, the radio on as my companion, I listen to the morning DJs do hilariously awlful pranks on unsuspecting listeners.

I am feeling good.

Then, a disc jockey says he can't believe that he just saw on TV a plane crash into the World Trade Center in New York.

I think: are they replaying some old news clip from long ago? I never heard about this. I don't always follow the news as closely as I should....

The disc jockey sounds upset. He says he can't believe that now a second plane is crashing into another tower.

Is this some kind of sick joke? I switch the station in disgust. What a rotten disc jockey. It is one thing to phone some unsuspecting listener and tell them you are calling from the dog pound, or a local auto dealer, or the courthouse, and tease them into thinking they are being fined or something. It is another thing to play a horrible joke about planes crashing into buildings.

As much as I love a good joke, this went too far.

But as I switch from station to station, I keep hearing more and more of the same thing. Two planes, two towers, New York City.

What is going on?

I don't want to listen anymore. This cannot be happening. I switch the channels on the radio faster and faster.

I no longer see the sunshine or the highway or anything else. The sun is still there, the day is still beautiful, but I can't see it, feel it, anymore.

By now, I know something wicked has happened. Something unimaginable. People on the radio are crying. Screaming. Confused. Even the disc jockeys and news people seem to be falling apart. Not today. Oh God, not today, not any day.

I finally arrive for my 10 o'clock appointment with Eileen. A few people are crying and people are going to an office upstairs to watch TV.

Eileen looks upset. We go into the room where she does her treatments. But today, she is not herself. Her brother lives in New York City and she can't get through to him. She doesn't know how he is. She starts my treatment, lowers her head and begins to sob. She prays out loud, asking God to please help those people suffering in those towers, people that could be dying or burning to death. She says there must be a reason I am there with her at this time. I don't say anything. I feel so confused.

Never in my life have I felt so torn between my own needs and the pressing needs of the larger world around me.

Tomorrow is the IVF I have waited for the past eight months. It is the IVF I am counting on to give me a baby and give my daughter a sibling. It is the IVF that I haven't stopped thinking about since last February. It is the IVF I have spent thousands of dollars preparing for. It is the IVF that has given me hope when all I felt was despair and rage.

I need Eileen to do a good job right now. I know I am selfish for thinking that. Then it hits me what is really happening to good wonderful people in those towers and I can't stay hidden from the truth anymore. The sadness hits me so hard. If I let my feelings descend any further, I am heading fast towards the brink of hysterical.

Eileen is not going to be able to focus. I know that. Her treatment was suppose to prepare my body to receive. I am trying to tell myself I can get pregnant whether this session with Eileen goes well or not. I tell myself this, but I know the timing of this cannot be worse for me.

Can I pretend this is not happening? Can I pretend that my country is safe and people in New York are going about their business as usual? Is it right to try and shut this out to save myself and my potential unborn babies? Or do I join everyone else and go insane? Do I hold tight to my sanity as a way to hold on to my chance of getting pregnant?

Eileen cannot continue. I am disappointed, but I understand. Dr. Deutsch comes in and does his treatment.

Driving home, I listen to the radio.

Oh my God, all my thoughts about tomorrow's IVF leave and I begin to cry. This is too horrible! Those poor people! I start screaming, sobbing, crying. Loudly, profusely. Getting ready for the IVF these past few weeks has made me feel very weary, but now everything feels unbearably sad like never before.

I get home and my husband is watching on TV a replay of what happened. Our daughter begins to cry. Does she understand what is happening?

I begin to watch the nightmare too...but it is too horrible. I cannot fall into the misery of this event. This is not happening, I tell my husband, it is not happening. It has never happened. I will lie to my body. I will trick my body and not let it know what unspeakableness has occurred today.

I cannot do this/I have to save myself/ My body will not get pregnant if it is laden down with sadness.

I ask my husband to shut off the TV. At first, he protests. He is sad, confused, needing to watch. I beg him, explaining that I can't take all the sadness. I can't take the whole IVF thing during an attack on my country. I wonder if we should even do the IVF tomorrow.
Will the hospital be blown up next? Is it safe to go to a public place tomorrow? Will there be a terrorist attack somewhere on the highway as we are driving?

There is no way I will can pregnant with the level of despair I am feeling. This is so crazy and unfair.

Just as it has been for months, I am completely alone in what I have to do--banished to some remote island where my reality has to be completely different than everyone elses. At a time when I have every right to wail and scream and cry, I'm not allowed. I have to stay disciplined, on track, focused.

Damn, this is too much.

Now the crazy, lonely, forbidden, desolate world I've inhabited in my head for the past few months is spreading out everywhere around me. I'm not the only one mourning, and it makes my pain more intense. It is like everything in my head is playing itself out in some dark national nightmare.

This is not happening. This is not happening. If I keep telling myself this is not happening, maybe it will go away. Please God, make this not be real.

Tonight, I lay in bed praying. Please God, help the firefighters, the people in the towers, the people on those planes, everyone.. I am in a tug-of-war: sad for the suffering of people I haven't met, sad for my babies that I haven't met, sad for myself, and hysterical for the people who have lost their lives and for their families.

It is all too much.

The world feels heavy tonight. Sad, heavy, and upside down.

I am trying to retreat into my own head, just as I have done for the past several months, but I can't. The reality of this is beyond what I can bear. I must sneak away to my own inside place or I'll never get pregnant and my daughter will end up without a brother or sister.

How can this be happening? How? To me! To the country where I live! To those innocent people in the World Trade Center! How? Why now?

I want to shut my eyes and block my ears. I am being robbed of my future babies. If I let them, my baby will be another casualty in this tragedy. Those terrorists are not going to steal my baby who I am suppose to conceive tomorrow. I won't let them take this one...I will get pregnant tomorrow!

I am suppose to have the transfer tomorrow, but the clinic doesn't guarantee it until the morning when they know for sure the embryos survived the transfer. Maybe all my embroys will die and I'll end up with no IVF tomorrow. I don't think I could take that right now.

God help us all tonight.

9/12 Day of IVF

Today, the day I have waited for since last February has finally arrived. The day I planned for, drept about, prayed day and night about, has finally arrived. Could I have ever imagined worse timing?

We got up and waited for the call from the nurse. I am getting panicky that maybe all my embryos have died.

Finally, we get the call that I have three viable embryos. Seven died. Man, all the things I did and still seven died.

My eggs aren't good quality. Will my three embryos die in a day or two also?

For a moment, I want to cancel the IVF.

Everything felt surreal on the drive to the clinic. I looked at the cars around me and wondered, are you the car carrying a bomb? I pray for safety. I pray for help. I don't know where to put my mind.

At the hospital, we head to the IVF floor.

The whole world feels upside down, and I think: how upside down is my world that my IVF falls on the day after one of the most horrific and heartbreaking national disasters of all time?

Everyone is acting differently today. The nurses are putting on a good face, trying to pretend that everything is normal, but nothing is normal.

I can't help but think: is this hospital the next target?

They tell me my eggs are showing lots of damage and they are a C quality. Great. Two eggs are rated poor quality and one fair. I wish they didn't tell me this. How in the world can I make a baby with such poor egg quality?

Dr. M does the transfer. She is positive, gentle, and says nice things. I try to be positive, but all I can think of is the poor quality of my eggs. I wish I didn't know that most of my eggs are considered a C or D. This is too weird, too science fictiony. I just want a baby, but knowing every little thing like egg quality, makes it all seem eerie, dark and impossible.

This time, after the transfer, I lay as long as I am suppose to. I drank less water than last time, so holding my pee isn't as bad.

We don't talk much on the way home. The world feels so heavy right now

Tonight's Explosion

It all came to a head tonight. An explosion of sorts. A dam-ready to burst.

It is the day after my transfer, and my husband decides he will go into work at 3 o'clock in the morning so he can come home early tomorrow to watch our daughter and give me a chance to a rest. His job sometimes allows him to make his own schedule.

He reasons that while me and my daughter are sleeping, he might as well work. The idea being, the more rest I have, the better chance I have of getting pregnant.

The plan seems good. Only somewhere around 3:30 p.m. my daughter wakes up crying. I rock her to sleep, but then I am left wide awake in the middle of a dark lonely night.

Such a dark lonely night.

The veil is lifted and it is all there. The World Trade Center, terrorism, planes flying into buildings, people dying, New York City under attack, my IVF.

I feel crazy, looney, thrust into some type of big screen terror flick, dozens of horrifying images playing out in my head. This seems like a bad movie gone wrong. I start to cry, a heavy, throbbing thundering cry. It is a cry I have cried before on my darkest of days, and I never forget when I cry this way. I fall to my knees and cry louder. I don't care that I have woken up my daughter. I don't care that she is crying now. I don't care, because my own sobs keep coming louder and louder and I can't stop. I am on my knees now, screaming for help, because the World Trade Center was attacked and the IVF I have waited so long for landed on the same week I can't stop crying. I cry and cry, and for a moment, I see myself in a snapshot of darkness and it becomes a permanent part of my memory, in the same way that those other times I have cried like this before have become.

I call my husband at work. Please come home, I beg. He is annoyed. He is tired of all my neediness. It is too much for him. He is ready to quit. He wonders why we are putting ourselves through this. He doesn't seem to care whether I get pregnant or not. He feels like he already did enough. Now, I am crying for more? I need him to come home. I need him to care for our daughter. I can't deal with her crying right now.

He reluctantly agrees to come home. He hates me, but I don't care. I just need him here. I don't care that he will have to go back to work later. I don't care about anything. I turn on the home and garden channel. My daughter calms down.

I hold her and try to pretend that the world is still as pretty as all those lovely homes on TV. I am scared and alone, and if the world falls apart tonight, I want my husband home with me, even if he hates me for it.

Red Alert

It has been a long, drawn-out, painstakingly agonizing ten days since my IVF. Pretty much, all I think about, except for my daughter, is that I have to be pregnant this time.

My mind runs in circles: Am I pregnant? I am pregnant! Yes, I know I am pregnant. I am so happy! I did it! No, I'm not pregnant. I am destroyed, depressed, a loser. I am not pregnant/ I have to be pregnant/I am not pregnant/I am/Am not/Am.

Am I pregnant? Yes, I am pregnant. My baby is on the way. My mood soars. No, it isn't going to happen. I am defeated, murdered, withered and grasping for breath. Please God."

On and on it goes.

There are moments of relief, of course, like when I look at my daughter's most beautiful face and I thank God for her existence. But the more I fall in love with her, the more frantic I become to get her a brother or sister.

Today, I hit an extreme low. All day, I feel sad and weird. Dr. Zhu gave me an herbal drink to help me get pregnant that I am suppose to take only once every few days. But today, I can't follow his instructions. Every few minutes, I go to the refrigerator and take a slug out of the bottle. I'm not suppose to do this, but I can't stop. I have to do something to make me get pregnant! I am drunk on Chinese herbs!

I also start slugging down liquid iron. I know I am not even suppose to take this, but I can't seem to stop.

I have to do something, take something...now I take a red raspberry herb. I took these when I was trying to get pregnant with my daughter...maybe they will help now.

Then I take two more vitamins.

Then I drink more of Dr. Zhu's herbs.

"You're not suppose to be doing that," my husband says. Ouch—I'm caught!

I try to convince him I know what I'm doing.

He says cut it out.

What a jerk.

I need to get away from him. I go outside to sit on the front steps and pray.

It is an incredibly beautiful sunny autumn day. In a few hours, we are going to a party at my cousin's house. I am not in the mood for a party. I am overcome by some new mutant breed of desperateness.

Being outside in the sunshine makes me feel a little better. Then my husband says it is time to get ready for the party. He is always bugging me. Good lord, just leave me alone.

He goes back in the house and I keep praying. The sun is beautiful and I feel close to God right now. I also feel a raw desperateness I hate feeling that won't let up for a moment and give me a break.

I feel overwhelmingly sad right now and I don't know why.

A few minutes later, I head into the bathroom to start getting ready for the party and I see exactly why I felt so desperate: blood.

No God, not after all this! No! Please God, no blood.

No Blood! I scream for my husband. When I tell him the blood has come, he looks so sad. I try tell myself that a woman can get her period and still be pregnant.

I phone the clinic's emergency hotline to ask them what they think I should do. A nurse calls back. I tell her I did an IVF and now I am bleeding

I ask her if I could still be pregnant despite the blood.

She is aggravated and instructs me to just come in for my pregnancy test in a few days. I start asking questions: could I still be pregnant? Is there any hope?

The nurse says little, yah, I could be pregnant. No, she can't tell me what chance there is. She seems angry. I don't care. I need answers.

At my cousin's party, I am quiet. I tell everyone I don't feel well. I sit in the kids playroom and watch my daughter play. I want to say: guess what everybody? I did an IVF two weeks ago and today I got my period. Chances are I blew this like I blow most things in my life.

No one could possibility understand how alone I feel right now, how this could mean that my dream of creating a happy family life for my child is disappearing.

Maybe I shouldn't have drank so many herbs. I can't think about that...can't deal with it being my fault. My husband wants to go down this road, but I won't let him. He has no idea how helpless I felt today, and compelled I was to drink and take things, and pray and take and drink again.

I don't even try to hide my glumness at the party. I sit, slumped in a big comfy old-fashioned recliner, watching my daughter play with other children. Thank God they have this playroom for the kids, or I would have been forced to socialize the whole night.

The pain inside me is so intense that hiding it is impossible.
Tonight I have absolutely nothing to say to anybody. I can only look at my beloved daughter and watch her play. Through her, I speak. Through her, I live. Through her, I glimpse a little of life's happiness. For myself, there is absolutely nothing left to say tonight.

I go to the clinic on Tuesday. I am clinging to the small slight hope that maybe I am still pregnant.

The blood is flowing and flowing. My red alert desperation tracking device worked loud and clear.

I guess when you've lost many, many times before, you get pretty good at
knowing when you are about to lose again.

Worst News

Today was my pregnancy test. I think I know the answer.

The nurse's called later that day: No, I'm not pregnant. I did, however, have a chemical pregnancy however and it did not continue. The words shake me to the core. What is this thing called chemical pregnancy?

Tell me everything, explain this to me, I ask. Why did this happen? Was it my eggs? Is it because of the quality of my eggs?

I am not trying to be a pain, but I need answers.

The nurse is annoyed. She barely answers my questions.

No, I am not crazy. I just want an explanation.

The nurse is cold, aloof, off-putting. As if I have no right to ask so many questions.

I dial the clinic again and get the voice mail for my nursing team. I leave a question.

A few minutes later, I call again. I leave another question. I call again 12 minutes later. I have more questions. I can't stop calling. I can't stop asking questions. I need answers. No one is giving me answers. No one is explaining why this happened. I dial again, and leave more questions. I need to know. Am I on the wrong medication?
What is going on with me? I need information.

If only I could understand this. Why isn't anyone telling me anything?

One nurse in particular is extremely rude to me. She acts as if I'm complaining about an order gone wrong at a drive through. She doesn't have time for me and I know she thinks I'm crazy. Maybe I am crazy. Yes, I am crazy today. Who can blame me? Who can blame me for being crazy? What am I suppose to be--rational after all this?

I dial again, and leave more questions. I can't stop even though I know I should. No one is answering me. No one is helping me. I feel compelled to act. Give me answers! Give me information! Please, tell me right now what went wrong and why.

Finally, a kind nurse calls me back. Her name is Chris and she is very sympathetic. She tries to answer my questions, but she doesn't have the answers.

I ask her if she thinks I'll ever get pregnant again. She tries to sound hopeful, without giving me false hope that could make the clinic liable. I appreciate her kindness and trying to answer my questions the best she could. She is so different from the other nurses.

I will never forget the kindness of this nurse who called me back.

I have so many questions. I need to make an appointment with my doctor to discuss everything about my treatment, from the amount of progesterone I am given, to my medication. Something is wrong. I can't believe this is happening. I feel a crazy inconsolable kind of anger and helplessness.

A few minutes later, a counselor from the clinic calls to see how I am doing.

Probably that mean nurse reported me, told the counselor to call the crazy woman leaving too many messages on the voice mail. I quickly get a grip and feign saneness while I talk to her. I'm frightened she will report that I am too nuts to go through another IVF.
I hate this counselor. She has to be the most insensitive, cruel counselor imaginable. She tells me some awful statistic on women my age getting pregnant. She goes on to list all the problems that can be expected at my age. Is that what she thinks is going to comfort me? What a freakin' idiot! I wish I could report her to someone, but if I do, she will label me as psychotic and they will kick me out of the clinic.

Someday I'll write a letter to the clinic telling them about the complete insensitivity of this supposed counselor. I wonder how many other woman she made feel hopless during their darkest moments. She has no right to hold this position, but I need to stay quiet right now and pretend I am okay.

I tell her I feel fine. Yes, I am disappointed, I say casually, but I'll get over it. She seems to accept that. The idiot can be tricked so easily. I thank her for calling. She asks if I want an appointment, and instead of saying no, I tell her I have my daughter to care for and getting a sitter is hard, but yes, eventually I would love to come in for an appointment.

What a stupid lady. She falls for it, hook, line and sinker. I hate playing this game with her, but she scares me. She is mean enough and lacks insight in such full measure that if I tick her off in any way, she will say I'm not psychologically fit to handle another IVF. So I pull myself together during this phone call and I act like I'm fine and okay about this pregnancy gone wrong, not a woman with any emotion, thank you.

My husband seems confused too. Has the possibility of having another baby already escaped us? I go crazy at the thought. I have a million questions and no answers. This was not at all what I expected.

Chemical Pregnancy Nightmare

Why didn't I get pregnant this time?

No one seems to be able to tell me why.

I have an appointment to talk with my doctor. I mailed her a letter with 20 questions, so that she can take some time and review my particular case before we meet.

Am I on the right medicine?

Am I getting enough progesterone?

Do I need some type of test to determine whether there is a virus in my body causing these problems? And if so, do I need a strong and swift antibiotic to be rid of this infection?

I hope sending the questions ahead of time will make it possible for her to thoroughly research all my questions.

I want everyone to just go away and leave me alone.

Devastating Meeting

Today was my meeting with Dr. M. I woke up excited. Finally! I'll get some answers! She has my questions and had lots of time to research them.

I have been reading about some new medications, and there are some medicines out there that seem to suit me. I am requesting a change.

I wore my red suit, with the idea that maybe, if I looked professional, she would take me seriously.

Boy, was I in for a surprise.

Instead of going over the questions, she immediately began talking about the number of messages I left on the nursing team's voice mail. She alluded to the fact that her nurses were aggravated with me.

Immediately, I knew this meeting wasn't going in a good direction.

I'm being tested right now, I thought, and I better remain cool if I ever want the chance to do another IVF at this clinic again.

I immediately apologized for my persistent phone calls, and explained that a first, I was very upset.

Then she asked if I was okay now, and if I felt I was able to take doing another IVF.

"I'm fine," I smiled convincingly "I was upset, but I'm over it. I understand these things happen."

Hah! I really wanted to say: Doctor, I'm still a basket case, but obviously, you, like everyone else around here, wants me to feel no emotion at all. You prefer me to be just
another quiet little number in the pecking order. Take my disappointment and shove it down. Ask no questions. Make no demands. Make no waves. Exactly what everyone wants out of women everywhere--to stay silent and just be good little soldiers who do as they are told without ever protesting or questioning or feeling. That's right ladies, you should feel nothing regardless of what you are going through. Say nothing, accept whatever is handed to you without any emotion at all. And you, being a women doctor, should know better, teach your nurses better, understand more. I expected more from you, but you are no different than the people who have wanted to silence women for years. I get it. I'm too much work, too much hassle, and you have no time to answer 22 questions. I understand the rules here: passion, sadness, hysteria, desperation, is in no way allowed. I understand. I am suppose to do this without feeling.

I'm suppose to take the bad news and cry silently alone, and never bother anyone with my pain.

Then she went on to suggest that maybe I take some test to determine my ovarian reserve and chances of getting pregnant. No way, I think, I am not taking some test so you can label me unable to conceive and then insurance will stop all my treatment.

I tell her maybe later, it sounds good, but I want to do another IVF first.

She looks at me quite seriously and tells me that because of the amount of medication I need, it looks as if my eggs are at the bottom of the barrel.

Everything stops for a minute. The little trickle of hope I had left oozes away. I didn't expect this.

She says for my age, I need way too much medication. She questions if I ever smoked, and I tell her I never even tried a cigarette in my life. She seems to not believe me, and asks again. I repeat that I've never even tried a cigarette in my life.

She now recommends that I look into donor eggs, and I think: no, I'm not doing that.

Then I tell her that despite all my problems, I think I still have a chance of having one more child. "All I need is for one egg to turn out right," I say, trying to sound reasonable, logical, defending myself against her attack, but most of all fighting the hopelessness building inside me.

"Maybe," she says, with an expression that means "keep dreaming dummy."

I ask her if she wants to go over any of my questions. She glances quickly at them. It is obvious she hasn't gone over them. She says they don't apply.

I ask about changing my medication. She doesn't want to consider it right now.

I rise to leave. We shake hands and I pretend I am okay.

I thank her for her time.

Once I get in the car, I feel wildly, frantically angry. I am stunned. I can't even cry. I drive home in a daze. Her words ring in my head: your eggs are the bottom of the barrel. Your eggs are bottom of the barrel...your eggs are bottom of the barrel."

I never realized it was this bad. Regardless of everything I've gone through, I never felt like my time was up.

My time can't be up! I need another baby--I need a baby for my daughter! I can't accept this...I can't live with this.

I start to pray. I pray and I pray and I pray, because I know under no uncertain terms that it will only be through God's help that I will ever get a baby now.

I am at such a desperate point. Her words have nearly broken my will and spirit. Thank God I know God. Thank God I can pray to God. If I didn't have God and His gift of prayer, I would give up right now.

After I pray, for some reason I can't explain, I stop on the way home at a big alternative supermarket in my area and go directly to their book section.

I am searching for hope.

I start reading a book on women's health written by Christine Northrup, "Women's Bodies, Women's Wisdom" and I
come upon her chapter on reproduction and fertility.

She writes that in other cultures, it is perfectly normal for women in their late 40s to have babies.

She thinks that some of the infertility problems in the United States are because women are told they are too old to have babies in their 30s. This is wrong, she says, and the problems stem primarily from lifestyle, eating habits and stress.

A little bit of hope returns, and I thank God for physicians like Dr, Northrup who give women hope, instead of ripping it away like Dr. M.

I had switched to Dr. M I assumed that because she was a woman, she would have more empathy and more of a bedside manner than Dr. S., but I was wrong.

First, she misdiagnosed me with a fibroid and now she calls my eggs bottom of the barrel.

She obviously doesn't like to be hassled or bothered, and someone like me, who asked too much of her nursing team and mailed her 22 questions, was obviously too much work.

When I got home, a neighbor who had undergone infertility treatments was visiting. She recommended I switch to her doctor, who was in the same clinic.

I went upstairs to call my mother. I desperately needed to talk to my mother. It is times like these that it is my mother's voice I need to hear above all others.

There are few people on this earth who you can always count on to provide you with hope, but I am fortunate enough to say regardless of whatever has happened in my life, my mother has always given me hope. My brilliant mother always understands that bottom line: hope will get a person through. If she didn't do this, I don't know if I would have ever gotten past some of the disappointments in my life.

 My mother is also very intelligent. She gave me this brilliant advice, "That doctor doesn't believe you can have a baby. I know you can. Change doctors. Do it today, immediately. If she is telling you this stuff, go to another doctor who is willing to work with you."

My mother was right. Why was I giving her opinion of my fertility so much power? My mother is right—let me see what another doctor has to say. I hung up with my mother, and immediately phoned the clinic to have my records transferred to Dr. G, my neighbor's doctor.

I set up an appointment for next week and mailed him the same 22 questions I had given Dr. M.

Dr. M has no idea what she did to me. If not for God and my mother, I might just give up on ever having another biological child.

What kind of monster is she? Who is this doctor that thinks it is okay to rip a person's heart out? Maybe in her mind, she really thinks there is no hope for me.

Maybe she thinks I'm so crazy, that it is better to remove all hope from me.

Well, maybe I am a bit crazy, but I'm not so crazy as to stop trying.

She took some of the fight out of me today. I went there looking for answers and instead I got put in my place. A demanding, out-of-control, strong-willed woman being put in her place, ironically, by another woman. Not at all what I expected when I chose this doctor.

Tonight, in bed, anger and rage came over me. I wanted to phone the clinic and leave 100 nasty messages about this doctor and her cowardly nursing team.

My husband stopped me.

"Give me the phone," I cried. "They all deserve to be told off! She deserves me to tell her what I think of her!"

"No, don't blow it," he warned.

"I don't want to ever go back to that clinic. I want to go to another clinic. She deserves to be told off," I say.

"Don't do it. If you do, you can't go back there. Just do another IVF and see what happens," he says reasonably.

"I can't stand it. I have to tell her off," I cry.

"Paula, don't blow this. If you tell them off, they will think you are crazy and they won't let you do another IVF. Not there, and maybe nowhere else either. Just do the IVF and maybe you'll get a baby next time," he says this with such reassurance that I calm down.

"You are right," I said. "But when I have my next baby, I am going to march into her office and say, "SEE YOU JERK! SEE THIS BEAUTIFUL BABY! THIS IS WHAT BOTTOM OF THE BARREL LOOKS LIKE!!!"

Jealous and Ashamed Of It

I am turning more and more inward, Being with people, particularly certain people, is getting harder and harder.

Tonight was a case in point.

A friend of ours got married last year to a wonderful girl, and now They are moving back to her hometown next week. We invited them over for a farewell dinner.

A few days ago, we also found out she is pregnant.

Tonight, I could hardly stand the way they joked about the surprise of it all. Surprise? What is it like to get a baby as a surprise? No work, no heart break...just SURPRISE!

Every jealous bone in my body came popping out.

Right now, I can hardly stand knowing that some people just make love and get pregnant. Of course, I know that happens all the time, but to have someone in my house, joking about getting pregnant, not understanding that in my world, pregnancy is accompanied by lots and lots of shots, lots and lots of blood tests, lots and lots of calls from nurses, and lots and lots of nos, is hard.

My friend's wife comes from a family of eight kids. She is 28 years old. They've been married barely over a year.

When I hesitated to let her have chocolate, remembering that chocolate is not recommended for high risk pregnancies, she ate it anyways without a care in the world. What is that like? Having babies is going to be no big deal for her. She said she definitely wants at least one more baby. And she said it in a way that you know she could have whatever number of children she wanted. One more, three more, six more..she will have the choice in creating whatever size family she wants. What is that like?

It was hard hearing about how they are going to living right next door to some of her siblings, who also have lots of kids. Great...lots of ready-made friends and cousins for her baby!

It was also hard hearing how excited her sisters are for her, while I am feeling so alone right now, my daughter without cousins and without a sibling.

Finally, I couldn't stand it anymore. All I kept thinking was: I should be pregnant. Not her. What did she do to earn this pregnancy? What suffering has she done? I know this is a terrible way to think, but I couldn't shake the feeling of how unfair it is that some people can get pregnant without hardly even trying.

I told everyone that I was sick and took my daughter and went up to bed.

When I got to the top of the stairs, I felt such relief. Ah, escape!

Right now, the only place in this world I feel safe is in my bedroom, alone, faraway from reality.

After they left. I told my husband I wished he never invited them over.

He didn't understand and scolded me for being a lousy friend.

I am not in the mood for his lectures.

Ever since that stupid Dr. M. decided to crack my will in half, I am sad beyond words.

I am only happy when I'm with my daughter, but there is a constant ache inside me that maybe no more children may be coming to me. How dare Dr. M steal my hope away. What now? What next?

I felt so trapped in my own house tonight--trapped with two people that in any other circumstance I would love spending time with--but in the world I'm inhabiting right now, when all that matters is getting pregnant, I couldn't stand being with them.

I was jealous of her nausea and had no stomach for her stories about morning sickness.

Give me the nausea. Give me the morning sickness. Give me the baby. Give me the opportunity to choose the number of siblings my daughter has.

All I want to do right now is be alone with my daughter and feel sorry for myself.

Fair Time

A darkness has come over me I am trying to conjure up the optimism and hope I had last spring, when I was in full throttle healing mode, but I can't.

It isn't that easy to get revved up again. Where did all that healing get me? No pregnancy and a bad diagnosis from my doctor?

What if I took that awlful test she recommended and the results were that my chances of ever getting pregnant were zero? What do I do then?

If I think too long, a scream builds in my throat. How wrong it would be if my biological clock is up.

I don't want to talk about this with anyone. It seems that beneath the smiles and nods, people mostly agree with my doctor. My husband joins me in the world of miracles and prayer. He is ready to believe despite the physical evidence around us, and right now, except for my parents, he is the only one I can trust with this.

I understand that I am extremely fortunate to have my daughter, but it is because of my love s for her that I desperately want to give her a sibling. Am I asking too much? Is it so wrong of me to want for her what millions and billions of other children around the world have? A sibling to grow up with, a lifelong friend, someone to share her childhood with?

I am not giving up just because my doctor says I should. My daughter deserves better from me than that.

Today was a big fair in our area. We planned to take our daughter and meet up with some friends. My heart was barely in it. While I was excited for my daughter to try fried dough and see elephants and ponies, it hurts to be with lots of people right now.

I don't know why, but it seems everyone we ran into at the fair was there with their adult brothers and sisters.

We ran into one friend who was there with her younger brother. When her brother walked away, she whispered about the surprise anniversary party she was throwing him and his wife. Normally, this wouldn't bother me, but today, anything related to siblings hurt a lot.

Then I ran into a friend who is pregnant with twins, already has two children, and four siblings of her own. How lucky can one person get? I am jealous. What is it like to be surrounded by family and able to give this gift to the next generation?

Then some of my husband's cousins met up with us. Of course, they arrive two brothers with their sister. Fairs must bring out some sort of family togetherness thing or something. I can't wait to go home and hide in my bedroom.

But when we get home, a bunch of our friends from the fair come over too. Our friend who lives in our basement complains that it is too hot in the house, and I say that I am cold. Then (he definitely picked the wrong day to say this) he says, "ah, the sister I never wanted."

Wow—bad timing. I took my daughter and marched up to my bedroom.

Being referred to as an unwanted sister was not exactly what I needed to hear today.

I can't let my daughter down. She deserves to have the safety of a brother or sister that all those people I saw today have.
God help me, what if my time is up? What if my eggs are mostly gone and the ones left are so damaged that no baby can ever come from them? What then....?

I pray and I pray and I pray, because prayer is all I have left.

Phone Conference With New Doctor

Today was my first meeting with my new doctor. I didn't feel well, so I phoned the clinic to see if our first conference could be on the telephone. Surprisingly, the doctor agreed without a hitch.

I immediately felt better when I heard the doctor's voice. He was kind. He
wasn't rushed and he had answers to almost all of my 22 questions. He agreed that it was time to change medications, and had already been thinking of the medication I requested.

Let me say it again: he was already considering the new medication I was requesting What a good sign! We were on the same page. So different from Dr. M who wouldn't even consider trying a new medication on me!

Then, as we talked, he said,"considering everything, I see no reason why you can't have another baby."

Hallelujah!

Give that doctor a gold star, a medal, some type of award!

His words gave me hope!

Now that is what a doctor is suppose to do!

We agreed I would phone his nurses on Day One of my next period. Thank God, and my mother, that I changed doctors. What a difference!

If I had stayed with that other doctor, she would never have changed my medication, and because she saw no hope for me, she would not have done anything to help me.

In contrast, this doctor was open and willing to try something new.

Was didn't Dr. M. consider changing my medicine? Did a patient like me, who wanted to try again and again, threaten to screw up the statistics that made her the most successful infertility doctor in New England?

My new doctor sees hope for me! I hate caring so much what authority figures think, but considering he is on my side, I am pretty excited.

Could this make the difference? I hope so.

Riding the See-Saw

A few days ago, I got an e-mail from a friend who said pregnancy at 34 was difficult for her, and that made me slightly depressed all day.

A friend in my department at work just announced she is pregnant. She is 42+ and I am elated--there is hope for me too!

My moods go up and down all day just like that, based on information I receive on pregnancy.

A friend confides that his girlfriend is 42 and doctors predicted they couldn't have children. But she had a baby boy last month! Score another for hope!

Up and down, up and down. It is hard to be constantly riding the see-saw of hope and despair.

We took my daughter to the park today and it was beautiful. The air warm. The leaves a color feast. Sometimes at the park I feel lonely.

So many people come and go, and we say hi to them all, but chances are we'll never see them again.

I sometimes wish I could make friends with all of them, that somehow more people would come into my life. I feel sad when I see my daughter so much wanting to connect with children who are either too shy or already have a set of friends/cousins/siblings/whatever to meet their social/emotional needs.

It is hard to talk about this with most people. When people say things like, 'if God wants you to have another baby, you will." My question is: what if God doesn't want me to have another baby? What then?"

 Then I want to say: "Why would God dislike me so much that He wouldn't want me to have another baby?'

A part of me wants to say, "Shut up! Of course God wants my daughter to have a sibling. Cut the crap." No one would ever dare tell a cancer victim fighting for their life, "If God wants you to live, you will." But in the world of infertility, people still feel they have some right to make you feel like maybe God isn't in with you on your plans.

A Ride to Maine with Leah

   Leah and I both had appointments with Dr. Deutsch today, and so we drove up to Maine together. She moved back from Portland—thank God!

On the way up, Leah asked me how do I know I will get pregnant again. She asked in a positive let's-have-some-heartfelt-talk kind of way.

Usually, I love when she asks me these kind of questions. Normally, the more we talk, the better I feel.

But for the first time in my life, I didn't want
discuss anything to do with fertility.

Something inside me wanted to stay silent and shut.

Somehow, I know that if I let the words start pouring out, they are not going to be positive, productive words.

They are going to be words of fear, of a foreboding that perhaps I am really not going to have another baby.

If I let the feelings that live inside my body form themselves into words, they are going to turn into words that drag my body down even further, maybe even permanently.

This time, I don't want to talk. I just want to win. I don't want to be comforted, soothed, or given advice.

I just want to win.

If I started in on a long discussion with Leah about having another baby, I would have to reveal how I am living off the faith that lives in my head. I would have to let it be known that I am ignoring the statistics, ignoring the facts, and creating my own reality based entirely on faith.

I am doing the most that medical science offers, but the bottom line is that I could not do this without believing in an alternative reality based on miracles and faith.

I pray God helps me have another baby, and I believe He will help me. I believe He wants my daughter to have a sibling to love.

I could tell Leah was hurt when I said that I did not want to talk about getting pregnant, but I just couldn't put into words the reality I am living right now.

Getting Ready for the Next IVF

I have my whole IVF planned. I am going to Dr. Deutsch three times next week. Once, the day before my eggs are retrieved. A second time the day before they are implanted, and then the day after they are implanted. Once I get pregnant (no ifs here) I am going to see him once a week to keep my body on track.

My husband hates the idea of traveling so far every week, but he hated the idea last time and look what happened.

Preparing to Conceive

Dr. Deutsch says I'm ready. He says my body is ready to conceive.

Eileen and I continue working on removing difficult memories from my body.

I have been getting my shots every night.

When my husband gives me the shot, it is an oddly tender and tense time between us.

Sometimes, I adore him for his skill and experience in administering the shots. I love him for his ability to give the shots so quickly. But if he pricks me or hits a wrong spot, I get super annoyed at him--like I think I would punch him if I could.

I am not making any plans because I expect to be pregnant soon all I want to do is incubate myself to help my baby survive.

Chapter 30: How to Maximize Your Chances For Conception The Days Before and After An IVF

Before

• Consider additional acupuncture treatments close to the time you are doing an IVF. Ideally, increase the number of acupuncture treatments the week of the IVF to two to four. If you can, have one also done the day before the procedure. Perhaps if you go once a week, consider increasing your appointments to two to three times within the seven days before an IVF. Research has shown that acupuncture improves blood flow to the ovaries and uterus, relaxes uterine spasms, and relaxes the nervous system.

• In the weeks prior to an IVF, make sure you are eating well. This is not the time to splurge on foods with lots of sugar, trans fats, msg, or white flour. Consider increasing the amount of vegetables you take in, such as spinach and garlic.

• Green tea is linked to increased fertility. The polyphenols and hypoxanthine in green tea can increase the percentages of viable embroyos. Some studies suggest drinking treen tea can also help eggs become more fertile.

• Increase the amounts of healthy fat you consume. In a recent study, women who ate avocados, a healthy monounsaturated fat, were more likely to conceive a child after IVF. Other healthy fats include olive oil. Avoid saturated fats and trans fats as much as you can, ideally entirely, for two to four weeks before IVF.

- Be aware of the help certain supplements can provide, such as coenzyme Q10, which in some studies have shown to improve egg quality. Some studies have shown that women taking coenzyme Q10 had higher fertilization rates in IVF than women who weren't taking the supplement. Some studies also show that coenzyme Q10 deficiency can sometimes cause miscarriage.

- Increase your time spent in the sunshine to 30 minutes a day if you possibly can. Even if it is cold out, try to be in the sun more than usual amount of time. Perhaps bundle up and sit outside. Sunlight increases levels of Vitamin D, which is key to balancing sex hormones in women and improving sperm count in men, according to various researchers. In cold northern countries, the rate of conception increases during the summer months, according to some studies. If you are doing an IVF in the summer and you live near a beach, park or lake, consider spending more than the usual time outside in the sun.

- Pineapple contains a proteolytic enzyme called bromelain which reduces inflammation, improves uterine lining and breaks up proteins that prevent embryo implantation. Eating pineapple core a few days before an IVF cycle can help implantation. Cut the core into round sections and eat after embryo transfers to help implantation. Note: Stop eating pineapple after any IVF or IUI or if you think if there is any chance you might be pregnant. While pineapple helps implantation, it is not recommended for pregnancy.

- Close to the time of transfer, cut out all sugar and white flour products if you possibly can.

- Make sure your guy is eating garlic, raw pumpkin and sunflower seeds, walnuts, almonds, and oysters. Reduce his amount of dairy and fat.

- Stop all coffee and caffeine products close to the time of conception. Ideally, perhaps a week or two before an IVF.

- Make sure you are taking a prenatal vitamin and folic acid.

- About two weeks before the IVF, stop the late bedtimes and give yourself added sleep.

- Do whatever you can to start to relax. Spend more time in nature, knit, crochet, listen to soothing music, get a massage. Take a break from thinking about all your problems. As much as you can, get your body out of fight or flight mode.

- If it is summer and you live near a beach, consider a week-long beach vacation a week before your IVF and a week after the IVF. The time spent relaxing, in the sunshine, might help your body prepare for pregnancy.

After the IUI/IVF:

- For a few days, make sure you get adequate sleep and try to keep stress levels down. Whatever you can do to promote a deep feeling of relaxation, do it. If that means, spending a day just sitting by the ocean, singing, or doing some art work that relaxes you. The goal is to let yourself feel peace. I know this is easier said than done, especially when so much is riding on the outcome of an IVF. And to be frank, many women get pregnant stressed or not, so don't get into a doomsday mode if you simply can't relax. The human body is strong and can often conceive even in bad circumstances. But whatever you can do to relax and reduce stress levels, be open to doing. Knit, crochet, watch something funny that makes you laugh. Spend time in nature, whether at the beach, a lake, a beautiful park, your backyard or just sitting outside in a driveway.

- Make sure you continue to get adequate amounts of sunshine each day.

- If you can plan a getaway, not too far from your home, during the wait time after an IVF, that might help. A getaway to a local beach, lake, something relaxing that doesn't take a lot of planning or travel time. Do not go away if travel in any way makes you feel stressed or overwhelmed. Something within an hour's drive might be ideal.

- If you can, take a few days or even a week off of work to just be home, rest, listen to music, and have fun.

- Continue to eat foods that promote fertility. Olive oil, avocado, spinach.

- Stay away from screens as much as you can.

- Ask your doctor about progesterone and if you might need it to help implantation.

- Don't drink coffee.

- Avoid hot baths.

- Keep positive and see yourself as pregnant. Try to keep a hopeful, happy outlook. Repeat affirmations like: I welcome you baby.
Life is beautiful.
I am pregnant.
My body is comfortable receiving.
It is safe for me to be pregnant.
 It is safe for me to have a baby.
I give myself permission to be pregnant.
I am allowed to get pregnant.
I am ready to be pregnant.

Write, say and sing these words as often as you can.

Diary Excerpt: Sunday Retrieval

Today was the egg retrieval.

We got to the hospital about 6 a.m. A kindly nurse at the desk welcomes us. For a moment, the whole place feels different—a fantasy island of fertility where surgical procedures are pink and beautiful. For a few minutes, I am lulled into actually believing this might turn out to be fun.

We were the ones on the floor that morning and we are put in a room at the end of the hallway. It is so quiet. I am not deceived by the wallpaper anymore. Now, it all feels very serious and very real, just like it did the other two times. I pray and pray. I always feel a measure of fear when I'm going under anesthesia. And heaviness. I feel a heaviness when it comes time to do an IVF, as if the weight of the world is on me.

Finally a young man comes to wheel me down to the OR. I have seen him before. He has wheeled me to several operations and procedures. He doesn't remember me, but I remember him. He must see a thousand like me each month.

In the waiting area, I am put me in front of station 3.
Three? Could it mean..a sign that I am going to have triplets!!!!!

I let myself get a bit giddy imaging that this IVF will result in triplets. Triplets....Imagine! The instant large family of my dreams! My little girl suddenly blessed with three siblings! Three sisters? Oh my God, four girls!!!! Or maybe two girls and a boy? Oh my God, a family of three girls and one boy! Two boys and a girl? Then I would have two girls and two boys! Four children would be a lot of work at first, but my kids would never be lonely. I am imagining our family photo twenty years from now. All four kids and then someday all their kids will have babies and their kids will have lots and lots of cousins. In my old age, I'll always have a child to be with. I'll be busy with kids until I'm 58 years old!

I let this fantasy play out in my head and I am feeling happier and happier.

Triplets!

A few minutes later, I am wheeled into the operating room. The anesthesioligist is kind, and very quickly, I am asleep.

I wake up, I don't know how much later, in that horribly awlful waiting recovery area. But good news—I am told retrieved ten eggs! Ten! Oh my God! Ten!

All my hard work trying to get healthy paid off. I can't believe this. I probably will end up with six good eggs, and then there is a good chance that three of those six will take, and I will have triplets!

Can you imagine? My daughter will never be lonely. She will always have at least one sibling in the house to play with.

In three days, my eggs will be implanted back in me. Ten! I'm betting triplets are on the way!

Day of Transfer

Today was the transfer of the embryos, where they implant the eggs mixed with my husband's sperm back into me.

I ended up with three eggs, not ten, but three.

Dr. M, the one who so devastated me a few months ago by saying my eggs were bottom of the barrel, was ironically, the doctor on hand for the procedure. As always during procedures, she was kind, generous and nurturing. I've figured out that she is good at handling tests, but not to have as the primary doctor on your case. Maybe she likes the non-pressure of just stepping in for a procedure, without the pressure of having to follow-up and figure out what is going on.

Dr. M. said it was wonderful that I did everything the clinic asked of me, submitted to all the tests they recommended, including a balloon test known as a hysterosalpingogram that was not too pleasant. I just smiled, pretending to be laid back about the whole thing. She never could have guessed how much she devastated me a few months ago. She seemed to have no anger or resentment over the fact that I dumped her and switched to another doctor. Maybe she is so busy, she didn't even notice that I had switched doctors at all. Or she was just relieved to be rid of a patient who was creating too much work for her.

Anyways, as she was just about to do the transfer, she said it was bad luck to have the same doctor do a transfer twice, especially since the last transfer she did didn't work out. So she went to get another doctor to insert my eggs. I was grateful for her sensitivity, especially since she was the one whose words made me feel so hopeless.

Before she went to get the other doctor, she took an ultrasound picture of my eggs and said, "Let's hope this is a first baby picture." Hopeful and kind words, and made me feel good. Imagine if this was my baby's first picture. She smiled kindly at me, and for a minute, I think I can forgive her for the pain she caused me.

The other doctor came in, did the transfer, and now I must wait and hope my baby comes soon.

Worn Out and Tired

It has been two days since the embryos were put into my body.

Most of the time, I am on my knees in prayer, asking God to send an angel to guide my embryos to life, to give this baby the breath of God. If He wants to empower my tired old eggs to turn into a baby, He can and will.

And I'm tired. So very tired.

Praying and Waiting

It is 5 o'clock in the morning. A light snow decorates the earth outside my window, and there are three embryos inside me fighting to live.

After changing doctors, eating according to blood type, taking two shots a day of some pretty powerful infertility drugs, going to acupuncture once a week, a myofascial release expert and a kinesiologist twice a month, I ended up with three fair-to-poor quality embryos.

If I have one baby, I will be glad. No, ecstatic. Overjoyed. Full of bliss and gratitude. Yet, there is a part of me who wants three babies, an instantly large family by today's standards.

I am trying not to be stressed. I am trying not to think negatively. I am trying not to hate myself, but right now, self-hate is roaring through my body. It seems no one in my life realizes how absolutely helpless you can feel when you've done everything medically possible both in conventional medicine and in alternative medicine and still end up with only three embryos.

Earlier this week, I made a collage representing pregnancy.

I got a giant poster-size paper and cut and glued pictures of babies and mothers and words like 'revel in your ripeness' 'miracle' 'prayers' and 'mom knows cool.' My collage is beautiful and I hung it in my office.

I love this collage. I look at it and think: 'it is possible. I could make a baby.'

For now, however, I'm going to cheer my little embryos on.

"Dear Embryos,

I don't know you yet. One of you, or all of you, may end up being one of the most important persons in my life. You may end up being the answer to my prayers. I may someday get to hold you and love you.

You may grow and become more than I ever imagined. Right now, know I love you. I love you if you make it and I love you if you don't make it. I am cheering for you. I am trying to give you the best parts of me. I am your mother and you are my children, and I'm hoping we can take that connection into the physical realm. Take what you need to take from my body. Feed off me. Ignore my tired, cranky spirit. Ignore the self-hatred looming inside of me. Ignore all the mixed emotions that are stirring around in my head. Just hear this: you are loved. You are wanted. You will be given as much as I can give. Your sister Amber needs you. Your Daddy Chris is praying for your continued growth. I, your mother, sit nervously and tenuously, hoping Dec. 20 comes quickly and the answer is yes. Please, please, please, let the answer be yes."

I Am Pregnant

Today, I got the call: I am pregnant.

I was happy for a moment. Then I ran into the bathroom to check for blood.

The phone call came at 10 o'clock. When I got the news, I thought: "If I can make it to 5 o'clock with no blood, then I'll feel good."

Pregnant. For now. I keep going to the bathroom and checking

Tonight, I thought: one day down, nine months to go.

One Month Pregnant

It is January and I have been pregnant for a month. I am happier than I would have been if I was not pregnant, but being just one month into my pregnancy, I live each day with fear and a bucket of sadness I can't shake.

Since the day I learned I was pregnant, I have not once gone to the bathroom without immediately checking for blood, holding my breath every time I wipe myself, and feeling waves of relief each time I see no blood.

I am ever vigilant about everything, from where I go, to what I eat, to how long I sit or stand. There are moments I feel relief, like Mondays when we go to the library storytime and visit my mother, or when I'm reading to my daughter and I sink into the in-love feeling I have for her, but other than that, my life feels very hard right now. I have a lot of faith, and a strong part of me feels that God would not have taken me this far to let me fall. If I did miscarry, I would never blame Him, nor would I give up.

I told Leah the other day that I feel weary in a way I never felt before.

When I visualize what is happening within me, I see a girl wearing an ugly brown vest over a once white and beautiful dress. She is laying on the floor and can't walk--she has no legs. She crawls instead and her hair is messy. This girl's inability to walk, in many ways, reflects how tired I feel, how completely worn down I am by the last few months events. This is in no way a relaxed, comfortable pregnancy. It is a pregnancy where I am crawling all the way to the finish line.

But there is another part of me. A woman who stalks the forest deliberately and carries my daughter on her back. She swings through trees, swims through rivers, and seems to be the one capable of doing the hard stuff now. She loves my little girl more than anything, and she keeps her on her back no matter what. She carries a knife, and will fight off bears, lions, anything that tries to get near her baby. It is a good feeling to visualize her now.

She doesn't seem as forlorn and scared as she once was.

Every week, we drive the hour and a half to Portland, Maine to see Dr. Deutsch. One week, he looked down at me with a very concerned expression and said, "it is good you came this week." He didn't say anymore and I thought: I wonder if he knows that if I didn't come, my body would have miscarried." Dr. Deutsch doesn't always say a lot, but I could sense by his tone that something serious was going on. As usual, he did his thing to strengthen my adrenals, thyroid, and whatever else was off whack, weak, or out of alignment. I thank God for this man's ability to help me. He has become a key part of my journey this pregnancy.

April and Still Pregnant

It is April 6 and I am still pregnant. After almost two straight years of infertility hell for the second time around, I am now entering my fifth month of pregnancy.

I had mistakenly thought infertility hell would end the moment the nurse announced over the telephone that yes, I am pregnant.

But after so many disappointments, the hell only intensified: now I really had something I had to fight and pray to hold on to. Now I had something I could lose.

For a long time, it was a hell to hear that no, I was not pregnant, but a different type of hell ensued once the answer was yes. Now, a dream coming true is within my shaky reach, but could be yanked away by something crazy like poor egg quality or hormone imbalance.

So the hell has continued these five months...so much so, that I could barely write this journal.

The first day I found out I was pregnant went by oh-so-slowly. I looked at the clock a million times. Was my baby still growing? Could I carry to term? Would I miscarry and start bleeding any minute? I remember looking at the clock that day at exactly 5 o'clock thinking: one day down, nine months to go.

I have not gone to the bathroom once during these past five months where I didn't hold my breath, look at the toilet paper for signs of blood, and at the blessed sign of no blood, say a quick prayer of thanks to God for helping my baby to survive.

The first month of pregnancy, intensified by high doses of progesterone shots adminstered every night, was an exercise in mental torment and hellish frustration. I woke up every night about midnight, and would stay wide awake until 4 or 5 o'clock.

I pray a lot. I pray very specifically: asking God to please, don't let me eat anything that could hurt my baby. Please, don't let me contract anything that could hurt my baby, like fifth disease. Please, please, please. Prayer is always at the tip of my lips.

It has been an odd pregnancy, not blissful like my daughter's, but fraught with the potential for great hurt. I feel like a young girl who has finally won the boyfriend of her dreams, only to know that the head cheerleader is after your guy, and no matter how hard you try, she is always right there smiling and tossing her wavy blonde pony tail.

In my third month of pregnancy, my wisdom tooth got infected, and I spent a few hysterical days imagining that the infection would kill my blossoming fetus. I tentatively went to the oral surgeon to have the tooth removed. Only, right before he was about to start, something inside me knew I shouldn't have this procedure. After much questioning, the oral surgeon finally admitted there were no guarantees that the novacaine would not hurt my baby.

I walked out. Pencillion got rid of the infection and Dr. Deutsch agrees that I probably did the right thing in not having the tooth removed.

I found out last week I was having a boy, which brought with it a host of joyful feelings. I was ecstatic: me, having a boy, my old and tired body actually producing a boy.

Relief...Thanks...Amazement.....

My daughter speaks fondly of her brother, and often asks me why he can't come out now. "YES I WANT TO TAKE HIM OUT TOO" I want to tell her. I want to feel his beautiful cheeks against my cheeks and I want to kiss him and say thank you God, thank you baby, for finally arriving!!!"

I am on a medical leave from work, and it is tough not having this emotional outlet. I miss chocolate so much I dream about it. I have informed my husband that the moment Dr. Lirrette removes the baby from my body, that he is to present me with a box of Godiva chocolates, Mrs. Field's chocolate chip cookes and Chinese food (which I also can't have.)

I am also not allowed to eat a lot of fish, and I miss tuna fish. I often think longingly about a D'Angelo's tuna fish sandwich.

Yet, the other day at the ultrasound, I got a reward for all my discomfort: a large, beautiful, glossy ultrasound picture of my son.

My son...what marvelous words I thought I would never speak. He looked so cute! Adorable! Incredibly handsome like some Greek Adonis or something. The ultrasound technician, who was very kind, zoomed in to show me a close up of my son drinking my amniotic fluid.

When I saw his mouth moving, gulping in the fluid that
Only my body is able to give him, my heart turned upside down and I fell crazy in love.

The day I found out I was having a boy, I looked in the
mirror and for the first time in months, I felt pretty. Don't ask me why, but I suddenly saw something different in myself that I hadn't seen for awhile.I don't know why finding out I was having a boy made me feel pretty, but I did.

Now I wait. Four and a half, perhaps five, months to go. I start the emotional training it will take to turn myself over to this little human who will need the best, kindest and most significant parts of me.

A journey has begun that I have needed for a very, very long time.

Today's Main Theme: Fear

Today is one of those days when fear seems to be the main theme running through my day.

Actually, I shouldn't say today is one of those days, when the reality is, during this pregnancy, every day is a day full of fear.

This morning, we went to the library with my mother for a story time and puppet show. Usually, this is one of my favorite times during the week. Yet today storytime wasn't so fun, because moments after we got to the library, I started to feel pain in my buttocks and with the pain came fear.

Lately any type of mild pain elicits fear in me. Pain: is something is wrong with my baby? Pain: (hell even mild discomfort)—am I about to lose my baby? Pain: Did I do something to hurt my baby?

So the rest of the time at the library, I asked my mother to watch my daughter. I sat down and didn't move, because I was afraid that too much movement would hurt my baby.

Tonight, I am left thinking: Was there ever a time in my life when my body was free to do what it wanted without fear? Was there really a time when I could move any way I wanted without worrying that I was moving too fast or too something?

After the library, we went to Friendly's, a favorite of my daughter. I desperately wanted the cheese quesadillas, but I read that soft cheese isn't safe during pregnancy, and although quesadillas are made with hard cheese, that information on soft cheese has made me very weary of cheese in general, and throughout this pregnancy, cheese has been something I eat with suspicion.

Another blow to freedom. I ate onion rings instead, as I am afraid to eat chicken, hamburger, or any type of meat at restaurants (what if they undercook the meat and that hurts my unborn child?)

I admit: I am paranoid. Had I had my babies in my 20s and never gone through infertility, I'm sure I would have heartily enjoyed cheese quesadillas and a hot fudge sundae today.

I am antsy. I am bored out of my mind. I want to stay up all night and drink wine with friends. I want to eat mounds of chocolate, piles of cheese quesadillas, and loads of hamburgers. I want to be able to go to the library on Monday, and run as wild and free as my daughter, and not for a minute worry about pulling a muscle or doing something to hurt my unborn baby.

Instead, it is 7:26 p.m. and I will probably be asleep in half an hour. I cherish this little boy inside me. So much so, I am a walking advertisement for what happens after lots of reproductive trauma, and so I forgive myself kindly and when this little boy arrives, I am going to smother him in an absurd number of kisses.

Then I am going to ask my husband to please pass the cheese quesadillas.

Wishing For Popcorn and Molasses

Right now, I want to the calendar to say 1982 again, and I'm back at my parents' house doing my homework on the couch as my mother surprises me with a big white plastic bowl of popcorn smothered in butter and molasses that she popped on our brown stove in a regular frying pan.

Last night, a horrible thunder and lightning storm ruined my evening.

Then today I had severe stomach pains and
I thought something was wrong with my baby. I ended up going to see my ob/gyn for an ultrasound.

The baby was fine, thanks to God. Now I'm just tired, and craving the safety that once existed when I was young and able to eat my Mom's molasses and butter popcorn. Why does life have to turn out so hard sometimes?

June: Feeling Overwhelmed

It arrived in the mail the other day. The date for my caesarean has been scheduled. I'm not crazy about the date, and so when I go to my doctor this week, I might ask for another date. But seeing a definite date written on paper, scheduled in somebody's appointment book, makes me happier than one can imagine.

We have lots of ideas on how to help my daughter adjust to her new brother. We are going to buy her a beautiful, beautiful, beautiful (did I say beautiful?) dress and give it to her the morning of my caesarean so she can wear it to the hospital for her first official meeting with her brother.

We are also going to give her a gift a day for the first two weeks after the baby is born...wrapped with pretty paper and lots of bows.

Nothing too expensive mind you, but small things, like a book, a Barbie, maybe a game or two, a t-shirt that says, "I'm A Big Sister Now", a cake with a picture of her and her new little brother on it.

I want the day of his birth to arrive now.

Countdown to August. Here it comes...

Last Day of June

Today is the last day of June. In 52 days, my son will be born. I am moving closer and closer to that long awaited day of his birth, but I still feel like I am a 100 miles away from a much needed glass of water on a scorching July day.

I can't let myself relax into this pregnancy, can't let down my guard for a moment, because if I do, there is always the fear that something could go very wrong.

My life has gotten very small this pregnancy.

I don't go many places.

Sometimes, when I hear a song from my past, I start to cry: was there ever really a time in life when I was so free and without fear constantly accompanying me? It seems impossible.

These nine months have seemed like 20 years, slow, terrible, every step a warning. I don't feel normal very often anymore.

There have been joyous moments too. Each week, when I get my ultrasound, and see my son growing, surrounded by plenty of healthy placenta and fluid to keep him well-fed, I feel a slight relief.

Each time I leave Dr. Lirrette's office, I marvel that I was able to find such an outstanding doctor.

18 Days To Go

I am 18 days away from giving birth. It still feels like a million years from now, 20 years at least. A year when I'm feeling good.

I am still nervous. Still paranoid. Not as fearful as I was, say, six months ago, but still not as relaxed as I should be. I know the odds are in my favor, but still, I've never been one to find comfort in the odds.

I pray a lot. I pray that God protects me and my baby from fifth disease, bacterial poisoning, car accidents, listeria, anything and everything that could hurt my baby.

I am excited about my son's birth, but not fully comfortable allowing myself to feel happy just yet.

Countdown To My Son

I am in countdown mode. Two weeks until my scheduled c-section. It still feels like a million light years away.

This journey has been long, grueling, sometimes unbearable. It has included six IUIs, three IVFs, and 9/11 occuring the day before my second IVF.

Getting pregnant also included a weekly hour and a half drive to a chiropractor/kinesiologist, a weekly visit to an acupuncturist, several hundreds of dollars spent on homeopathy, visits to an herbal expert where I bought bags of herbs each week that had to be boiled into tea and hours and hours spent at the bookstore researching the topic of infertility.

Achieving this pregnancy also included having two shots a day in my thigh, stomach or butt for three weeks in preparation of my IVF cycle and progesterone shots that made me slightly crazy every day for six weeks once I became pregnant.

Could this hell really be almost over?

Even though I'm nearing the finish line, I feel safer keeping up my guard.

The other day, we went shopping at a big baby store and there was this little blue outfit that said, "Thank heaven for little boys." Just seeing those words made me start to cry.

When I got home, I started eating watermelon. Wham--without ten minutes, I was vomiting profusely, wondering where this vomit was coming from, since I felt no pain or nausea.

Of course, since this never happened to me before, I was scared and phoned Dr. Lirrette.

The poor man must have cringed when he saw my name on the beeper, since at least once every two weeks I have gone in for an emergency appointment or called in because of this pain or that pain. But being the great doctor he is, Dr. Lirrette called back within 10 minute. All I can say is, thank God he is my doctor. Most doctors would have kicked me to the curb by now.

The rest of the night, I became whiny, asking my husband to please, go buy me an almond slush, please, please massage my back and legs, please, could he juice me some garlic and lemon (in case I had a stomach bug).

My daughter kept asking, "Mom, why do you like garlic lemonade so much?"

Two Hours To Take-Off

In two hours, I will be going to the hospital to have my c-section.

Two hours..have I really made it this far? I am still praying to God that nothing happen to my baby...can you imagine...even at this point, fear still looms. I feel undeserving of this miracle.

One would think by now I would feel at ease, full of hope that everything was going to be all right, and yet I am afraid to let myself be happy.

I am more than thankful that this nine months of hell is almost over.

Two hours. Did I really make it this far? Me? Me who usually messes up and fails?

Right now, so many emotions are churning inside me, from fear to worthlessness to awe.

I am waiting.

The Birth Of My Son

A month and three days ago, my son was born. It seems like forever and a day ago that I was wide awake at 2 a.m., waiting anxiously for morning so the birth of my son could begin...my darling prince could finally arrive.

Where do I start in flashing back to one of the most momentous and long-anticipated moments in my life.

To start, I am not the same person I was a month and three days ago.

Back then, I still boiled constantly with fear that something would go wrong and my son would not come to me.

August 22 began early for me. I was scheduled for my c-section at 7:30--ironically the same time as my daughter's c-section, and I could hardly wait for this day to get started.

Instead of being relaxed, I was still worried that something terrible would go wrong and take my baby away from me.

I was up the whole night before my son's birth, too excited to sleep, so excited for it all to begin, I did not want to miss a moment. I felt like I was waiting for this moment all of my life. A son! A son coming to me! Me! Actually me! I refused to sleep all night.

I would not be absent for a moment of this moment.

Finally, finally, 5 a.m. arrived and I could begin the day.

"Can you believe the day is here?" I whispered to my husband, who was still half asleep.

"You made it," my husband said.

"Don't say that," I cringed, still in fear that something might go wrong at the last minute. I loved him for trying to boost me up, but I didn't feel safe letting myself completely relax yet.

It was damp that morning, a slight chill in the air, surprisingly after the long hot summer. I wanted to look beautiful to meet my son, but I had avoided salons for nine months, because of fear of chemicals, so my hair was long, unruly, a big knot in the back. I had tried to cut my own hair about five months before, which resulted in an even bigger mess. Still, I applied my make-up carefully, and put my hair up to hide the mess it had become.

Now I was done showering, doing my make-up and hair. I put on the purple top and shorts that was one of only three pregnancy outfits I wore these past months.

The first day I learned I was pregnant, I spent the day checking myself in the bathroom every hour to make sure I was not bleeding. To be in my bedroom that morning, dressing to go the hospital with a full living baby thriving inside me seemed almost too much, too good, too impossible, to be true.

Then it was time to wake our daughter. We spent a lot of time thinking about how we could make this transition easy on her. We bought her a beautiful flowered white satin dress to wear to the hospital and several new toys to be given to her over the next few weeks. "Honey, today is the day your baby swims out," I said.

She smiled sleepily. We couldn't wait any longer, and we gave her the first of her presents: an Enchanted Forest Barbie with storybook.

Now we were all dressed, and headed downstairs to be with my parents, who had stayed over the night before. I took out my camera and was snapping pictures of this and that, trying oh so hard to capture the moments before my son arrived.

Like many mothers before me preparing for the moment of their baby's birth, I knew I was stepping into one of life's timeless moments and I wanted it all on film.

Then we drove to the hospital. Once inside, I went up to the third floor maternity ward, the same one where my daughter was born. I got a picture of my husband holding my daughter, standing next to my parents, going up in that elevator. Everyone looks serious, tired, happy. I love that picture.

At the hospital, I was escorted into a room to be prepped. The two nurses assigned to me were kind, funny, and nice. They had a hard time getting my IV in, but looking back, even the discomfort of the IV wasn't bad. I was lucky that my doctor, Dr. Lirrette, inserted the catheter that I was so dreading. He is a gentle and kind man, who I feel amazingly safe and comfortable with.

He was one of the few aspects of my pregnancy where I did feel completely safe. Every woman on earth preparing to give birth should be so fortunate as to have a doctor like Dr. Lirrette.

Then it was on to the operating room for the C-section. Dr. Lirrette walked me and my husband down to the room.

My husband had to leave for the epidural. During the epidural, Dr. Lirrette held my hand to get me through it and kept saying things like, "You can do it" and "You're the best" and "think of your beautiful baby" in such a confident and gentle way that the epidural barely hurt. In fact, I can't even remember it because Dr. Lirrette's reassuring voice overshadowed any fear or pain in that moment.

But once the epidural was done, another drama had begun. I was numb--even my mouth was numb. People were running in and out of the OR. Time seemed to drag on. I was so nervous.

"Why do you like playing cards?" I asked my husband, because I wanted to distract myself, as my stomach was being cut open. I waited for what seemed like a long, long time.

"Paula, look, the baby is here," Dr. Lirrette called out.

"I can't look," I said, in fear that if I looked, I would see my cut-open stomach.

'Look!" and the sheet came down and I could see the very long umbilical cord attached to this golden beautiful boy. My boy...my boy....here.

It was all so surreal, that even now I can't totally focus on that moment without a fuzzy blur of heaven opening up and my son coming to me surrounded by clouds of white. It was almost like a light surrounded my son, a culmination of a dream that I didn't feel totally deserving of and still doubted even when the reality hit.

I looked at him, and thought, "He looks like an angel...he looks just like an angel." He was golden, completely golden, and perfect.

Then he was ushered away for shots and a clean-up, and I was on my way to recovery.

A few minutes later, in the recovery room my parents came in with my daughter.

"He looks strong honey," my father said.

Then I went to my room, and waited for what seemed like hours for the nurse to bring my son.

During those first moments together with my son I remember only two things: he was beautiful and I immediately liked his personality. I sensed a goodness and kindness about him. I remember him rooting immediately, and staring at me, as if playing that tape to him each night with my voice paid off, because he seemed to recognize my voice. I was surprised that he wanted to breast feed so easily and so soon.

So much happened during those five days in the hospital...there are flashes of memories that come and go..me ordering chocolate cake from the cafeteria, delighted that finally I could eat chocolate again...my daughter crying hysterically on the last night of my stay at the hospital that she missed me...me breast feeding in front of visitors and not at all caring who saw my breasts and me feeling incredibly proud that my son wanted so desperately to drink milk from my tired and sagging old breasts.

There is one particular incident, however, that best summed up my son's birth.

Two days after my son was born, a cafeteria worker found my son's alarm on the floor. The alarm on my son's leg that was suppose to protect him from being abducted had fallen off. To say I was upset was an understatement, and the more I tried to get an explanation, the more the nurses, aides and everybody else went into defensive mode. They insisted security was not violated, and I insisted that it was.

"Could someone have walked off this floor with my baby?" I wanted to know.

"No" they contended. I didn't buy their explanation.

Night came, and I was still feeling scared, restless, full of trepidation that I had come so far, delivered a healthy baby, only to lose him somehow at the hospital because of a security glitch. I almost checked out of the hospital early because of fear that security at the hospital was poor. All kinds of scary scenarios played out in my head. My husband insisted we stay, which probably was for the best, but I still felt uneasy.

Around 8 o'clock, I started missing my son terribly. The nursery was a long walk down the hallway, but I decided I was going to see him regardless. Walking was still hard for me. Any movement at all was hard and I was in great pain, but I kept walking. I'd inch a few feet, stop, inch a few more.

I finally got to the nursery, wearing a blood-stained nightgown, but not really caring that I was a mess.

I walked in the nursery, took one look at my son in his incubator, and burst out crying. I hated him being away from me. I hated that I was too weak to care for him at night.

"I just miss him so much," I said. "I am so worried that he's not safe."

The nurses were cold to me, one even saying I must be hormonal because it was my third day after birth. My guess is that they feared getting in trouble over the missing alarm. I hobbled back to my room, sad, but proud that I had forced myself down that long hallway to see my son. He was here, a part of who I was, and there was no turning back.

That image of myself; a ragged, disheveled woman, wearing a blood-stained night gown, and who looked like a neurotic mess and probably was a bit over the top, is who I am most proud of. She was the mother warrior who walked me through the years of infertility treatments, who dared to defy the doctor who said the game was over and no more children would be coming to me because of my old and dwindling number of eggs.

It was that crazy lady who dragged herself to appointment after appointment, test after test, and who tried everything from homeopathy to acupuncture, to get this much desired baby. And in that craziness, in that mother lion, was a strength, a love, and a complete willingness to look like a fool if it would someday bring my beloved child to life.

Only a nut keeps trying when it looks hopeless...only a nut..and so if the nurses thought me a bit quirky and weird, so be it. If the only way I could arrive at the nursery to see my son was to hobble down the hallway wearing a very icky blood-stained night gown because I was too tired to change, so be it.

Today I hold my son and he is here. Crazy nuts who do not give up are sometimes not so crazy. Prayers are indeed answered. Thank you Father in heaven. Amen.

The Beginning: A New Journey Has Begun

I am now a mother of two children. I say these words with pride, trepidation, and a feeling that unless you've gone through infertility, it is a statement that could sound deceptively ordinary and mundane.

Two children, 'that's nice, so what', could be the reaction of someone whose children arrived unexpectedly, without much effort or planning, after a wonderful night or two of love making.

But for a woman who has endured four years of infertility treatments, 16 IUIs, four IVFs, two shots a day month after month, and who once put two chocolate donuts on her stomach as an incentive to get her through a painful test, being able to say she has two children is perhaps the most amazing, the most momentous achievement one can imagine.

I might have well been elected the first female president, or climbed Mount Everest, or written 'Gone with the Wind'.

For someone like me, being able to say I have two children is like being able to say that your craziest, wildest, most important dream actually came true.

I might have well won ten million dollars, or flown to the moon alone, or found the cure that would have allowed Christopher Reeve to walk.

Something that seems so regular and so ordinary is anything but ordinary to me, and that is both the beauty of suffering with infertility and the curse of suffering with it.

I cherish my children in a way that is slightly different, because I know from bitter experience how tough it can sometimes be for a sperm and egg to successfully join together and make it through the nine months to transform into a healthy baby.

I've seen science up close, in a way I sometimes wish I never saw it, but in a way that makes every new baby I see seem like the greatest invention ever.

I sometimes look at my children, during the most ordinary of moments, and I think, "Good God, it all worked out. Somehow, it all worked out."

And often, in those moments, I feel a sort of survivors' guilt, because I know for many women, it doesn't work out, and I get angry and sad all at once. I want to tell them 'don't give up! never give up hope! Don't listen to the doctors who tell you your eggs are too old' don't listen to well-meaning friends and relatives who say crazy, stupid things like, "maybe God doesn't want you to have a child." I want them to know that infertility is not a result of being flawed in some way, or cursed in some way, but it is a sickness, a disease, just like breast cancer, heart disease or the common cold.

It is a physical problem, and sometimes all the relaxing in the world won't make a baby.

When I look back, over the past five years, and I analyze closely the step-by-step process of getting pregnant, staying pregnant, and giving birth, I get depressed and then tired. It was too much. Too hard, too long, too painful--and thank God I didn't know that at the time and thank God I experienced all of it. Thankfully, as I walked that road, I never knew how long and how hard it would be. As a young teen, I learned the poem, "inch by inch, life's a cinch. Yard by yard, it is hard. Mile by mile, it is a trial" and sometimes when everything got too hard I'd say to myself, 'inch by inch' and I kept slowly inching forward towards my goal.

At one point, when I so desired my second baby, I would wake up each day, open my appointment book, and write a list of what I could do that day to move me closer to my goal. Sometimes it was doing things like eating lots of salad, avoiding coffee, or making an appointment with my acupuncturist.

Sometimes it meant going to swimming, listening to my relaxation tapes, and of course praying. Always praying. I was a woman at war, and every day I had to pull together my strategy.

Now I am a mother. A new journey has started for me.

I have the little girl I yearned for, and the son that I so wanted to complete my family.

My daughter is not an only child, and in seeing her with a brother, I see all the advantages I had being the only one, and all the disadvantages I had.

It has made me cherish my childhood even more, and at the same time, I am profoundly thankful that their lessons will be different than mine.

What has the experience with infertility taught me? First, on a practical level, I firmly believe that infertility clinics should be taking advantage of all that is offered by holistic and alternative practitioners. Sadly, eastern and western medicine refuse to come together. Holistic practitioners often discount the power and effectiveness of conventional medicine.

Some of the holistic and alternative practitioners I worked with recommended that I stop using the medicines and techniques available at the infertility clinic. Had I listened to them, I doubt my two children would be here today. Conventional medicine has made great and daunting strides in helping women have children, and to not take advantage of all the science available would be foolish. I know that without the IUIs and the IVFs and all the medication I took, my children would not be here. To not tap into these powerful medications and procedures would have probably meant not meeting the two most awesome people I ever imagined.

At the same time, there no denying that there is a lot that alternative medicine has to offer, as it can sometimes uncover the subtle reasons, not so easily detected on standard tests, why a woman is having a problem getting pregnant, reasons that conventional doctors all too easily label and dismiss as 'unexplained infertility.' There are millions of women who can't get pregnant for specific reasons never uncovered by conventional medicine. There are also millions of women who miscarry again and again, and no explanation is offered.

Alternative medicine delves into these murky, difficult-to-understand areas. It looks at things like the impact of emotions on a women's reproductive system, the condition of the adrenal glands, thyroid, kidney and liver that can impact conception and pregnancy, and the role nutrition may play in the body's readiness to conceive.

My question is: why isn't acupuncture available at all the infertility clinics as part of the treatments, as a compliment to standard treatment?

Why aren't women undergoing infertility treatments told to stop the coffee, cut out the white flour and sugar, and get themselves on a healthy diet? Why do infertility clinics allow coffee to be served in their waiting rooms?

Why isn't there a massage therapist available to stressed out infertility patients--especially before procedures like IVF and IUI, as a means of helping patients relax?

Isn't it time that alternative medicine and conventional medicine come together to help struggling infertility patients. The two should not see each other as the enemy. I would be willing to say that many more women could successfully have babies if conventional infertility treatments and alternative medicine joined together.

Isn't it time the battle over infertility be fought on all grounds--rather than two opposing teams who really need to be allies.

I know that this experience took away a feeling of carefreeness I once had. I'm more cautious, more serious, wounds leftover from a lady scarred in the battle, but somehow one who survived this fertility war.

I am stronger now, different, even thankful for this tumultuous and sometimes painful journey. It molded and sculpted me into a mother and was probably the best preparation for parenthood I could have asked for.

My journey now is using what I learned to help others, and somehow putting it all to good use as a mother. I'll remember the words of my dear friend Chelsea Lowe, who said, "For some women, this comes easily. For you, it is a long and difficult road. It doesn't mean you can't eventually have what others have, but it does mean you have to travel down a different road."

So I walked that road, unfair as it was, and I came to the destination that many women ultimately come to: I am a mother.

Amazing.

The walk was hell, but oh, the destination sweet.

www.ingramcontent.com/pod-product-compliance
Lightning Source LLC
Chambersburg PA
CBHW060300230426
43663CB00009B/1534